EXERCISE FOR SPECIAL POPULATIONS

PEGGIE WILLIAMSON, MS, CHES, CPT, CFT

Professor
Anatomy and Physiology and Nutrition
Central Texas College
Killeen, Texas

Wolters Kluwer | Lippincott Williams & Wilkins
Health

Philadelphia · Baltimore · New York · London
Buenos Aires · Hong Kong · Sydney · Tokyo

Acquisitions Editor: Emily Lupash
Product Manger: Andrea M. Klingler
Marketing Manager: Christen Murphy
Designer: Teresa Mallon
Compositor: SPi Technologies
Printer: C&C Offset

First Edition

Copyright © 2011 Lippincott Williams & Wilkins, a Wolters Kluwer business

351 West Camden Street   Two Commerce Square, 2001 Market Street
Baltimore, MD 21201   Philadelphia, PA 19103

Printed in China

Library of Congress Cataloging-in-Publication Data
Williamson, Peggie.
    Exercise for special populations / Peggie Williamson.
        p. ; cm.
    Includes bibliographical references and index.
    ISBN 978-0-7817-9779-5 (alk. paper)
    1. Exercise therapy. 2. Chronic diseases—Exercise therapy. 3. People with disabilities—Rehabilitation. I. Title.
    [DNLM: 1. Exercise Therapy. 2. Disabled Persons—rehabilitation. 3. Exercise. 4. Physical Fitness.
WB 541 W732e 2011]
    RM725.W55   2011
    615.8'2—dc22

                                                                              2010000514

DISCLAIMER

Care has been taken to confirm the accuracy of the information present and to describe generally accepted practices. However, the authors, editors, and publisher are not responsible for errors or omissions or for any consequences from application of the information in this book and make no warranty, expressed or implied, with respect to the currency, completeness, or accuracy of the contents of the publication. Application of this information in a particular situation remains the professional responsibility of the practitioner; the clinical treatments described and recommended may not be considered absolute and universal recommendations.

The authors, editors, and publisher have exerted every effort to ensure that drug selection and dosage set forth in this text are in accordance with the current recommendations and practice at the time of publication. However, in view of ongoing research, changes in government regulations, and the constant flow of information relating to drug therapy and drug reactions, the reader is urged to check the package insert for each drug for any change in indications and dosage and for added warnings and precautions. This is particularly important when the recommended agent is a new or infrequently employed drug.

Some drugs and medical devices presented in this publication have Food and Drug Administration (FDA) clearance for limited use in restricted research settings. It is the responsibility of the health care provider to ascertain the FDA status of each drug or device planned for use in their clinical practice.

To purchase additional copies of this book, call our customer service department at (800) 638-3030 or fax orders to (301) 223-2320. International customers should call (301) 223-2300.

Visit Lippincott Williams & Wilkins on the Internet: http://www.lww.com. Lippincott Williams & Wilkins customer service representatives are available from 8:30 am to 6:00 pm, EST.

9 8 7 6 5 4 3 2

CCS0912

IN LOVING MEMORY OF SIERRA

In the past, experts considered exercise to be contraindicated for special populations—groups of individuals who exhibit medical conditions that impair health and functional ability. Many thought that the added strain of organized physical activity would further disable those already suffering from debilitating physiological conditions. Moreover, since certain preexisting conditions increase the risk of complications or injury during exertion, these experts assumed that routine exercise would do more harm than good. Thus, to prevent further decline in functional capacity, physicians and other health care providers discouraged special needs groups from participating in structured exercise.

Recent research, however, indicates that exercise is beneficial for most populations. In fact, health professionals now believe that physical activity not only reduces the risk of chronic disease but also promotes the health and well-being of those already coping with long-term health issues. Clearly, each person, whether healthy or not, requires an individualized exercise prescription. Experts, however, can categorize people with similar symptoms into specific special populations and prescribe *general* exercise guidelines appropriate for each group.

This book addresses populations in which symptoms are common among all sufferers. It does not address populations in which symptoms, functional ability, and required adaptations are too varied and complex to make general guidelines. Additionally, because it is beyond the scope of any book to address every existing special needs population, this book focuses on groups who most frequently seek the services of fitness and health professionals. When working with clients who suffer from multiple conditions, health and fitness professionals should consider the cumulative limitations imposed by each condition and modify exercise prescriptions accordingly. The good news is that those with special needs do not have to avoid exercise; instead, they require specialized modifications, guidance, and instruction when participating in physical activity. Input from medical personnel and other qualified health care providers is crucial to minimize risk and optimize benefits. Because people with special conditions are now encouraged to exercise, personal trainers and other fitness professionals must be prepared to address their needs. This book will serve as a comprehensive course supplement and resource guide for personal trainers, students enrolled in personal training programs, and students pursuing health/fitness professional degrees.

ORGANIZATION

Chapter 1 discusses the variables that contribute to overall health and fitness. It also summarizes exercise recommendations for the general population, since several special populations may follow these same basic guidelines. Chapter 2 provides an in-depth anatomy and physiology review for readers who want to reacquaint themselves with the 11 different body systems. It is designed to promote understanding of the changes that occur in the various systems as disease develops. Chapters 3 through 12 provide background information about certain special populations which were chosen because members of these populations frequently seek the services of fitness and health professionals. Each chapter describes anatomical and physiological changes associated with the condition, important precautions during exercise, reasonable expectations about outcomes, general exercise recommendations, and basic nutritional considerations.

Each chapter is intended to stand alone so that this book can serve as a ready reference for practitioners working with the specific group addressed in any given chapter. Consequently, some information may be repeated in two or more chapters. This format minimizes the amount of time needed for a full understanding of each special population. The terms "trainer," "instructor," "fitness professional," and "health/fitness provider" are used interchangeably to refer to anyone who develops exercise programs for those with special needs.

FEATURES

Exercise for Special Populations has been designed to help readers get the most out of the information presented. **Quick References** are small boxes placed throughout the text that emphasize interesting facts, exercise tips, and important information. **Definition Boxes** explain some of the more difficult terminology. **Highlights** offer additional information on topics related to those presented in the book. **Sample Exercise Sections** provide examples of exercises suitable for a given population, show pictures of starting and ending positions, and provide step-by-step instructions on how to perform the exercise. **Case Studies** are short real-world scenarios followed by questions that require readers to assimilate information given in the text. Finally, **Thinking Critically Questions** are designed to stimulate thought and evaluate basic understanding of key points in the chapter.

SUPPLEMENTAL RESOURCES

Exercise for Special Populations includes additional resources for both instructors and students, which are available on the book's companion website at http://thepoint.lww.com/Williamson.

Approved adopting instructors will be given access to PowerPoint presentations for each chapter, answers to the Thinking Critically questions, and an Image Bank. Students who have purchased *Exercise for Special Populations* have access to Exercise Handouts and Appendices.

In addition, purchasers of the text can access the searchable Full Text Online by going to the *Exercise for Special Populations* website at http://thePoint.lww.com. See the inside front cover of this text for more details, including the passcode you will need to gain access to the website.

This book is designed for anyone attempting to attend to the physical welfare of the special needs populations presented within. Overall, it provides readers with information, principles, and guidelines that make working with special populations easier, enjoyable, and more productive—for health professionals and for their clients.

Peggie Williamson

Kristie Abt, PhD
Assistant Clinical Professor
Department of Health and Physical Activity
University of Pittsburgh
Pittsburgh, Pennsylvania

John Alvarez, PhD
Associate Professor
Delta State University
Cleveland, Mississippi

Nicki Anderson, CPT NASM
President Reality Fitness, Inc.
Author/Columnist
Naperville, Illinois

Lisa Blum, BS (IFPA)
Certified Personal Trainer
York, Pennsylvania

Karrie L. Hamstra-Wright, PhD, ATC
Clinical Assistant Professor
Assistant Director, Undergraduate Studies
Department of Kinesiology and Nutrition
University of Illinois at Chicago
Chicago, Illinois

William E. Harrell, CPRP
Aquatics and Fitness Director
Student Affairs
Virginia Wesleyan College
Virginia Beach, Virginia

Sarah Harrison, DPT
Physiotherapy Associates
Havre de Grace, Maryland

Michael R. Kushnick, PhD
Associate Professor of Exercise Physiology
School of Recreation and Sport Sciences,
  Exercise Biochemistry and Physiology
  Laboratories
Ohio University
Athens, Ohio

James J. Laskin, PT, PhD
Associate Professor
School of Physical Therapy & Rehabilitation
  Sciences
The University of Montana
Missoula, Montana

Gail Sas
Fitness Trainer
Fitness Therapy Certified
Buellton, California

Christine B. Stopka, PhD, ATC, LAT, CSCS, CAPE, MTAA
Full Professor
Adapted Physical Activity, Exercise Therapy, &
  Medical Terminology
Department of Health Education & Behavior
College of Health & Human Performance
University of Florida
Gainesville, Florida

Carena Winters-Hart, PhD, MPH
Assistant Professor
Physical Therapy and Exercise Science
Chatham University
Pittsburgh, Pennsylvania

ACKNOWLEDGMENTS

Any book or instructional manual of this type is the result of a team effort. A number of people at Lippincott Williams & Wilkins were indispensible to the writing of this book. I would like to give a special thanks to Emily Lupash, acquisitions editor, for her belief in this project and for guiding me through its early stages; and to Andrea Klingler, product manager, who offered invaluable suggestions, wrestled with deadlines, and was dedicated to creating the best product possible.

I would also like to thank my family and friends for their encouragement and support throughout this and many other life journeys. I am grateful to my parents for everything they have done to get me to this point in my life; to Steve who has always believed in me and pushed me to reach new heights; and to Mike whose confidence and faith in my abilities have never wavered.

C O N T E N T S

THE IMPACT OF EXERCISE AND NUTRITION ON HEALTH AND FITNESS

1

Numerous variables contribute to overall health and fitness. *Nonmodifiable factors*, such as age and gender, are programmed into genes and therefore may not be changed. Other factors, however, such as diet, activity level, cigarette use, alcohol consumption, and exposure to toxins, are controllable. Appropriately manipulating these *modifiable* variables can enhance both quality and quantity of life. This chapter focuses on two modifiable risk factors: exercise and diet.

BENEFITS OF EXERCISE

Years of research have demonstrated that a physically active lifestyle enhances **health** and maintains **fitness.** Requirements for optimizing fitness, though, are slightly more strenuous than those for improving health. The distinction between activity for health versus activity for fitness is why recommendations, particularly suggestions for exercise, are so confusing. One leading expert, for example, might advise 60 minutes of *continuous* physical activity on 3 to 5 days per week. Another might suggest accumulating 30 to 45 minutes of *noncontinuous* activity on most days of the week—perhaps in three separate 10 to 15 minute bouts of exercise per day. Which one of these suggestions is most beneficial? Well, they both improve health and reduce the risk for cardiovascular disease, stroke, diabetes, and many other diseases. However, the continuous activity of longer duration and higher intensity develops performance and fitness more than the shorter duration, less-intense, noncontinuous activity.[1-4]

Five measurable components of fitness are muscular strength, muscular endurance, cardiovascular endurance, flexibility, and body composition. Fitness professionals initially assess each of these components in new clients to establish baseline data to which

> **Health**—the ability to perform normal activities of daily living without undue physiological or emotional stress. A higher level of health decreases the risk for chronic diseases such as coronary heart disease, diabetes, hypertension, osteoporosis, and obesity.
>
> **Fitness**—characteristics that allow optimal functioning of the body. Improves and maintains balance, agility, speed, power, muscular strength and endurance, cardiovascular functioning, flexibility, and body composition.

they compare future measurements. As their clients continue to exercise and make improvements, the fitness professional monitors and documents progress in each of these areas.

> ## QUICK REFERENCE
> According to the U.S. Department of Health and Human Services, individuals who perform at least 150 minutes of moderate-intensity exercise per week experience the greatest health benefits.[4]

DEVELOPMENT OF MUSCULAR STRENGTH AND ENDURANCE

When muscles are challenged with progressive workloads (as occurs during progressive resistance training), they develop as they learn to overcome increasing amounts of stress. Although strength training affects all muscle fiber types, it has the greatest influence on fast fibers. With training, fast fibers grow in size primarily because the number of myofibrils increases. An increase in the number of myofibrils translates into a larger cross-sectional area, a stronger force of contraction, and ultimately greater strength, power, and speed. Additionally, the trained muscle fiber stores a larger quantity of **glucose** and calcium, substances essential for muscle contraction. With these products readily available, the muscle fiber is prepared for action. Moreover, training improves **recruitment ability**. In fact, this neuromuscular adaptation is one of the major contributors to strength gains observed during the first few weeks of resistance exercise training. In essence, as the body becomes accustomed to a new activity and load, communication between the nervous system and the muscular system improves. Better communication means better neuromuscular control. Better neuromuscular control results in greater strength during maximal exertion. Lastly, increased strength also improves joint stability, a factor that can reduce the risk for joint injury.

Like strength training, cardiovascular exercise affects all fiber types; however, it has the most profound effect on slow oxidative fibers (red fibers). With aerobic training, slow fibers develop more capillaries, **myoglobin**, and **mitochondria**—structures that improve their ability to contract. Expanding capillary networks allow the heart to deliver more glucose, fat, and oxygen to working muscles. A greater amount of myoglobin ensures a readily available oxygen supply within skeletal muscles to enhance the aerobic synthesis of ATP. And a greater number of mitochondria facilitates ATP production because the aerobic synthesis of ATP occurs within this organelle. Lastly, **lactic acid threshold** increases with continued aerobic exercise, which means that muscle fibers become better at producing ATP aerobically for a longer duration before having to convert to anaerobic glycolysis. Ultimately, all of these changes result in more efficient muscle metabolism, improved endurance, and greater resistance to fatigue.

QUICK REFERENCE

The precise causes of muscle fatigue are unknown; however, it likely results from both psychological factors (the loss of desire to continue an activity) as well as physiological factors (the inability of a muscle to contract even though a stimulus is present). Experts once believed that lactic acid accumulation within a working muscle was the major contributor to physiological fatigue; however, studies now suggest that lactic acid plays a greater role in psychological fatigue rather than physiological fatigue. The physiological inability of a muscle fiber to contract when stimulated likely results from ion imbalances within the muscle itself. These imbalances occur when sustained, vigorous exercise causes small tears in the sarcoplasmic reticulum of the muscle fiber (see Chapter 2 for more information on muscle fiber structure). This allows calcium to leak into the sarcoplasm. The presence of excess calcium desensitizes the muscle and makes it less responsive to stimulation.[5] Additionally, the loss of potassium from within a muscle fiber might also inhibit contraction despite continued stimulation from the nervous system.

ENHANCED CARDIORESPIRATORY HEALTH

The cardiorespiratory system, which includes the heart, blood, blood vessels, and lungs, functions better with consistent aerobic exercise training. Routine exercise is associated with lower blood pressure, decreased resting pulse rate, improved ratio of

Glucose—a monosaccharide used to produce ATP in muscle fibers. The storage form of glucose is glycogen. The liver stores one third of the body's total glycogen, while skeletal muscle stores the remaining two thirds.

Recruitment ability—the number of muscle fibers stimulated to contract during an all-out exertion. The greater the recruitment ability, the stronger the force. Average recruitment ability in an untrained person is 50%. In a trained athlete, recruitment ability reaches 90% or more.

Myoglobin—an organelle exclusively found in muscle fibers that binds and stores oxygen to be used by muscle fibers during the aerobic production of ATP.

Mitochondria—called the "powerhouses" of cells because a large amount of ATP is produced in them. Slow twitch muscle fibers contain many mitochondria.

Lactic acid threshold—also known as the onset of blood lactate (OBLA). Lactic acid is a natural by-product of anaerobic glycolysis, which produces small amounts of ATP to support short-term, high intensity energy needs. The cardiovascular system transports most lactic acid to the liver where the liver converts it back into glucose. During sustained activity, however, LA production exceeds the liver's ability to recycle it, so it begins to build up. As lactic acid accumulates, it alters muscle pH. Optimal muscle pH is about 7.1—the level at which muscles contract most efficiently. As levels of lactic acid rise, pH drifts to 6.5 at which point local pain receptors are stimulated and burning develops. Typically, lactic acid is removed within 1 hour following exercise cessation.

HIGHLIGHT   LDL and HDL

Contrary to popular belief, there is only one type of cholesterol in the body. Cholesterol is primarily transported by two different types of carriers—LDL and HDL.* A high blood level of low-density lipoprotein, or LDL, is associated with an increased risk of cardiovascular disease. This is not because the cholesterol contained within LDL is different from any other cholesterol in the body. Instead, LDL's *structure* is the primary reason why high levels are so dangerous. Imagine LDL as a hay cart that has a flat bed and railings but is open on top. Rather than carrying hay, LDL carries cholesterol, but the cholesterol is not secured within the LDL molecule. Therefore, as it travels through blood vessels, LDL spills its cholesterol leaving it to accumulate on arterial walls. As cholesterol builds up, it entraps other substances and begins to impede blood flow.

High-density lipoprotein molecules, or HDL, actually decrease the risk of cardiovascular disease. Again, this has nothing to do with the cholesterol that HDL carries since all cholesterol in the body is the same. Instead, a high level of HDL is healthy because of HDL's structure; in other words, HDL holds onto cholesterol without spilling it. Imagine HDL as a vacuum where the contents are tightly enclosed and not able to spill. In addition, imagine that the hose or nozzle of the vacuum suctions up cholesterol lost by LDL. In essence, HDL cleans up cholesterol deposited by LDL. What does HDL do with all of this cholesterol? It transports the cholesterol to the liver where the liver breaks it down and uses it to make bile or other substances. Thus, a high level of HDL actually reduces the risk for cardiovascular disease and is therefore considered a negative risk factor.

* HDL and LDL are lipoproteins, lipids that contain varying amounts of triglycerides, phospholipids, cholesterol, and protein. Fifty percent of an HDL molecule is protein; the remaining 50% is mostly cholesterol with smaller amounts of phospholipids and triglycerides. The greater proportion of protein is what makes this molecule dense. LDL, on the other hand, is 50% cholesterol. Only about 20% of LDL consists of protein; the rest is made up of phospholipids and triglycerides. Additional lipoproteins include chylomicrons, intermediate density lipoprotein (IDL), and very low-density lipoprotein (VLDL). Chylomicrons are the largest and least dense because they contain so little protein and so many triglycerides. Their primary role is to transport dietary triglycerides through lymph and make them available for cells. As they lose triglycerides, chylomicrons become smaller and smaller. The liver ultimately removes them from circulation and recycles the parts. The liver also assembles VLDL and releases these molecules into body fluids. VLDL consists of approximately 50% triglycerides, 40% other lipids, and about 10% protein. They, like chylomicrons, deliver triglycerides to body cells. As they lose triglycerides, their relative cholesterol content increases until they are eventually called IDL. The liver removes and recycles some IDL, but most of it travels through body fluids to deliver more triglycerides. Eventually, these molecules become LDL. Cholesterol plays some important roles in the body. For instance, body cells stabilize themselves by incorporating cholesterol into their cell membranes. Additionally, cholesterol is the basis for substances such as vitamin D, testosterone, estrogen, aldosterone, and cortisol; without it, these substances cannot be synthesized. Interestingly, the liver produces 800 to 1,500 mg of cholesterol per day—far more than what the average person obtains from the diet.

low-density lipoprotein (LDL) to high-density lipoprotein (HDL) levels, and less central fat stores—all of which reduce the risk for cardiovascular disease. In addition, the body develops more capillaries, red blood cells, and hemoglobin, which together improve the efficiency at which the cardiovascular system delivers oxygen to body cells. Like skeletal muscle fibers, cardiac muscle cells adapt to progressive workloads and are able to handle greater demands without undue stress. Tidal volume and VO_{2max} also increase with exercise, and the efficiency of gas exchange across the **alveoli** improves. Overall, these changes decrease the risk for life-threatening cardiovascular events during periods of rest as well as during exertion.[2,6–8]

INCREASED FLEXIBILITY

Flexible joints are necessary to perform common tasks such as bending down to tie a shoe, reaching overhead for a glass, or buckling up a seat belt. Some experts also believe that flexible joints decrease the risk of injury—during normal daily activities and during exertion. Since joint flexibility diminishes significantly with inactivity, exercises that move joints through a full range-of-motion help maintain the pliability of the muscles and connective tissues that form the joint. Thus, aerobic, strength, and stretching exercises positively influence joint function.[2]

IMPROVED BODY COMPOSITION

A healthy body consists of both fat and lean mass. Stored fat insulates, surrounds, and protects many internal body organs, and provides a concentrated source of energy to support metabolism. Therefore, maintaining adequate fat stores is critical. Unfortunately, the average person stores much more fat than necessary. Excess fat is dangerous because it strongly correlates with several chronic conditions.

A higher proportion of lean mass (which includes muscle and bone tissue) promotes overall health and well-being and reduces the risk for several chronic conditions such as diabetes and heart disease. Resistance training is the best way to increase muscle mass and bone density because it applies progressively greater loads that stimulate tissue development. Because muscle is so metabolically active, a person with greater muscle mass burns more kilocalories than one with less muscle mass. As metabolism increases, body fat stores—particularly in the abdominal area—begin to dwindle. Since excessive abdominal fat correlates with an increased risk of numerous chronic conditions, this loss of central fat decreases overall risk.

Aerobic training also improves body composition. As frequency, duration, and/or intensity of aerobic exercise increase, the body loses excess body fat as it burns a greater number of total kilocalories.

Despite the known benefits of physical activity, 60% of American adults fail to meet the minimum recommended amounts of exercise, while nearly 25% are completely sedentary.[3] Some estimates suggest that nearly 70% of Americans are not even remotely active during their leisure time.[9]

Low-density lipoprotein (LDL)—a carrier that transports cholesterol throughout the body.
High-density lipoprotein (HDL)—a carrier that transports cholesterol to the liver.
Alveoli—microscopic air sacs in the lungs; sites of oxygen and carbon dioxide exchange. Each lung has millions of alveoli.

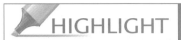

HIGHLIGHT Body Mass Index

Body mass index, or BMI, is a measure of weight in relation to height. It is a reliable tool for assessing risk for disease; however, it does *not* reflect body fat percentage—nor does it provide any information about fat distribution. Because it is inexpensive and easy to use, many health professionals use it to determine client health status. In most cases, health practitioners collect additional information, such as health history, activity level, waist measurement, skin-fold thickness measures, etc., for a comprehensive assessment of a client's overall health.

BMI values can be determined using metric or standard measures. The formulas are as follows:

$$BMI = \frac{kg}{m^2} \text{ or } BMI = \frac{lb \times 703}{in.^2}$$

Sample calculation: A 5′9″ woman weighs 145 lb. What is her BMI?

Multiply weight in pounds by 703:
145 × 703 = 101,935

Convert height into inches:
5′9″ = 69″

Square the inches:
69 × 69 = 4,761

Divide to determine BMI:
BMI = 101,935 ÷ 4,761 = 21.4

BMI is *not* a measure of body fat percentage. Instead, it is a ratio of weight to height and acts as an *indicator* for potential health risks. Use the following guide to determine overall risk for chronic disease:

BMI	Classification
<18.5	Underweight
18.5–24.9	Normal weight
25–29.9	Overweight
≥30	Obese

According to the Centers for Disease Control and Prevention, adults and children can use the same formula for calculating BMI. For those aged 20 and older, the classification chart is the same for all ages and both sexes.[9]

For those under the age of 20, BMI is both age-specific and sex-specific. Therefore, BMI-for-age percentiles for boys and girls, aged 2 to 20, show how one child's measure compares to that of other children of the same age and sex. As an example, a BMI-for-age percentile of 91% means that the child's weight is greater than that of 91% of other children of the same age and sex.[9] This measurement suggests that the child is overweight and has the potential of becoming obese later in life. Consequently, steps should be taken to minimize weight gain and increase activity level. Parents of overweight or obese children, however, should never put them on weight loss diets without consulting a physician.[9] See Appendix C for CDC's body mass index-for-age percentiles, boys and girls, aged 2 to 20.

Underweight	<5th percentile
Healthy weight	5th percentile to 85th percentile
Overweight	85th percentile to <95th percentile
Obese	≥95th percentile

BENEFITS OF NUTRITION

Over the years, the focus of nutrition research has shifted from preventing nutrient deficiencies to preventing **chronic diseases**. Chronic diseases develop slowly over time and tend to persist. Their likelihood of developing is directly related to the **risk factors** present. Since the number of risk factors usually increases over time, most people develop chronic conditions with advancing age. In fact, nearly 80% of Americans over the age of 65 have *at least* one chronic health condition. Although diet has little or no impact on certain chronic conditions, it is directly related to the presence (or absence) of others.

QUICK REFERENCE

Diseases such as scurvy, pellagra, rickets, and beriberi are associated with nutrient deficiencies. Scurvy develops from insufficient vitamin C, pellagra from lack of niacin, rickets from inadequate vitamin D during childhood, and beriberi from thiamin deficiency. Fortunately, nutrient deficiency diseases are no longer common in the United States. Unfortunately, the incidence of chronic conditions, often associated with excess saturated fat, cholesterol, trans-fats, and kilocalories, is on the rise.

The presence of risk factors does not guarantee the development of a chronic disease, nor does the absence of risk factors assure freedom from a disease. However, people with several risk factors are much more likely to develop chronic diseases than those with fewer risk factors. Several risk factors for chronic disease are related to diet. These include the intake of cholesterol, fiber, and total kilocalories, as well as the relative proportions of saturated, trans, and omega-3 fatty acids.

QUICK REFERENCE

The number one modifiable risk factor for chronic disease is cigarette smoking.

To survive, the human body needs carbohydrates, protein, fat, vitamins, minerals, and water. Carbohydrates and fats are major energy nutrients that can be used immediately or

Chronic disease—a condition that develops gradually and slowly over the long term. Chronic diseases are now the leading causes of death in the United States. They include heart disease, cancer, stroke, chronic lung disorders, diabetes, and arthritis.

Risk factor—a behavior or condition that increases the likelihood of developing a chronic disease. Although risk factors are not causal, they are strongly correlated with disease development. The number one modifiable risk factor for chronic disease is cigarette smoking. Other modifiable risk factors include diet, exercise, and alcohol consumption.

stored for future use. Excess dietary fat is easily stored as **adipose**. Excess carbohydrates, on the other hand, fill up glycogen stores in the liver and muscles first; then they form adipose. Unlike carbohydrates and fats, proteins perform various body functions. In addition to forming body structures, they transport substances in body fluids, maintain acid-base balance, regulate water movement, catalyze reactions, function as antibodies, and form the basis of some hormones. Although proteins also provide energy, they are insignificant energy molecules compared to carbohydrates and fats. Excess protein, however, is stored as adipose—not as protein.

QUICK REFERENCE

Excess kilocalories—whether from carbohydrates, protein, or fat—are stored as adipose in the body.

Vitamins and minerals are crucial for metabolism. Although they do not supply energy themselves, they facilitate the metabolic reactions that release energy from carbohydrates, fats, and proteins. Many vitamins act as **coenzymes** in these chemical reactions, while several minerals function as **cofactors**. Additionally, vitamins and minerals transport substances, form structures, and maintain water distribution across cell membranes.

Water, which makes up 60% of the average adult body, is a part of almost every reaction that occurs in the body. If it is not a product or a reactant, it is the medium in which reactions occur. Water is also important in maintaining normal body temperature because it has a high **heat capacity**. As body temperature increases, water in the form of sweat evaporates from the surface of the skin and carries a tremendous amount of body heat with it.

Adequate intake of the six nutrients over time ensures optimal functioning of body systems. Although all people require the same nutrients, the amounts needed to sustain health differ depending upon general body condition. The remaining chapters describe the specific needs and nutrient concerns of individual special populations.

QUICK REFERENCE

Numerous vitamins and minerals are thought to have protective effects when taken in excess of current recommendations. Consider vitamin D. Current recommendations suggest a daily intake of 200 to 600 IU, but researchers believe that as much as 1,000 IU per day is necessary to reap all of the benefits of this vitamin. See the highlight in this chapter for further details. The National Academy of Sciences/National Institutes of Medicine suggests an upper limit of 2,000 IU per day for vitamin D.

State laws closely regulate the dissemination of nutrition information and in most cases restrict nutrition counseling to registered dieticians (RDs). An RD has an undergraduate or graduate degree in nutrition, has completed an American Dietetic Association–approved internship program, has passed a national licensing exam, and accumulates continuing education credits to maintain licensing. Because of these strict regulations, personal trainers and other health professionals need to be cautious when offering nutrition advice to clients or patients. Although nonlicensed individuals are usually restricted from offering specific nutrition prescriptions to clients, it is still important that they understand the unique nutritional requirements of their clients. Why? Nutrition is important for anyone trying to improve or maintain health, and those who exercise need to balance their activity level with healthy food choices and adequate energy intake. Since clients routinely request nutrition advice from their trainers, trainers should be prepared to offer general comments regarding diet quality. In addition, fitness instructors must be able to discern when it is necessary to refer clients to RDs. The more nutrition knowledge fitness professionals have, the better equipped they are to refer their clients to appropriate experts.

CURRENT GENERAL EXERCISE GUIDELINES

Several different organizations offer recommendations related to the frequency, intensity, duration, and type of activity to support health and fitness in the general population. For example, the U.S. Surgeon General suggests that all adults participate in moderate activities such as brisk walking or raking leaves for a minimum of 30 minutes per day. If time is a factor, 15 to 20 minutes of a more strenuous activity such as jogging provides the same health benefits but is associated with a higher risk for exercise-related injury. Although exercise intensity need not be vigorous to improve conditioning, the Surgeon General recognizes that routine, longer duration, higher intensity exercise provides more health and fitness benefits than shorter duration, less intense activities. Like all other organizations, the Surgeon General advises caution when initially beginning an exercise program. Beginners should start with 5 to 10 minutes of exercise during each session and slowly progress to longer bouts as conditioning develops.[3] Overall, some activity is better than no activity, and improvements in health and fitness generally increase with increased frequency, intensity, and duration of activity.[10]

The American College of Sports Medicine (ACSM), which sets the accepted standards for exercise testing and prescription, and the American Heart Association (AHA) offer suggestions for cardiorespiratory, strength, and flexibility training.[1,11,12] Resistance training should be performed with control and through a full range of motion on at least 2 to 3 days per week. Optimal intensity varies for different people, but it should stimulate increases in strength. The duration should be 8 to 12 repetitions of 8 to 10 exercises that target all

---

Adipose—a type of connective tissue that stores excess fat.

Coenzyme—an organic cofactor; often formed from vitamins. Examples include NAD (nicotinomide adenine dinucleotide) and FAD (flavin adenine dinucleotide), which are necessary for cellular respiration. NAD transports hydrogen ions and their electrons to the electron transport chain. It requires the B vitamin niacin. FAD transports hydrogen ions and their electrons to the electron transport chain. It requires the B vitamin riboflavin.

Cofactor—a nonprotein molecule that enables an enzyme to function; may be a metallic ion (such as potassium or calcium) or an organic coenzyme (such as niacin or pantothenic acid).

Heat capacity—the amount of heat required to raise the temperature of one mole or gram of a substance, in this case water, by one degree Celsius.

HIGHLIGHT   Vitamin D: A Miracle Worker?

Scientists have long known how important vitamin D is to bone health. Vitamin D, found in eggs, fish, and fortified milk, is necessary for calcium absorption in the small intestine. Without it, calcium passes through the GI tract unabsorbed. Since calcium is the major constituent of bone matrix, the ability to maintain healthy bone tissue is contingent upon calcium intake *and* calcium bioavailability (the extent to which the body can absorb the nutrient).

Ninety-nine percent of the body's total calcium is found in bones and teeth—in fact, it gives this tissue its strength and flexibility. Calcium, however, is even more critical for processes such as muscle contraction and neuron functioning; therefore, even though only 1% of the body's calcium supply is in blood, the body maintains this blood calcium level even if it must destroy bones to do so. In other words, if dietary calcium intake is low, the body strips calcium from its huge reservoir in the skeleton. After all, a person can live with demineralized bone but not without muscle contraction and neuron functioning. Unfortunately, it is not enough to ingest recommended amounts of calcium. To ensure that dietary calcium is actually absorbed into the body, vitamin D levels must also be maintained.

Recent research suggests that vitamin D might also protect against conditions such as cancer, hypertension, and several autoimmune disorders.[13–19] The amount necessary to reduce risk for these disorders, however, is much higher than the average person could obtain from dietary sources alone. Therefore, supplemental vitamin D might be required to increase blood serum vitamin D to a level that actually reduces risk.

What exactly does the research suggest with regard to cancer? One study in which women older than age 55 took 1,000 IU of supplemental vitamin D per day found a significant decrease in the risk for all cancers.[14] Another study found a slight decrease in the risk of breast cancer among a large group of postmenopausal women who took a daily supplement that contained at least 800 IU.[16] A daily intake of 1,000 to 2,000 IU of vitamin D was associated with a reduced incidence of colorectal cancer according to a metaanalysis of existing research.[13,20] Studies in which the subjects took lower amounts of vitamin D, such as 400 IU per day, found that the risk of cancer was not significantly reduced.[18]

Some existing data suggests a link between vitamin D deficiency and cardiovascular disease. Subjects in the Framingham Offspring Cohort who had low serum levels of vitamin D experienced hypertension, myocardial infarction, angina, stroke, and transient ischemic attacks more often than those who had normal vitamin D serum levels. However, whether supplementing the diet with vitamin D reduces the risk is still not known. More research is needed before recommendations can be made.

Many studies have noted that subjects with higher vitamin D serum levels had low risks of developing type 1 and type 2 diabetes. This was true for both children and adults. Diabetes results in an elevated blood glucose concentration because the body is unable to transport this glucose into cells. It appears that adequate calcium and vitamin D levels help optimize the body's ability to metabolize glucose and might, therefore, normalize blood glucose levels.[21]

(continued)

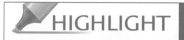

HIGHLIGHT | Vitamin D: A Miracle Worker? (*continued*)

Surveys indicate that vitamin D intake in the United States is far below recommended levels. In fact, nearly half of all middle-aged and older adults have a deficiency of this vitamin.[22] Based on recent research, some experts suggest that Americans increase their dietary intake of vitamin D and consider vitamin D supplements to achieve the potential benefits of high blood serum levels.

An inactive form of vitamin D stored within dermal blood vessels can be activated upon exposure to UV radiation. As little as 10 to 15 minutes of exposure on 2 to 3 days per week is usually adequate. Keep in mind, sunscreen, which helps protect the body against the damaging effects of UV radiation, also interferes with the body's ability to activate vitamin D. In other words, it reduces the amount that is produced from sun exposure; however, since the risk of skin cancer increases proportionately with exposure of unprotected skin to UV radiation, it is not the intent of this highlight to discourage readers from wearing sunscreen.

major muscle groups. Effective resistance training might use bands, free weights, stability balls, weight machines, or exercises that employ body weight (such as pull-ups and push-ups).

Cardiovascular training includes continuous aerobic activity that uses large muscle groups. Moderately intense aerobic activity should be performed for a minimum of 30 minutes on at least 5 days per week. Vigorous aerobic activity need only be performed for a minimum of 20 to 25 minutes on at least 3 days per week. A combination of moderate and vigorous activity should be performed for a minimum of 20 to 30 minutes on at least 3 to 5 days per week. Examples of aerobic exercises include running, bicycling, elliptical training, swimming, group-fitness aerobics classes, water aerobics, tennis, and volleyball. Those desiring to lose weight—or those trying to maintain weight loss—probably need to participate in 60 to 90 minutes of moderate aerobic activity on most days of the week. Stretching exercises should target all major muscle groups. They should be performed 2 to 3 days per week for ≥4 repetitions per muscle group. Examples include static stretching, dynamic stretching, **proprioceptive neuromuscular facilitation,** yoga, and tai chi.[1,11,12]

Proprioceptive neuromuscular facilitation—an advanced form of stretching that involves contraction and stretching of the targeted muscle. Do a light warm-up to prepare the muscles for this intense stretching. To begin, get into position for the stretch. Have a partner slightly stretch the targeted muscle. Then contract this muscle group against the immoveable resistance created by the partner (or a towel). Contract for 5 to 6 seconds. Relax. Have the partner stretch the muscle group for about 30 seconds. Completely relax the muscle group for 30 seconds to allow for recovery. Repeat the contraction and stretching phases two to four times.

QUICK REFERENCE

ACSM suggests that the general population participate in resistance training on at least 2 to 3 days per week at an intensity that permits 8 to 12 repetitions of 8 to 10 exercises that target the major muscle groups (chest, shoulders, abdomen, back, hips, legs, and arms). Duration should be two to four sets per exercise. ACSM suggests moderate aerobic activity (40% to 60% VO_{2R}) for at least 30 minutes on at least 5 days per week, or 20 to 25 minutes of vigorous aerobic activity (≥60% VO_{2R}) on at least 3 days per week, or a combination of moderate and vigorous activity for at least 20 to 30 minutes on at least 3 to 5 days per week. Additionally, ACSM advises that all populations engage in flexibility training targeting all major muscle groups on at least 2 to 3 days per week with ≥4 repetitions per muscle group. Static, dynamic, or proprioceptive neuromuscular facilitation (PNF) improve flexibility. Hold static stretches for 15 to 60 seconds. During PNF, follow a 6-second contraction by a 10 to 30 second assisted stretch.[1]

Inherent in any exercise program is the risk of injury and even the possibility of death; accordingly, fitness professionals must screen clients, obtain medical clearances, and offer exercise testing when necessary. These precautions are even more important when working with special populations since the characteristics of individuals in any given special needs group predispose them to risks that might not be associated with the general population.[1]

BENEFITS OF EXERCISE FOR SPECIAL POPULATIONS

Special populations include a broad and diverse group of people who have conditions and needs different from the general population. In some cases, a person belongs to a special population for a finite time. Pregnant women, for example, have special exercise and dietary considerations during gestation to ensure optimal maternal health and fetal development. These particular requirements, however, become unnecessary once the baby is born or is no longer breast-feeding. In most other cases, once special needs develop, they remain for a lifetime. Consequently, individuals with special needs demand special lifelong exercise prescriptions and dietary modifications to ensure health, safety, and effectiveness.

QUICK REFERENCE

Regular physical activity provides health benefits for most special populations, including seniors, youth, and those with disabilities.[4]

Most authorities now recognize that special populations receive the same benefits from routine exercise as the general population (see Table 1.1). In fact, the Surgeon General suggests that those with conditions such as heart disease, diabetes, or obesity begin exercising once they receive physician clearance. With regular exercise, participants can

TABLE 1-1   HEALTH BENEFITS OF EXERCISE, ACCORDING TO THE U.S. SURGEON GENERAL

- Reduced risk of developing high blood pressure
- Maintenance of a healthy blood pressure in those with chronic hypertension
- Reduced risk of developing type 2 diabetes
- Reduced risk of death from coronary heart disease
- Reduced risk of osteoporosis
- Maintenance of pain-free range-of-motion at joints
- Increase in and preservation of muscle mass
- Maintenance of a healthy weight
- Decreased body fat
- Relief of symptoms associated with anxiety and depression

improve functional capacity and future health outcomes, and as long as safety guidelines are followed, the benefits far outweigh the risks.

SUMMARY

Evidence suggests that a combination of increased physical activity and improved nutritional intake enhances growth and development in all populations. Furthermore, it minimizes the rate of body system decline for practically everyone regardless of their current health status. Therefore, it is important to challenge the heart, muscles, and bones throughout life to encourage optimal functioning of each body system and to manage or reduce the risk for chronic disease later in life. Although one special population might respond to exercise differently from another, each can still reap many benefits. Trainers, therapists, health professionals, and anyone else involved with designing exercise programs should tailor programs to meet individual needs. Not only does activity influence current health status, it also improves self-image, mood, body composition, and self-efficacy. By adhering to the guidelines presented throughout this book, health professionals can ensure that their clients participate in safe exercise programs that can be continued for a lifetime.

THINKING CRITICALLY

1. Explain the difference between exercise for health and exercise for fitness. Give a brief description of an exercise routine that would fall into each category.
2. How does recruitment ability change after doing resistance training?

VO_{2R}—oxygen consumption reserve; the difference between resting and maximal VO_{2max}.

3. Describe some of the physiological changes that occur with continued cardiovascular training.
4. Differentiate between LDL and HDL in both structure and function.
5. Explain the relationship between chronic diseases and risk factors.
6. Name the six categories of nutrients and explain the importance of each.
7. Who is legally permitted to develop nutrition prescriptions? Explain the role of the fitness professional as related to nutrition.
8. Differentiate between the "general population" and a "special population."
9. Explain some of the benefits of exercise for both general and special populations.

REFERENCES

1. American College of Sports Medicine. ACSM's Guidelines for Exercise Testing and Prescription, 8th Ed. Philadelphia: Lippincott Williams & Wilkins, 2010.
2. Harvard Health Letter. The best prescription money can't buy. January 2006. http://www.healthy.harvard.edu
3. National Center for Chronic Disease Prevention and Health Promotion: Physical Activity and Health. A Report of the Surgeon General. http://www.cdc.gov/nccdphp/sgr/adults.htm
4. United States Department of Health and Human Services. 2008 Physical Activity Guidelines for Americans. www.health.gov/PAGuidelines
5. Bellinger AM, Reiken S, Dura M, et al. Remodeling of ryanodine receptor complex causes "leaky" channels: a molecular mechanism for decreased exercise capacity. The Proceedings of the National Academy of Sciences, February 11, 2008.
6. Barlow CE, LaMonte MJ, Fitzgerald SJ, et al. Cardiorespiratory fitness is an independent predictor of hypertension incidence among initially normotensive healthy women. Am J Epidemiol 2006; 163(2):142–150.
7. Lee IM, Sesso H, Oguma Y, et al. Relative intensity of physical activity and risk of coronary heart disease. Circulation. 2003;107:1110–1116.
8. Tanasescu M, Leitzmann MF, Rimm E, et al. Exercise type and intensity in relation to coronary heart disease in men. JAMA 2002;288: 1994–2000.
9. Centers for Disease Control. www.cdc.gov
10. Healthy People 2010: Understanding and Improving Health. U.S. Department of Health and Human Services. http://www.healthypeople.gov/
11. American Heart Association. www.americanheart.org
12. Haskell WL, Lee IM, Pate R, et al. Physical activity and public health updated recommendations for adults from the American College of Sports Medicine and the American Heart Association. Circ J Am Heart Assoc 2007;116:1081–1093.
13. Gorham E, Garland C, Garland F, et al. Optimal vitamin D status for colorectal cancer prevention: a quantitative meta analysis. Am J Prev Med 2007; 32(3):210–216.
14. Lappe J, Travers-Gustafson D, Davies KM, et al. Vitamin D and calcium supplementation reduces cancer risk: results of a randomized trial. Am J Clin Nutr 2007;85(6):1586–1591.
15. Pittas A, Lau J, Dawson-Hughes B, et al. The role of vitamin D and calcium in type 2 diabetes. A systematic review and meta-analysis. J Clin Endocrinol Metabol 2007;92(6):2017–2029.
16. Robien K, Cutler G, Virnig B, et al. Vitamin D intake and breast cancer risk in postmenopausal women: the Iowa Women's Health Study. Cancer Causes Control 2007;18(7):775–782.
17. Schumann S, Evigman B. Double-dose vitamin D lowers cancer risk in women over 55. J Fam Pract 2007;56(11):907–910.
18. Wactawski-Wende J, Kotchen J, Anderson GL, et al. Calcium plus vitamin D supplementation and the risk of colorectal cancer. N Engl J Med 2006;354(7):684–696.
19. Lind L, Wengle B. Reduction of blood pressure during long-term treatment with active vitamin D (alphacalcidol) is dependent on plasma renin activity and calcium status. A double blind, placebo-controlled study. Am J Hypertens 1989;2(1): 20–25.
20. Garland C, Garland F, Gorham D, et al. The role of vitamin D in cancer prevention. Am Public Health 2006; 96(2):252–261.

21. Mathieu C, Gysemans C, Bouillon R, et al. Vitamin D and diabetes. Diabetologia 2005;48(7): 1247–1257.
22. Crawford-Faucher A. Commentary: Does vitamin D deficiency increase risk of cardiovascular disease? Am Fam Physician. 2008;78(8):1.

SUGGESTED WEBSITES

American College of Sports Medicine. http://www.acsm.org

Healthy People 2010: Understanding and Improving Health. http://www.healthypeople.gov

2 ANATOMY AND PHYSIOLOGY OF BODY SYSTEMS

Each of the eleven body systems consists of two or more organs that cooperate to achieve a common purpose. For example, the digestive system includes the mouth, esophagus, stomach, and small intestine which work together to break down food, absorb nutrients, and eliminate wastes. The urinary system, which consists of the kidneys, ureters, and urethra, systematically processes blood to form urine to rid the body of metabolic wastes.

Although fitness professionals can successfully create exercise programs for clients without thoroughly understanding all body systems, practitioners usually find it helpful to understand basic organization and function (Table 2.1), particularly when working with special needs groups. Understanding how systems *should* work provides the foundation for understanding what goes awry in those with special conditions. This chapter is for readers who are unfamiliar with the body systems and want a firmer foundation before delving more deeply into specific special populations.

INTEGUMENTARY SYSTEM

The integumentary system includes the epidermis, dermis, hypodermis, hair, hair follicles, nails, nail beds, **sebaceous glands**, **sudoriferous glands**, and nerve endings. In general, it keeps harmful substances out of the body, regulates internal body temperature, produces a usable form of vitamin D in the presence of UV radiation, and provides **cutaneous sensations**.

QUICK REFERENCE

The term *skin* refers to both the epidermis and the dermis. It does not include the hypodermis, also known as the subcutaneous layer or superficial fascia.

Intact skin acts as a nearly impenetrable barrier partly because it consists of multiple layers. Additionally, the outermost cells of the epidermis contain keratin, a protein that toughens the skin. Together, the multiple layers and the keratin inhibit the entry of most **microbes** and protect underlying tissues from harsh chemicals. If a **pathogen** happens to gain entry by way of a break in the skin, **Langerhans cells** located in the

TABLE 2-1 MAJOR BODY SYSTEMS	
Body System	**Function**
Integumentary system	Protects; regulates body temperature; supports sensory receptors; eliminates wastes; helps produce vitamin D
Skeletal system	Provides body framework; protects soft tissues; provides attachment for muscles; produces blood cells; stores minerals
Muscular system	Powers movement; maintains posture; produces heat
Cardiovascular system	Heart creates the force to move blood through blood vessels; blood components deliver oxygen and nutrients and help protect against disease
Respiratory system	Permits inhalation and exhalation; provides oxygen and eliminates carbon dioxide; regulates pH balance; produces sound
Endocrine system	Regulates body activities by producing and releasing hormones
Nervous system	Regulates body activities by initiating and propagating nerve impulses that control muscle and glands; detects, interprets, and responds to stimuli
Digestive system	Receives, digests, and absorbs food components; eliminates wastes
Lymphatic/Immune system	Returns excess interstitial fluid to blood; transports fats from GI tract to venous system; protects against disease
Urinary system	Filters blood to form urine; eliminates wastes; maintains water and electrolyte balance; stores and transports urine
Reproductive system	Produces and maintains gametes; produces and releases sex hormones

Sebaceous glands—also known as oil glands. They produce and release sebum, an oily mixture composed of protein, lipids, and cell fragments. Most sebaceous glands attach to hair follicles and release sebum into the follicle where it moisturizes and protects the hair from breakage.

Sudoriferous glands—also known as sweat glands. There are two types. *Eccrine sudoriferous glands* are more common and are active throughout life. They regulate temperature by releasing sweat—a mixture consisting of water plus a small amount of dissolved substances—when body temperature increases. *Apocrine sudoriferous glands* become active at puberty and release a combination of water and lipids during times of fear, stress, or sexual arousal. When bacteria on the skin surface metabolize this product, they create body odor.

Cutaneous sensation—sensory perceptions in the skin such as hot, cold, pressure, touch, tickle, etc.

Microbes—microscopic organisms such as bacteria, fungi, protozoa, or viruses. Many microbes are pathogenic, or disease-causing.

Pathogen—an agent that causes disease; usually refers to an infectious organism such as a bacterium, virus, or fungus.

Langerhans cells—a type of white blood cell that engulfs, dismantles, and inactivates foreign particles that enter through the skin. UV radiation easily destroys Langerhans cells. Langerhans cells are phagocytes, cells that are discussed in more detail in the section on the lymphatic/immune system.

deeper epidermal layers usually engulf and destroy them before they cause damage. **Melanin**, a pigment that protects epidermal DNA from UV radiation, is also present. Deep epidermal cells produce melanin and transfer it to surrounding cells where it accumulates on the sunny side of the nucleus and shields DNA from sunrays. Lastly, glycolipids fill the spaces between cells in the more superficial epidermal layers and thereby prevent excessive loss of body fluids.

Normal metabolic reactions continuously produce heat as a by-product; therefore, metabolically active organs release large amounts of heat that can threaten the homeostasis of body temperature. To prevent dangerous increases in body temperature, which can occur during exercise as skeletal muscle becomes more active, the body activates sweat glands and dilates superficial blood vessels. When activated, eccrine sudoriferous glands release sweat onto the surface of the body. As this sweat evaporates from the skin surface, it carries large amounts of heat with it and allows body temperature to normalize. The activity of sweat glands declines as body temperature returns to normal through a process called negative feedback. Blood vessel dilation reduces internal body temperature by permitting the radiation of heat. Although the epidermis is **avascular**, the dermis contains an elaborate network of blood vessels. As internal body temperature rises, these dermal vessels dilate. Blood flow to dilated vessels increases, which means that blood flow to deeper vessels decreases. This brings warm blood from deeper tissues closer to the skin surface where heat radiates into the surrounding environment. As body temperature drops, vessel diameter returns to normal, blood flow to the skin surface decreases, and heat loss decreases.

The hypodermis, which is the third layer of the integument, also influences body temperature. This layer contains adipose, which insulates and protects against heat loss.

QUICK REFERENCE

Water has a high heat capacity; this means that it takes a lot of heat to change the temperature of water. Because the human body contains a significant amount of water, extreme temperature changes are rare, so body temperature remains relatively stable.

The primary metabolic function of skin is to form active vitamin D. Cells within the small intestine convert some dietary cholesterol into 7-dehydrocholesterol, or provitamin D. This inactive form of vitamin D is then stored in dermal blood vessels. Exposure to UV radiation activates provitamin D by converting the modified cholesterol molecules within dermal blood vessels into calcitriol, the body's most active form of vitamin D. Vitamin D then stimulates the formation of calcium transporters in the digestive tract to allow the body to absorb dietary calcium. Without vitamin D, cells cannot absorb calcium.

> *QUICK REFERENCE*
>
> Vitamin D is necessary for dietary calcium absorption. It travels in the blood to the small intestine where it stimulates the production of a calcium-binding protein necessary for the movement of calcium from the digestive tract into body cells.

A final function of the integumentary system is to transmit sensory information about the external environment to the central nervous system (CNS). Each layer has a rich supply of sensory receptors that detect pain, pressure, touch, heat, and cold to protect it from prolonged exposure to potentially damaging stimuli.

SKELETAL SYSTEM

The skeletal system is composed of bones, cartilage, and ligaments. It provides a structural framework that supports the body, supplies attachment points for muscles and tendons, protects internal organs and other soft tissues, serves as a lever system that permits muscles to act across joints, stores and releases minerals as blood levels fluctuate, and houses red bone marrow, the site of **hemopoesis**.

The two types of bone tissue are compact bone and spongy bone. Compact bone is the major type of bone tissue in the femur, tibia, humerus, radius, and other long bones. It also forms the outermost layer of all bones. It is essentially composed of calcified rings of matrix with very little space inside. Spongy bone, found in the ends of long bones and in the center of flat, irregular, short, and sesamoid bones, is composed of **trabeculae**, branches of bone tissue surrounded by spaces filled with red bone marrow. Because spongy bone has so much space inside, it is lighter in weight than compact bone.

Somewhat surprisingly, bone is not an inert tissue. Instead, old bone tissue is continuously replaced with new bone tissue through a process called remodeling. To facilitate this continual turnover, a bone has a huge network of blood vessels that supply it with oxygen and nutrients. The two major types of cells involved with remodeling are osteoblasts and osteoclasts. **Osteoblasts** are bone-builders that deposit bone tissue in response to

Melanin—a pigment produced by melanocytes in the deepest layer of the epidermis. Melanin contributes to skin color. Melanocytes produce melanin from the amino acid tyrosine and transfer it to surrounding cells where it accumulates on the sunny surface of the nucleus— there it absorbs UV radiation to prevent DNA mutations.
Avascular—lacking blood vessels.
Hemopoesis (hematopoesis)—the formation of blood cells.
Trabeculae—branches of bone tissue surrounded by large cavities containing red bone marrow. The matrix of spongy bone is arranged in trabeculae.
Osteoblasts—bone-building cells that secrete the matrix in which calcium salts are deposited.

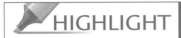

HIGHLIGHT   The Importance of Calcium

In addition to forming the basic structure of bone tissue, calcium serves several other crucial roles in the body. For example, nerve cells, called neurons, require calcium to release neurotransmitters. Neurotransmitters are important communicators between neurons and their effectors (which include muscle and gland tissue). If communication between a neuron and its effector is interrupted, the effector cannot respond. This can then disturb homeostasis. In addition, calcium is essential for muscle contraction. When calcium levels are either too high or too low, muscle fibers cannot generate force normally. Calcium is also necessary for normal blood clotting. Insufficient calcium delays blood clotting and increases the risk of hemorrhage.

Because of calcium's critical roles, the body maintains blood calcium levels within a narrow margin. If dietary intake is insufficient to meet demands, the skeletal system sacrifices its calcium reserves so that blood levels return to normal. Consequently, people must conscientiously consume foods high in calcium to preserve bone tissue and slow bone loss. Excess depletion of calcium from bones diminishes bone mass, which increases the risk for bone fracture.

mechanical stress. Osteoblasts also initiate calcification, or the hardening of bones as mineral salts are deposited. **Osteoclasts** are bone-destroyers that attack and break down bone tissue to clear a way for new bone growth. Additionally, the action of osteoclasts allows bones to serve as a reservoir for calcium to ensure optimal blood calcium levels. Obviously, a balance between the activities of osteoblasts and osteoclasts is critical if bone mass is to remain stable.

Several different hormones influence the rate and extent of bone remodeling. Calcitonin and parathyroid hormone (PTH), for example, dramatically affect bone mass. Their primary function is to maintain blood calcium levels, but while ensuring adequate blood levels, they indirectly affect bone density. The thyroid gland releases calcitonin in response to excess calcium in the blood (which occurs after consuming foods rich in calcium). Calcitonin inhibits osteoclasts and stimulates osteoblasts, factors that increase calcium deposition in bones. When blood calcium levels drop, the parathyroid glands release PTH to stimulate osteoclasts and inhibit osteoblasts. PTH also slows down the removal of calcium via urine, while it stimulates the kidneys to activate more vitamin D. Vitamin D then enhances calcium absorption in the small intestine. See Table 2.2 for a summary of these hormones and their actions.

Estrogen and testosterone also affect remodeling. These hormones stimulate osteoblast activity and thus increase calcium deposition in bones. Human growth hormone stimulates the lengthening of long bones by acting on the **epiphyseal plate**. As this cartilage layer grows and moves out, the bone lengthens. Thyroxine from the thyroid gland stimulates the pituitary gland to release additional hGH, so thyroxine also promotes the lengthening of long bones. However, since thyroxine stimulates the ossification of the epiphyseal plate, it ultimately inhibits bone lengthening.

TABLE 2-2 HORMONES THAT INFLUENCE BONE REMODELING

Hormone	Effect of Hormone
Calcitonin	Released by the thyroid gland when blood calcium levels increase. Inhibits osteoclasts and stimulates osteoblasts, which leads to increased calcium deposition in bone.
Parathyroid hormone	Released by parathyroid glands when blood calcium levels decrease. Stimulates osteoclasts, inhibits osteoblasts, slows the removal of calcium via urine, and stimulates the kidneys to activate more vitamin D.
Estrogen/testosterone	Both stimulate osteoblast activity and thus increase calcium deposition in bone.
Human growth hormone	Stimulates the lengthening of long bones by acting on the epiphyseal plate. As this plate grows and moves out, the bone lengthens.

QUICK REFERENCE

Because of remodeling, most spongy bone in the body is completely replaced every 3 to 4 years. It takes nearly 10 years to replace most compact bone. The rate of remodeling, however, varies in different bones.

The epiphyseal plates, which allow bones to grow in length, typically ossify between the ages of 19 and 25, at which time a bone's ability to lengthen ceases. Since bone growth in width does not depend upon a cartilage plate, bones can theoretically continue to grow in width whenever mechanical stress stimulates osteoblast activity.

Dietary intake and exercise dramatically affect the quality of bone remodeling. Healthy bone tissue forms when mechanical forces are applied to the bone and adequate calcium, vitamin D, protein, and other nutrients are present. Weight-bearing exercises, including walking, running, and resistance training, stimulate osteoblast activity along lines of mechanical stress. Osteoblasts ultimately deposit bone tissue to withstand the new forces applied.

Joints exist wherever two bones meet, so they are technically a component of the skeletal system. Although some joints in the body are immoveable or only slightly moveable, the freely moveable joints are most important relative to exercise (Fig. 2.1).

A double-layered joint capsule surrounds moveable joints. The articular cartilage, a layer of hyaline cartilage found on the articulating surfaces of bone, essentially resists wear and tear of bone tissue and acts as a shock absorber to prevent articulating bones from being crushed during impact. The joint capsule consists of an outer fibrous

Osteoclasts—bone-destroying cells that release acid and enzymes to dissolve bone matrix.
Epiphyseal plate (growth plate)—found at the ends of long bones like the femur and humerus; composed of hyaline cartilage; remains until the ages of 19 to 25. Bone continues to grow in length as long as the epiphyseal plate is present. Bone ceases to grow in length when this cartilage layer ossifies into the epiphyseal line.

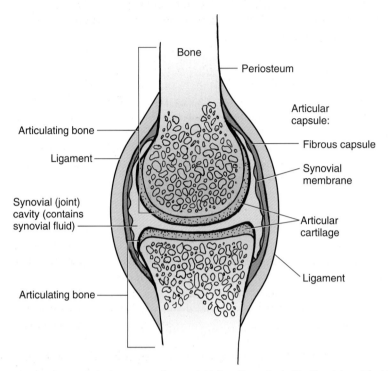

FIGURE 2.1 ■ General structure of a synovial joint. (From Oatis CA. Kinesiology. The Mechanics and Pathomechanics of Human Movement. Baltimore: Lippincott Williams & Wilkins, 2003.)

capsule—strong enough to resist pulling forces yet flexible enough to permit movement—and an inner synovial membrane that produces synovial fluid. Synovial fluid not only reduces friction between two bone ends, but it also supplies nutrients to the articular cartilage and contains cells that eliminate debris and microbes within the synovial cavity. Synovial fluid is similar in texture and appearance to egg whites. When joints are immobile, synovial fluid becomes almost gel-like, which limits joint mobility. Anyone who has experienced stiff joints in the morning upon getting out of bed knows what this feels like! With activity, synovial fluid thins and warms, which improves joint mobility.

Several additional structures help stabilize joints. They include tendons, ligaments, menisci, bursae, and tendon sheaths. *Tendons* attach bones to muscles and thereby allow low-level muscle contractions to stabilize and strengthen joints. In fact, this low level contraction, called muscle tone, is the greatest contributor to joint stability. *Ligaments* unite bones to bones and further stabilize joints. Ligaments typically firmly attach to the outer lining of bone and prevent excessive movements that might damage joint tissue. *Menisci* are pads of cartilage found between the articulating surfaces of some bones. The menisci in the knee, for example, increase stability by permitting a better fit between the femur of the thigh and the tibia of the leg. *Bursae* are simply bags of lubricant that act as ball bearings to reduce friction in joints such as the shoulder and the knee. *Tendon sheaths* are similar in structure to bursae; however, they wrap around tendons in areas that are prone to stress—such as the wrist and ankle.

Range of motion, or the flexibility permitted by a joint, is the range through which the bones of a joint can move. Flexibility and stability are inversely related. As stability increases, flexibility tends to decrease; as stability decreases, flexibility tends to increase. Factors that affect range of motion at a joint include the structure or shape of articulating surfaces; the tension of associated ligaments; the arrangement of the muscles acting on the joint; and the use of a joint.

As mentioned, the closer the fit between two bones, the more stable but less mobile the joint. Consider two ball-and-socket joints. The shoulder joint, formed between the humerus and the scapula, is the more flexible joint because the head of the humerus fits loosely into the shallow glenoid cavity of the scapula. Because of this extensive range of motion, however, this joint is not very stable and is prone to injury. The hip joint, on the other hand, formed as the head of the femur articulates with the deep acetabulum of the coxal bone, is much more stable. This extra stability impedes range of motion because the two bones fit so snuggly together. Although still freely moveable, the hip joint is less flexible than the shoulder joint.

Tension within associated ligaments also affects range of motion. Ligaments are taught when joints are in certain positions and flexible when joints are in other positions. Consider the anterior cruciate ligament of the knee joint. When the knee is flexed, the anterior cruciate ligament is taught and more restrictive; however, when the knee is extended, it is loose and less restrictive. The more pliable the ligament, the more range permitted at that joint.

Muscle tension affects flexibility of a joint as well. For example, knee extension limits hip flexion as the hamstrings muscles are lengthened and the quadriceps femoris muscles contract. Knee flexion, on the other hand, enhances hip flexion as the hamstrings contract and the quadriceps femoris muscles relax.

Lastly, the more frequently a joint is used and moved through its full range of motion, the more mobile it remains. In fact, consistent use keeps muscles, tendons, and ligaments pliable and encourages synovial fluid production.

MUSCULAR SYSTEM

The major functions of skeletal muscle are to maintain posture, provide stability across joints, permit locomotion, and maintain body temperature. The characteristics that enable them to perform these functions include excitability, extensibility, elasticity, and contractility. *Excitability*, or responsiveness, is a muscle fiber's ability to receive and respond to **stimuli**. The stimulus can be chemical (such as a neurotransmitter released by a neuron) or mechanical (as when tendons are overstretched). *Extensibility* refers to a muscle cell's ability

---

Stimulus—a change in the internal or external environment that initiates a response by the nervous or muscular system.

to stretch up to three times its normal length *without breaking*. Several other body cells rupture when subjected to such force. *Elasticity* refers to the muscle cell's ability to recoil, or return to its normal length after extension or contraction. *Contractility* is the muscle cell's ability to generate force. An isotonic contraction occurs when a muscle generates enough force to overcome a resistance. The *concentric phase* of an isotonic contraction is the positive phase where the entire muscle shortens as its force exceeds the force of the resistance. The *eccentric phase*, or negative phase, results when the same muscle lengthens as resistance begins to exceed muscle force; this occurs as a weight is lowered. Consider a flat bench press. The concentric phase of contraction occurs as the weight is pushed up; the eccentric phase occurs as the weight is lowered. When a muscle generates force, but that force is insufficient to overcome the resistance, the muscle undergoes an isometric contraction. In isometric contractions, the entire muscle does not shorten even though force develops.

Skeletal muscles are composed of long tubelike structures called fascicles that are separated from one another by a connective tissue layer called the perimysium (Fig. 2.2).

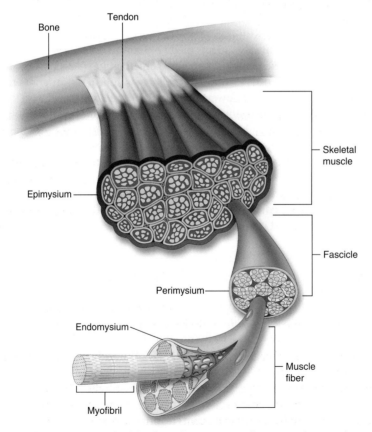

FIGURE 2.2 ■ Structure of a skeletal muscle. (From McArdle WD, Katch FI, Katch VL. Essentials of Exercise Physiology, 2nd Ed. Baltimore: Lippincott Williams & Wilkins, 2000.)

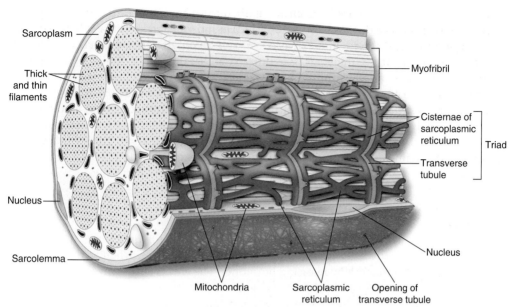

Sarcoplasm

Thick and thin filaments

Nucleus

Sarcolemma

Myofibril

Cisternae of sarcoplasmic reticulum

Transverse tubule

Triad

Nucleus

Mitochondria

Sarcoplasmic reticulum

Opening of transverse tubule

FIGURE 2.3 ■ Structure of an individual skeletal muscle fiber. (From McArdle WD, Katch FI, Katch VL. *Essentials of Exercise Physiology.* 2nd Ed, Baltimore: Lippincott Williams & Wilkins, 2000.)

Within each fascicle are 10 to 100 elongated cells called muscle fibers. Each individual muscle fiber is surrounded by a connective tissue layer called the endomysium, which wraps around the **sarcolemma** (Fig. 2.3). The fibers are packed with nuclei, **mitochondria**, **myoglobin**, and **glycosomes**. They also contain **myofibrils**, which form from various proteins including actin, myosin, tropomyosin, and troponin. Actin and myosin are contractile proteins that enable muscle fibers to generate force.

Surprisingly, people are born with the maximum number of muscle fibers they will ever have. This means that growth and development do not result from **hyperplasia**, or

> **Sarcolemma**—the cell membrane of a muscle fiber; the structure that separates the inside of the muscle fiber from the outside.
>
> **Mitochondria**—the powerhouse of a cell; the site of the Kreb's cycle and electron transport chain that complete glucose oxidation to produce large amounts of ATP. Mitochondria are abundant in slow twitch fibers.
>
> **Myoglobin**—a red-pigmented protein that stores oxygen. Found only in muscle tissue; abundant in slow twitch fibers.
>
> **Glycosomes**—organelles that store glycogen. Abundant in fast twitch fibers.
>
> **Myofibrils**—tubular organelles in which actin and myosin filaments are arranged in sarcomeres. Sarcomeres are the contractile units of muscle fibers.
>
> **Hyperplasia**—an increase in cell number. Fat cells increase in number; muscle cells do not.

an increase in the total number of muscle fibers. Instead, muscle fibers grow by the process of **hypertrophy** where the cross-sectional area of individual muscle fibers increases. Fast fibers, for example, develop more glycosomes and myofibrils when subjected to progressive overloads that force the fibers to perform at higher intensities. An increase in myofibrils translates into a greater muscle fiber diameter and improved muscle strength, power, and speed. Slow fibers, on the other hand, which have a limited ability to grow in size, develop more blood vessels, myoglobin, and mitochondria with long-term aerobic training. Although these factors do not significantly increase power, speed, or strength, they allow the slow fiber to contract without fatigue for a longer duration. Therefore, different methods of training benefit different muscle fiber types.

NERVOUS AND ENDOCRINE SYSTEMS: THE REGULATORY SYSTEMS

The nervous system and endocrine system regulate all other body systems. The nervous system controls body activities by propagating nerve impulses, whereas the endocrine system exerts its influence by releasing hormones. The effects elicited by the nervous system occur immediately and subside relatively rapidly. Those elicited by the endocrine system, on the other hand, generally take several minutes, hours, or even days to develop, but they tend to last longer.

Neuroglia and neurons are the two principal cell types found in the nervous system. Six types of neuroglial cells actively assist neurons. They have varied shapes and functions, but overall they supply nutrients to neurons, provide structural support, maintain the appropriate chemical environment for neuron activity, clear away debris, increase the rate of impulse propagation, and regulate what actually enters the Central Nervous System (CNS). Although they do not propagate impulses themselves, neuroglial cells are essential for neuron functioning. Neurons are the impulse-generating cells of the nervous system. They respond to stimuli; convert stimuli into impulses; control effectors such as muscles and glands; and allow people to sense, think, remember, and have emotions.

The two major structural divisions of the nervous system are the CNS and the peripheral nervous system (PNS). The CNS includes the brain and spinal cord, two organs physically connected and intimately tied to one another. The PNS includes all nervous tissue outside the CNS, such as cranial nerves, spinal nerves, and specialized sense organs like the eye and ear. Tissues of the brain and spinal cord are somewhat fragile, so these organs are protected by the meninges, cerebrospinal fluid (CSF), and bone. The meninges consist of three layers of connective tissue that surround and protect the CNS. CSF, found in between two layers of the meninges as well as in spaces within the brain and spinal cord, forms as neuroglial cells filter blood. It provides buoyancy to these organs and transports nutrients, oxygen, and wastes to and from neurons. Cranial bones provide additional protection by acting as physical barriers for the brain, while the vertebrae physically protect the spinal cord.

Although there are different types of neurons, each type has three basic parts—dendrites, a cell body, and an axon (Fig. 2.4). The dendrites are the receiving portions of the neuron; they detect stimuli. The cell body receives and integrates incoming information

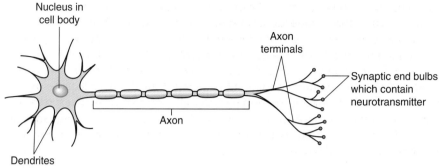

FIGURE 2.4 ■ Structure of a basic multipolar neuron.

and then decides whether to store the information or respond to the stimulus. The axon is the part of the neuron along which an impulse travels. An impulse itself consists of a series of action potentials that move along small segments of the neuron until they reach the synaptic end bulbs found at the end of the axon. Once the impulse reaches the synaptic end bulbs, it stimulates the release of neurotransmitters from vesicles. Neurotransmitters are chemicals used by neurons to communicate with effectors. If enough neurotransmitter is released, the effector is either stimulated or inhibited (the actual action depends upon several factors including the type of receptors present). In the case of skeletal muscle, the effect of sufficient neurotransmitter release is always contraction of the skeletal muscle fiber. Consequently, if adequate neurotransmitter is released at the junction between a skeletal muscle fiber and a motor neuron, contraction occurs.

The endocrine system works with the nervous system to control all body activities. The organs of the endocrine system are glands and collections of glandular tissue located throughout the body. Consequently, the endocrine system participates in various activities. It maintains the chemistry of the internal environment, controls metabolic reactions, establishes the biological clock, influences smooth and cardiac muscle contraction, and regulates growth and development.

Glands release **hormones** that ultimately enter blood vessels and travel to all areas of the body. Although exposed to all cells, hormones only affect **target cells**, or cells with receptors specific for them. A small amount of hormone can have tremendous effects due to amplification—the process where one hormone molecule triggers the action of

---

Hypertrophy—an increase in the cross-sectional area of a muscle fiber as the number of myofibrils increases. Both skeletal muscle fibers and adipocytes hypertrophy.

Hormones—usually steroid or protein molecules that exert an effect on target cells; target cells have receptors that bind specifically with a given hormone. Hormones then alter the metabolic processes of a cell by changing an enzyme's activity or altering the rate of transport of specific substances into a cell.

Target cells—cells throughout the body that have receptors for a given hormone.

thousands of enzymes. As long as the hormone is present, the effect occurs. Enzymes in the body, however, eventually break down hormones to limit their action.

CARDIOVASCULAR AND RESPIRATORY SYSTEMS

The cardiovascular and respiratory systems work together to ensure adequate oxygen delivery to and carbon dioxide removal from body cells. In the cardiovascular system, the heart is the pump that forces oxygen-containing blood through blood vessels. In addition to transporting oxygen, the cardiovascular system transfers nutrients and wastes.

Blood consists of plasma and formed elements. Plasma is the fluid portion of blood that contains water and dissolved substances such as ions, glucose, hormones, and gases. The formed elements include red blood cells, white blood cells, and platelets. Red blood cells contain hemoglobin, molecules that bind to oxygen. Their biconcave disc shape gives them an extensive surface area, a factor that facilitates the exchange of oxygen and carbon dioxide. White blood cells are primarily involved with immunity. Some travel through blood and lymph; others reside in lymphatic tissue. Platelets are actually cell fragments that participate in blood clotting and coagulation. They are important for preventing hemorrhage.

A healthy heart ejects enough blood to supply tissues with oxygen and nutrients. It easily adapts to increased demands such as those that result from exertion. **Cardiac output** measures the amount of blood pumped per minute; it is the product of **heart rate** multiplied by **stroke volume**. In general, a healthy heart has a high cardiac output as a result of a large stroke volume. This explains why heart rate decreases as cardiovascular health improves. In other words, a healthier heart does not have to work as hard as an unhealthy heart to deliver oxygen and nutrients to working tissues.

The respiratory system includes the nasal cavity, pharynx, trachea, lungs, bronchi, and bronchioles. The trachea branches into left and right primary bronchi, each of which travels to one of the lungs and divides many times to ultimately form **terminal bronchioles**. At the end of each terminal bronchiole is a small air sac called an **alveolus**. Numerous pulmonary capillaries surround each alveolus, so the lungs are richly supplied with blood vessels. In essence, this intimate relationship between the alveoli and their capillaries facilitates gas exchange. Lung tissue, therefore, is composed of alveoli, blood vessels, and branches of the bronchi, so it is rather spongy in texture.

The major function of the respiratory system is breathing or ventilation, the process that replenishes venous blood with oxygen while it removes accumulated carbon dioxide. Several structures and organs enable normal breathing. They include the internal and external intercostal muscles, the diaphragm, elastic fibers in the lungs, the sternum, and the ribs.

Respiration includes ventilation, external respiration, internal respiration, and cellular respiration. *Cellular respiration* occurs at the cellular level within organelles called mitochondria. It requires oxygen and produces carbon dioxide as a by-product. In the mitochondria, the chemical bonds of carbohydrates, triglycerides, and proteins are completely broken to yield large quantities of **ATP**. Oxygen is required because oxygen acts as the final electron acceptor at the end of the electron transport chain. If insufficient oxygen is available, the aerobic production of ATP slows. Therefore, metabolically active cells require a continual supply of oxygen to meet energy demands.

Internal respiration involves the exchange of oxygen and carbon dioxide between body cells and red blood cells. Bound to hemoglobin in red blood cells, oxygen travels through blood vessels and easily diffuses into metabolically active body cells. As mentioned, carbon dioxide is a by-product of cellular respiration; therefore, as cells produce ATP, carbon dioxide accumulates. Carbon dioxide, however, easily diffuses from body cells into the blood while oxygen diffuses from the blood into body cells. This exchange of oxygen for carbon dioxide is called internal respiration.

Since excess carbon dioxide alters blood pH, the respiratory system continuously removes it. Blood vessels facilitate this by transporting carbon dioxide to the lungs where carbon dioxide easily diffuses from the blood into the alveoli of the lungs, while oxygen from the alveoli easily diffuses into the blood. This process is called *external respiration.*

Ventilation is simply the movement of air into and out of the lungs—the process that ensures oxygen availability and carbon dioxide removal. It includes both inhalation and exhalation. Inhalation is an active process that requires contraction of the diaphragm and external intercostals. Understanding the basic structure of the pleural membrane, the protective membrane surrounding each lung, helps explain the process of inhalation. The pleural membrane is a double-layered structure that surrounds and supports each lung in its corresponding pleural cavity. The inner layer firmly attaches to the surface of the lungs, while the outer layer firmly attaches to surrounding structures such as the diaphragm, sternum, ribs, and intercostal muscles. In between these two layers is serous fluid that causes the inner layer to stick to the outer layer. Because of this overall arrangement, anything that moves the diaphragm or rib cage also expands the lungs.

When relaxed, the diaphragm is a dome-shaped muscle that separates the thoracic cavity from the abdominal cavity. If the diaphragm remains relaxed, pressure inside the lungs equalizes to atmospheric pressure, so there is no net movement of air into or out of the lungs. When the diaphragm contracts, however, it flattens. Since the outer layer of the pleural membrane attaches to the diaphragm and since movement of the diaphragm pulls

Cardiac output—HR × SV; equals the amount of blood the heart pumps per minute.

Heart rate (HR)—the number of times the heart beats per minute.

Stroke volume (SV)—the amount of blood pumped out of the left ventricle per heart beat.

Terminal bronchioles—branches of the respiratory passageway that terminate into alveoli. The trachea branches into right and left primary bronchi; each primary bronchus branches into right and left secondary bronchi, which branch into tertiary bronchi, etc. As the walls of the respiratory passageways thin, bronchioles form and terminate into alveoli.

Alveoli—microscopic, thin-walled air sacs located in the lungs. They are the sites of gas exchange in the lungs. Each lung contains millions of alveoli.

ATP (adenosine triphosphate)—is a high-energy molecule that provides the energy for most cellular activity. ATP, however, is not the only high-energy molecule in the body.

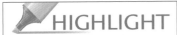

HIGHLIGHT   Deterioration of Lung Tissue

In cases of lung tissue damage, exhalation becomes an active process. When lung tissue loses its elasticity, the lungs tend to remain over-inflated, a condition that pushes on the thoracic wall, displaces the diaphragm and ribs, stretches lung tissue beyond its normal limit, and interferes with the functioning of synergistic muscles. All of these factors impede breathing. To counter some of these effects, the internal intercostals contract to depress the sternum and rib cage to force air out. Over the course of 10 to 20 years, the joints in the rib cage stiffen as fibrous tissue develops, a condition that inhibits rib cage range of motion. The result is rapid and shallow breathing. Eventually, accessory muscles for breathing, located in the upper thorax and typically only used in emergency breathing situations, are engaged. These accessory muscles include the sternomastoid and scalene muscles. This increased upper chest breathing coupled with the decrease in lower chest breathing results in the exaggerated alternating upward and downward chest movement associated with emphysema and other chronic obstructive pulmonary disorders. It also contributes to the development of the barrel-shaped chest common in patients with chronic obstructive pulmonary disease.

on this layer, the lungs expand as the diaphragm contracts. At the same time, the external intercostals contract and elevate both the sternum and ribs. Since the external intercostals, sternum, and ribs also firmly attach to the outer layer of the lungs, contraction of the external intercostals also expands the lungs. As the lungs expand, pressure within the thoracic body cavity decreases thereby creating a pressure gradient. Air from outside the body now moves from an area of higher pressure (in the atmosphere) to an area of lower pressure (within the lungs). Since this process requires the contraction of muscles, and since the contraction of muscles requires energy, inhalation is an *active process.*

Normal exhalation, on the other hand, is a *passive process.* As long as lung tissue remains elastic and muscle tissue maintains contractile properties, exhalation occurs as the diaphragm and external intercostals relax and the elastic lung tissue recoils. These conditions increase pressure within the lungs and cause air to move from the lung space (an area that now has higher pressure) to the external environment (an area of relatively low pressure).

Much of the respiratory system is lined with a type of tissue that secretes mucus and has cilia. The mucus traps potentially dangerous particles, while the cilia beat in unison to move trapped particles and mucus away from the lungs and back into the mouth where they can be swallowed or spit out. Thus, mucus and cilia work together to protect lung tissue. Nicotine in cigarettes paralyzes cilia. As a result, smokers develop a chronic cough that essentially does the job of the cilia—it moves mucus and trapped particles away from the lungs.

LYMPHATIC/IMMUNE SYSTEM

The lymphatic system consists of a group of close-ended vessels that transport **lymph**. Lymphatic vessels, similar in structure to blood vessels, exist throughout the body. Lymph has a composition similar to blood; however, lymph lacks red blood cells and usually does not contain proteins. It is typically clear and contains water, electrolytes, and wastes. The major functions of the lymphatic system are to return interstitial fluid to the blood, transport fat-soluble substances away from the digestive tract, and engage in immune surveillance.

FORMATION AND REMOVAL OF INTERSTITIAL FLUID

Hydrostatic pressure and **osmotic pressure** are responsible for much of the movement across capillary walls. The pumping action of the heart moves blood through large arteries into smaller arteries and arterioles. The arterioles ultimately branch into capillaries, porous vessels that permeate most body tissues. The force exerted by blood against blood vessel walls is called hydrostatic pressure; it diminishes as blood moves further and further away from the heart.

Although hydrostatic pressure diminishes as blood moves farther away from the heart, it remains high enough at the arteriolar end of the capillary to force many plasma components through the leaky capillary walls into the **interstitial space**. Anything small enough to exit the capillary wall becomes part of interstitial fluid. This includes water, oxygen, carbon dioxide, glucose, small amino acids, fatty acids, hormones, and salts. If left to accumulate in the interstitial space, blood volume would dwindle and interstitial fluid would build up. This, however, rarely happens for reasons explained in a moment.

Osmotic pressure remains constant all along blood vessels since it is created by the presence of proteins in the blood and proteins are too large to filter through capillary membranes. Overall, the opposing forces of hydrostatic and osmotic pressure constantly act on the capillary and determine net movement. At the arteriolar end of the capillary, hydrostatic pressure exceeds osmotic pressure; therefore, there is a net movement of substances out of the capillaries. At the venular end of the capillary, hydrostatic pressure decreases while osmotic pressure remains the same. Ultimately,

---

Lymph—the fluid transported by the lymphatic system. Includes excess interstitial fluid, white blood cells, and fat-soluble substances absorbed into the small intestine.

Hydrostatic pressure—the pressure exerted by blood against the wall of blood vessels.

Osmotic pressure—the pressure exerted by solute particles on one side of a membrane that is permeable to water but impermeable to solute. Water moves across the semipermeable membrane to the area of lower water and higher solute concentration as a result of the pull of the solutes.

Interstitial space—extracellular space located in between cells. Contains a fluid called interstitial fluid.

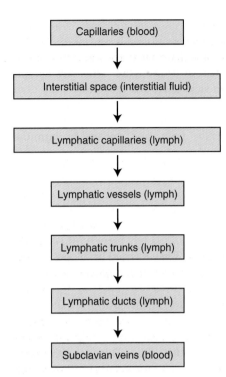

FIGURE 2.5 ■ Overall flow of fluid.

osmotic pressure exceeds hydrostatic pressure, thereby drawing some water and dissolved substances back into the blood vessels. This pressure, however, is not enough to pull all of the interstitial fluid back in, so as the heart continues to pump, interstitial fluid continues to accumulate. If left to accumulate in the interstitial space, **edema** develops. Edema, however, is largely prevented by the lymphatic system. As tissue fluid collects, it exerts pressure on surrounding vessels, many of which are lymphatic capillaries. The structure of these capillaries enables them to remain open even when the pressure against their exceedingly thin walls is great. Instead of causing lymphatic capillaries to collapse, the buildup of pressure actually forces them open so that fluid may enter. Once the interstitial fluid enters the lymphatic capillaries, it cannot escape back into the interstitial space. Instead, this fluid, now called lymph, travels toward the heart, passing through lymph nodes along the way. Ultimately, lymph passes into one of two major lymphatic ducts and returns to the blood vessels at two points near the clavicles. Once it reenters blood vessels, the fluid is called blood again (Fig. 2.5).

TRANSPORT OF FAT-SOLUBLE SUBSTANCES FROM THE GASTROINTESTINAL TRACT

During digestion, large food particles are broken down into small components that pass through the digestive tract lining. The major site of absorption is the small intestine. The small intestine has a vast supply of both blood capillaries and lymphatic capillaries called lacteals. Water-soluble substances such as amino acids, glucose, minerals, and most vitamins pass into the blood capillaries. Medium-chain to long-chain fatty acids and fat-soluble vitamins, however, do not enter blood capillaries. Instead, they initially enter lacteals and travel via the lymphatic system until they are ultimately delivered to the blood.

IMMUNE SURVEILLANCE

Organs of the lymphatic system include the red bone marrow, thymus gland, lymph nodes, and spleen. *Red bone marrow* is where both red and white blood cells form. Various white blood cells protect the body from pathogens. B cells and T cells are two types of white blood cells intricately involved with immunity. After they form, B cells remain in red bone marrow to mature. Once mature, they either travel in body fluids or reside in the lymph nodes or the spleen. Immature T cells travel to the *thymus* where they mature and learn self-tolerance. Once mature, T cells leave the thymus and either travel through body fluids or reside in lymph nodes or the spleen. Another type of white blood cell important in immune system functioning is the **macrophage**. Macrophages are active **phagocytes** that engulf and destroy pathogens before they are able to cause harm. Phagocytes also travel through body fluids and reside in lymphatic tissue.

The principal lymphatic organs are the lymph nodes. More than 600 of these bean-shaped organs cluster near the body surface where lymphatic vessels form trunks. They are particularly prevalent in the cervical, axillary, mammary, and inguinal areas. Lymph nodes contain macrophages that filter lymph, destroy microbes, and remove cellular debris before returning the fluid back to blood. This limits the spread of potentially damaging agents. In addition, local T and B cells monitor lymph, mount an attack against pathogens, and activate the immune system so that it can effectively and efficiently destroy harmful invaders.

Unlike lymph nodes, the spleen filters blood rather than lymph. It contains two types of tissue, white pulp and rep pulp, that enable it to function. Residing in the white pulp of the spleen are macrophages, B cells, and T cells, all of which monitor incoming blood for pathogens. The red pulp, on the other hand, contains large veins filled with blood. In the red pulp, macrophages destroy worn-out red blood cells, whereas B and T cells destroy pathogens. Together, B and T cells effectively disarm most invaders. Because several B and T cells exist in lymphatic tissue, the lymphatic system is a crucial component of immunity.

The immune system consists of both nonspecific (innate) resistance and specific (adaptive) resistance. The components of nonspecific resistance provide *immediate* and *general*

Edema—accumulation of excess interstitial fluid in the interstitial space. Excess tissue fluid leads to redness, swelling, pain, and sometimes itching.

Macrophage—a type of white blood cell involved with both specific and nonspecific defense. Macrophages are important phagocytes.

Phagocyte—a cell that engulfs and destroys potentially harmful substances including microorganisms, foreign particles, cellular debris, and aging cells. After ingesting their prey, phagocytes release powerful enzymes that digest the foreign substance.

TABLE 2-3   MECHANICAL AND CHEMICAL BARRIERS TO PATHOGENS

Mechanical Barriers	Chemical Barriers
■ Multiple layers found in epidermis and dermis	Tears and saliva which contain lysozyme, a substance that kills pathogens
■ Tightly packed cells of the epidermis	Sebum that contains a bactericide
■ Keratin in epidermis	Mucus which traps foreign particles to prevent entry into deeper tissues
■ Melanin in epidermis	
■ Glycolipids in between epidermal cells	
■ Sloughing off of superficial layer of epidermis	

protection against various pathogens. It consists of **mechanical barriers** designed to prevent microbe entry; **chemical barriers** to effectively weaken or destroy pathogens (see Table 2.3); reflexes to quickly remove or expel pathogens before they enter deeper tissues; and additional components to immobilize pathogens that actually gain entry into the body.

Mechanical barriers include intact skin and mucous membranes, which are major deterrents to microbes. The general characteristics of skin make it a formidable physical barrier. As mentioned earlier, skin consists of multiple layers that protect deeper tissues from the external environment. The cells in the outer layer of skin are also packed with keratin and surrounded by glycolipids. The keratin makes it more resistant to damage and penetration, while the glycolipids waterproof it. Additionally, skin contains melanin, a pigmented protein that protects cellular DNA from UV radiation. Lastly, as sweat drips from the skin and as layers slough off, pathogens on the body surface are carried away.

Chemical barriers consist of substances produced by cells that form the mechanical barriers. Tears and saliva contain **lysozyme**, an enzyme that destroys pathogens. Perspiration, gastric juice, and vaginal secretions are all low in pH, and since some pathogens cannot reproduce in an acidic environment, these secretions effectively inhibit pathogen proliferation. **Sebum** from sebaceous (oil) glands contains a toxin that directly kills certain bacteria. Mucus produced by mucous membranes traps foreign particles while associated cilia beat in unison to move the mucus and its trapped particles away from deeper tissues (see Table 2.3).

Reflexes include coughing, sneezing, vomiting, and diarrhea; they quickly and efficiently expel potentially damaging particles to prevent their entry into deeper tissues or organs. Additional nonspecific components activated if a pathogen breaches one of the aforementioned barriers include *phagocytes, inflammation, fever, natural killer cells*, and *protective proteins.*

As defined earlier, *phagocytes* are white blood cells that engulf foreign substances and break them down before they harm the body. Neutrophils and macrophages are the most active phagocytes. They often travel through blood and lymph, but some station themselves in specific tissues to monitor local conditions.

Although sometimes considered dangerous, *inflammation* is actually a normal, natural, and helpful process. Inflammation is triggered by infections from viruses, fungi, or bacteria; by physical trauma as a result of excessive friction, heat, or cold; or by exposure to irritating chemicals like acids or bases. The localized redness, heat, swelling, and pain are primarily a result of increased blood flow and capillary permeability in the affected area. Several factors contribute to this. Injured cells release histamine, kinins, prostaglandins, and other substances which dilate blood vessels in the area. Dilated blood vessels receive an increased blood flow which allows blood to move into the interstitial space. The result is that the area becomes red as blood accumulates. Local swelling actually helps dilute harmful substances, but it also creates pressure that stimulates local pain receptors. The area becomes warm because blood from deeper tissues is diverted to the area of infection. Traveling in the blood are additional macrophages and neutrophils sent to eliminate harmful agents. As they engulf pathogens and cellular debris, they die and become a part of the pus that begins to form. Consequently, pus, which is a normal part of the healing process, contains pathogens, dead phagocytes, and dead cells. Overall, inflammation walls off the area of infection to prevent the spread of damaging agents, disposes of cellular debris that results from dead or dying cells, and sets the stage for repair by delivering the components necessary for repair once the infection is controlled.

When a virus or bacterium invades white blood cells, the white blood cells release chemicals known as pyrogens (or interleukin-1). Pyrogens then act on the **hypothalamus**, the small part of the brain that establishes the set point for body temperature. Under the influence of pyrogens, the hypothalamus increases the set point for body temperature, which results in a *fever*. Fevers in children and high fevers in adults are dangerous because they **denature** body proteins, which interferes with their actions. Mild to moderate fevers in adults, however, seem to enhance the body's ability to disarm invaders. How? A higher-than-normal body temperature stimulates the

---

Mechanical barrier—a physical obstruction to entry; includes intact skin and mucous membranes.

Chemical barrier—includes substances such as tears, saliva, sebum, and mucus that are produced by cells that form the mechanical barriers.

Lysozyme—an enzyme contained in tears and saliva that digests and destroys pathogens.

Sebum—an oily product produced by sebaceous (oil) glands. It moistens the hair and skin to prevent cracking or breaking. It also contains a substance that is toxic to bacteria.

Hypothalamus—a small area in the brain with significant responsibilities. In addition to establishing the set point for body temperature, the hypothalamus contains eating, drinking, and satiety centers. It also regulates the release of many hormones.

Denature—to change the shape and subsequent function of a molecule. Denaturation often occurs when a molecule is subjected to extreme heat, agitation, or chemicals.

intensity of phagocytosis; speeds up metabolic processes to include those involved with tissue repair; and causes the liver to sequester iron, a mineral necessary for bacteria and fungi to multiply. Without adequate iron, bacterial reproduction slows and might cease altogether.

Natural killer cells are special types of lymphocytes that travel throughout blood and lymph. These cells are only involved with nonspecific resistance and are not phagocytic. Instead, they release **perforins**, cytolytic substances that essentially cause cancer and virus-infected cells to disintegrate. Additionally, natural killer cells release potent chemicals that enhance and stimulate the inflammatory response.

Various *protective proteins* either directly or indirectly enhance nonspecific resistance. **Interferons** are proteins produced by certain virus-infected lymphocytes and fibroblasts. Although the infected cell can do nothing to save itself, it can help protect nearby cells by releasing interferon. Interferon binds to uninvaded cells and stimulates them to produce proteins that interfere with viral replication. This seriously diminishes the damage that a virus causes. In addition, interferons enhance resistance by stimulating phagocytosis and mobilizing natural killer cells.

Complement proteins include a group of over 20 proteins that normally circulate in body fluids in inactive form. Once activated, complement proteins swarm to an infected area, lyse bacterial cell membranes, inactivate viruses by altering their molecular structure, enhance phagocytosis by clumping together antigens, and amplify inflammation to inhibit the spread of infection. See Table 2.4 for a summary of nonspecific resistance.

Adaptive resistance reacts more slowly to an initial encounter with a particular **antigen**. There are four characteristics of adaptive resistance: *specificity*, or the ability to recognize and respond to particular antigens; *systemic action*, or having widespread rather than local effects; *memory*, or the ability to "remember" an initial encounter so that future encounters with the same antigen stimulate a more rapid immune response; and *self/ nonself recognition*, or the capacity to distinguish between normal body cells and potentially

TABLE 2-4 NONSPECIFIC RESISTANCE IS PROVIDED BY MECHANICAL BARRIERS, CHEMICAL BARRIERS, REFLEXES, AND ADDITIONAL COMPONENTS

Resistance	Function
Mechanical barriers	Designed to keep pathogens out of the body
Chemical barriers	Produced by cells forming the mechanical barriers; their goal is to destroy pathogens prior to entry
Reflexes	Intended to expel pathogens as they try to enter deeper body tissues
Additional components ■ Phagocytes ■ Inflammation ■ Fever ■ Natural killer cells ■ Protective proteins	Target pathogens once they enter the body. Still provide immediate and nonspecific defense against various pathogens.

damaging agents. Adaptive resistance relies significantly on B cells, T cells, and macrophages.

B and T cells have different modes of action. Two types of B cells exist—plasma B cells and memory B cells. *Plasma B cells* are antibody-producing factories that respond to threatening pathogens by producing antibodies specific to the invader. Antibodies have various modes of action; for example, they can make pathogens vulnerable by clumping them together so that macrophages are able to engulf a large number at once. In addition, antibodies activate and enhance other methods of defense. *Memory B cells* remain after an initial encounter with a given antigen. Although dormant in an initial encounter, they proliferate immediately upon subsequent exposure to the same antigen.

The immune system produces four general types of T cells—cytotoxic T cells, helper T cells, regulatory (or suppressor) T cells, and memory T cells. In contrast to the plasma B cell's indirect mode of action, *cytotoxic T cells* directly attack and kill virus-infected cells and tumor cells. For instance, when cytotoxic T cells recognize an infected cell, they release substances called perforins and granulysin. These substances result in the formation of tubular openings in the infected cell's membrane—a condition that allows extracellular substances to enter the internal environment. Eventually, as extracellular fluid accumulates within the intracellular compartment, the cell **lyses**. Unlike cytotoxic T cells, *helper T cells* do not kill pathogens. Instead, they enhance the immune response by releasing chemicals that stimulate B and T cell proliferation. Although helper T cells do not protect against antigens directly, the immune system would not mount an effective attack against antigens without them. Thus, in the absence of helper T cells, the body suffers severely from—and likely succumbs to—invasion.

Regulatory T cells essentially moderate the immune response by turning off the activity of T cells when they are no longer needed. They provide an important "self-check" to ensure that responses do not magnify and continue unrestrained. *Memory T cells*, like memory B cells, remain dormant during an initial attack. They, however, rapidly mobilize

---

Perforins—a group of proteins that cause cell lysis (or cell bursting). They operate by causing the formation and insertion of tubes into the cell membranes of pathogens. Once present, these tubes allow intracellular materials to leak out of the pathogen.

Interferons—a group of proteins produced by virus-infected body cells. Interferon 'interferes' with the ability of the virus to replicate in nearby body cells.

Complement proteins—a group of proteins that circulate through body fluids in inactive form. They are activated by one of two pathways and significantly enhance both nonspecific and specific resistance.

Antigen—a substance that initiates an immune response upon entry into the body. This stimulates antibody production. Antigens include bacteria, viruses, toxins, and foreign tissues or organs.

Lysis—death of a cell by swelling and bursting

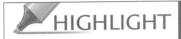

HIGHLIGHT   Helper T Cells and Human Immunodeficiency Virus

Mature helper T cells (along with a few other cells) express a surface protein called CD4. The human immunodeficiency virus (HIV), which causes acquired immunodeficiency syndrome (AIDS), attacks this CD4 receptor and renders the helper T cell incapable of functioning. To understand the importance of helper T cells, consider what happens to the immune system of someone with AIDS. The immune system is unable to fight off antigens that a healthy immune system could easily handle because helper T cells are not stimulating B and T cell activity.

and proliferate during subsequent attacks by the same antigens and thereby enable a stronger and more rapid attack during a secondary invasion.

DIGESTIVE SYSTEM

The major function of the digestive system is to convert food into products that can be absorbed into vessels of the cardiovascular or lymphatic system, while it passes undigested material out as feces. During the process of food breakdown, digestive organs release many secretions. The end products of digestion, along with water and other materials, are absorbed, while feces is compacted and stored before defecation.

Food passes through a series of organs called the **alimentary canal**. The alimentary canal, or gastrointestinal tract, consists of the mouth, pharynx, esophagus, stomach, small intestine, and large intestine. In addition to the alimentary canal, several accessory organs participate in digestion. These include the salivary glands, which empty into the mouth, and the pancreas, gall bladder, and liver, which empty into the duodenum of the small intestine.

The ingestion of food occurs at the mouth. The tongue manipulates food, mixes it with secretions from the salivary glands, and ultimately helps convert food into a semi-solid mass called a bolus. The surface of the tongue has numerous papillae, some of which contain taste buds. A strip of tissue called the lingual frenulum connects the tongue to the floor of the mouth to prevent the tongue from sagging and blocking the opening of the trachea. The boundary between the oral cavity and the nasal cavity is the palate. The front of the palate is made of bone and is called the hard palate. The posterior portion, called the soft palate, is made of skeletal muscle. A projection called the uvula hangs from the posterior edge of the soft palate. During swallowing, the soft palate and uvula lift to block off the nasal cavity and channel the bolus into the pharynx.

The major salivary glands connect to the mouth by ducts and produce a mixture of water, mucus, and enzymes. Saliva, which is 99.9% water and only 0.5% solutes, keeps the mucous membranes of the mouth and pharynx moist, cleanses the mouth and teeth,

TABLE 2-5   FUNCTIONS OF THE STOMACH

- Acts as a temporary storage tank for ingested food
- Undergoes churning to mix the bolus with stomach secretions
- Chemically breaks down proteins
- Converts the semisolid bolus into a semiliquid chyme
- Absorbs some water, ions, alcohol, and drugs

lubricates and dissolves food so that it can be tasted, and begins the chemical breakdown of carbohydrates.

Food passes from the mouth into the pharynx. Masses of lymph tissue called tonsils are located on the posterior wall of the pharynx. Like other lymphatic tissue, the tonsils assist in protecting the body from infection. Overall, the major role of the pharynx is to transport food from the mouth into the esophagus.

During swallowing, the epiglottis covers the opening of the trachea as the hyoid bone elevates the larynx. At the same time, the upper esophageal sphincter relaxes to permit the bolus to enter the esophagus. To transport the bolus to the stomach, the esophagus must pass through an opening in the diaphragm. Once it passes through this opening, the bolus enters the stomach as the cardiac sphincter, or lower esophageal sphincter, relaxes.

QUICK REFERENCE

Sphincters, which consist of smooth muscle arranged around a **lumen**, play an important role in many body systems. In the digestive system, sphincters are located at junctions between many gastrointestinal tract organs. When a sphincter contracts, it closes the lumen and prevents entry or exit of a substance. When a sphincter relaxes, it permits a substance to move into another organ or segment.

The stomach is an enlarged J-shaped sac where the first substantial digestive activity begins (Table 2.5). Two sphincters—one located at each end of the stomach—regulate the flow of substances into and out of the organ. One of these sphincters, the cardiac sphincter, was mentioned earlier. The other, the pyloric sphincter, is in the terminal portion of the stomach in a region called the pylorus. Together, these sphincters ensure that the

Alimentary canal—also known as the digestive tract or GI tract; includes all digestive organs that contact food and its breakdown products. Food particles pass through the opening in the center called the lumen.

Lumen—the inner space or cavity of a tubular organ such as the esophagus, stomach, or blood vessels.

bolus of food remains in the stomach long enough for the three layers of muscle in the stomach wall to actively mix it with hydrochloric acid (HCl) and the protein-digesting enzyme pepsin. This mixing process is called churning; it converts the semisolid bolus into a semiliquid chyme. Food usually remains in the stomach for 2 to 6 hours depending on the quantity and composition of the meal. Periodically, the pyloric sphincter relaxes to permit small amounts of chyme to enter the duodenum of the small intestine. The rate of chyme release into the small intestine is closely regulated to ensure that the small intestine has adequate time to complete digestion and begin absorption of all macronutrients before additional chyme enters. The stomach is capable of holding a large quantity because of its shape and the presence of large folds called rugae on its inner surface. Rugae enable the stomach to expand to accommodate a huge meal.

As mentioned, the acidic chyme in the stomach passes gradually into the small intestine. The first 25 cm of the small intestine is the duodenum. In the duodenum, products from the liver and pancreas combine with secretions of the small intestine to neutralize and chemically break down the acidic chyme that just entered from the stomach. Together, the secretions released into the duodenum perform most chemical digestion. Digestion and absorption continue in the jejunum and ileum, the final two segments of the small intestine.

The small intestine has a small diameter but is quite long; it averages about 3 m in a living person. The small intestine exhibits various adaptations that enable it to perform its functions efficiently. For example, the inner lining forms circular folds called plicae circulares that swirl the chyme as it passes through the lumen. In effect, this slows the movement of chyme and gives digestive enzymes time to break down macromolecules. Additionally, a series of fingerlike structures called villi project from the plicae circularis. Each villus is covered with tiny membrane extensions called microvilli. Together, the villi and microvilli increase the surface area for absorption. The microvilli also contain various intestinal enzymes necessary for digestion. In essence, the length of the small intestine coupled with the presence of plicae circulares, villi, and microvilli enable digestion and absorption in this organ.

Exocrine cells within the pancreas secrete pancreatic juice, a mixture of water, salts, sodium bicarbonate, and enzymes, which passes into the pancreatic duct prior to entering the small intestine. The sodium bicarbonate neutralizes the acidic chyme that has just left the stomach. This allows the enzymes, which include peptidases, lipase, and amylase, to chemically break down most of the carbohydrates, triglycerides, and proteins consumed.

The liver is the largest gland in the body. It has many functions related to blood homeostasis, detoxification, and nutrient conversions. Its major digestive function, however, is to produce and secrete bile. **Bile** is a **fat emulsifier** used to convert large globs of fat into smaller particles that are more vulnerable to enzymes. Bile also contains pigments produced from the breakdown of old red blood cells.

Bile produced by the liver leaves the liver via the common hepatic duct and backs up into the cystic duct to enter the gall bladder. The gall bladder, a small saclike structure located on the posterior surface of the liver, stores bile until fat-laden chyme enters the small intestine. When the cells of the small intestine sense the presence of fat, they release a hormone that stimulates contraction of the smooth muscle lining of the gall bladder. As the gall bladder contracts, it releases bile.

As mentioned, most digestion and absorption occur in the duodenum of the small intestine as bile and pancreatic fluid mix with chyme from the stomach. The remaining digestion and absorption occur in the jejunum and the ileum. Products that are not absorbed in the duodenum, jejunum, or ileum pass into the colon where further water absorption occurs. The ileum connects with the colon on the lower right side of the abdominopelvic cavity where the ileocecal sphincter controls the movement of chyme. The cecum is a part of the large intestine that projects inferior to this junction and attaches to the appendix. The appendix contains a small amount of lymph tissue.

> ### QUICK REFERENCE
>
> If the appendix becomes infected as in appendicitis and subsequently ruptures, the hole created in the wall of the cecum permits the colon contents to enter the abdominal cavity and cause a condition called peritonitis. Peritonitis is a potentially lethal condition because of the huge quantity of bacteria present in the colon contents.

The colon, or large intestine, is the terminal portion of the GI tract. Although shorter in length than the small intestine, the large intestine has a much larger diameter. What enters the colon is chyme; what leaves is feces. The colon is drawn into a series of pouches called haustra, which contain the contents of the colon. Haustral churning manipulates the haustral contents and allows the cells of the large intestine to absorb most of the remaining water prior to defecation.

Peristalsis is the alternating contraction and relaxation of the GI tract smooth muscle lining; it propels the contents along. Movement through the alimentary canal must occur slowly enough for enzymes to break down larger molecules into smaller ones, but not so slowly that excessive water is absorbed in the small and large intestines. If peristalsis occurs too rapidly, too much water remains in the feces—a condition called diarrhea. If peristalsis occurs too slowly, constipation results as the contents of the large intestine become more compact with increased water loss.

URINARY SYSTEM

The urinary system filters blood to form urine and then transports and stores urine prior to elimination. Overall, the goal is to eliminate wastes while maintaining fluid and electrolyte balance. The kidneys are the workhorses of the urinary system; they remove **nitrogenous waste products**, excess salts, excess water, some drugs, and other toxic

Bile—a mixture that contains bile salts used to emulsify fat in the small intestine.
Fat emulsification—a process that physically breaks down large fat globs into smaller fat globules.
Nitrogenous wastes—nitrogen-containing wastes such as urea, ammonia, uric acid, and creatinine.

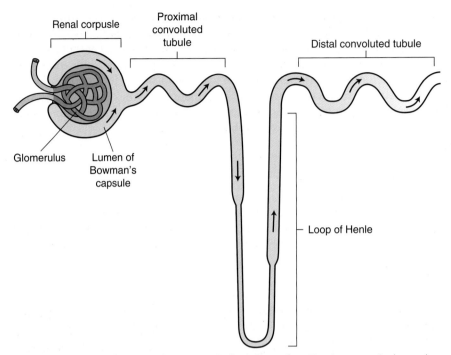

Glomerulus   Lumen of Bowman's capsule

FIGURE 2.6 ■ Structure of a nephron. *Arrows* indicate filtrate flow. Fitration occurs in the renal corpuscle. Reabsorption and secretion occur along the renal tubule.

compounds from blood. These waste products, collectively called urine, eventually leave the kidneys, pass through tubes called ureters, and enter the urinary bladder. The urinary bladder stores urine and expels it when its smooth muscle lining contracts. Urine then exits the body through the external urethral orifice.

Each kidney contains over a million filtering and processing centers called **nephrons** (Fig. 2.6). A nephron consists of a renal corpuscle and a renal tubule. Nephrons adjust blood composition through three main processes: **filtration**, **reabsorption**, and **secretion**. Blood is *filtered* in the region of the nephron called the renal corpuscle. The renal corpuscle consists of the glomerulus and the Glomerular (Bowman's) capsule. To understand the structure of the renal corpuscle, keep in mind that a renal artery branches many times after entering a kidney and ultimately forms an individual afferent arteriole to supply each nephron in each kidney. Because blood pressure in the afferent vessel is high, small plasma components are forced (filtered) from a round capillary bed called the glomerulus into a space called the Glomerular (Bowman's) capsule. The resulting fluid is filtrate.

The renal tubule consists of three segments: the proximal convoluted tubule, the Loop of Henle, and the distal convoluted tubule. The distal convoluted tubules of many nephrons empty into a collecting duct that ultimately empties into a structure called the renal pelvis. From the renal pelvis, urine passes through a ureter into the urinary bladder.

The filtrate that enters the proximal convoluted tubule is different in composition from the urine that enters the renal pelvis. This difference exists due to the processes of *reabsorption* and *secretion*, which occur along the proximal convoluted tubule, the loop of Henle, the distal convoluted tubule, and the upper regions of the collecting duct. Reabsorption returns water, salts, glucose, amino acids, and other useful material to the blood. Secretion moves additional nitrogenous waste products, excess salts, excess hydrogen ions, drugs, and some toxic materials into the kidney tubule. Overall, the composition of urine varies depending upon the relative intake of water and salt versus their loss by digestion, respiration, and perspiration.

REPRODUCTIVE SYSTEM

The purpose of the male and female reproductive systems is to produce **gametes**, to deliver sperm to an oocyte for fertilization, and to support and nurture a growing embryo/fetus. In addition, they produce hormones that ultimately affect muscle and bone health.

MALE REPRODUCTIVE SYSTEM

In addition to producing the male gamete, or sperm, the testes also contain cells that produce and release testosterone, the hormone that maintains sperm production, gland functioning, and secondary sex characteristics. Secondary sex characteristics include dense and thick facial hair, increased chest and axillary hair, greater muscle mass and strength, lower overall body fat, narrow waist, increased size of larynx and subsequent deeper voice, higher metabolism and red blood cell count, and denser bones.

FEMALE REPRODUCTIVE SYSTEM

The gonads in the female reproductive system are the ovaries. The ovaries produce the female gamete, or oocyte, which exists in a structure called a follicle. A female is born with the maximum number of follicles and oocytes that she will ever have. Interestingly,

---

Nephron—the microscopic filtering units found in the kidneys. Each kidney has over 1 million nephrons, which process blood to form urine.

Filtration—the process of forcing certain blood components through a series of membranes to remove water and small solutes. The removed substances become filtrate. Filtration occurs in the renal corpuscle of the nephron.

Reabsorption—a process that returns certain substances such as water, glucose, and salts to blood vessels after they have been filtered.

Secretion—a process that removes additional wastes including urea, drugs, and hydrogen ions from the blood. Removed substances become a part of filtrate (which eventually becomes urine).

Gametes—the female gamete is the oocyte; the male gamete is the sperm.

most of the oocytes that are present at birth actually die before the female reaches puberty. Each month after puberty, several follicles enlarge as their oocytes develop. Typically, one follicle dominates and becomes larger than any other follicle. The oocyte within this mature follicle is the one that will be ovulated. As the follicles enlarge, they produce and release more and more estrogen, which is discussed in the next section. Ultimately, ovulation occurs when the follicle bursts and releases its oocyte into the abdominopelvic cavity. The follicle then collapses inward and begins to produce progesterone.

Estrogen and progesterone maintain normal monthly cycles and prepare the uterine lining for implantation of an embryo if fertilization occurs. In a nonpregnant woman, the primary sources of these hormones are the follicle and the corpus luteum, structures found in the ovaries. The follicle develops as stated in the previous paragraph. The corpus luteum forms when the follicle collapses inward following ovulation; it produces and releases progesterone for at least two weeks postovulation to sustain the uterine lining in case implantation occurs.

In addition to maintaining female secondary sex characteristics, the different types of estrogen contribute to tissue strength and elasticity throughout the body. This is apparent when considering aging skin—the skin wrinkles as estrogen levels drop. In addition, low estrogen inflames the gums, loosens teeth, and causes throat dryness, hoarseness, and subtle changes in voice pitch. Estrogen and progesterone are also necessary to preserve bone tissue. They stimulate osteoblast activity and calcium deposition and inhibit osteoclast activity. In addition, progesterone normalizes blood glucose levels, helps eliminate excess body fluid that often accumulates because of estrogen, and promotes the use of fats for energy.

SUMMARY

This chapter presented a basic overview of each body system to clarify how physiological processes work in a generally healthy person. Armed with this knowledge, health and fitness professionals will have a better understanding of the conditions and disease states that occur in their special needs clients or patients. As mentioned earlier, trainers can typically design successful exercise programs for clients without thoroughly understanding each body system; however, they might be even more effective after being exposed to this foundational material. This chapter, therefore, is for those readers who want to know not only *which* modifications are important for certain special needs groups but also *why* these modifications are necessary.

THINKING CRITICALLY

1. Consider the functions of the integumentary system. Select three and explain their importance during exercise.
2. Define bone remodeling. Explain how exercise promotes healthy bone remodeling.
3. Explain how estrogen and testosterone influence bone health.

4. Muscles grow through what process? Explain how exercise stimulates muscle growth even though people are born with the maximum number of muscle fibers they will ever have.
5. Which two body systems regulate all other body systems? Explain how they perform this task.
6. Describe the intricate relationship between the cardiovascular system and the respiratory system.
7. Explain what happens to a person who abruptly stops intense cardiovascular training without cooling down first.
8. Define edema and explain how it develops.
9. In order, list the organs through which food substances pass as they move through the GI tract. Briefly explain the role of each organ. Specifically where does most digestion and absorption occur?
10. What three processes convert blood into urine? Briefly explain each and indicate where each occurs.

3

EXERCISE DURING PREGNANCY

The advantages and disadvantages of exercise during pregnancy are topics that warrant debate. Although routine exercise seems to improve health during pregnancy, there is concern that it might interfere with fetal growth and development. Consequently, researchers continue to investigate the impact of physical activity on fetal development. Most studies agree that exercise—at one time contraindicated during pregnancy—is generally safe for both the pregnant woman and her fetus. Granted, potential risks *do* exist whenever a pregnant woman exercises; however, the psychological and physiological improvements seem to outweigh the negative aspects in most normal pregnancies. A woman who regularly exercised prior to becoming pregnant can typically continue her activity during pregnancy with minimal risks. Although she probably needs to adjust the frequency, duration, intensity, and type of activity in which she participates, her trained body is already strong enough to handle the stresses related to physical training. Modifying her habits to accommodate pregnancy should be relatively simple. Even a previously sedentary pregnant woman may begin a moderate exercise program as long as she is generally healthy and has medical clearance. Making drastic improvements in health or losing a substantial amount of weight should not be the goal during this time. Instead, pregnant women should focus on developing muscle strength and endurance to alleviate some of the discomforts associated with pregnancy, labor, and delivery. Although exercise cannot guarantee an easier pregnancy or delivery for *all* women, it likely helps manage discomfort.

This chapter explores the many physiological changes that occur during a normal pregnancy and offers suggestions on how to meet the needs of the developing fetus while continuing to reap the benefits of physical activity. It not only provides exercise recommendations, but also explores the nutritional needs resulting from the combined demands of both pregnancy and exercise.

ANATOMICAL AND PHYSIOLOGICAL CHANGES DURING PREGNANCY

To provide an appropriate environment for the developing fetus, a woman's body undergoes dramatic changes as pregnancy progresses through the average 38 to 40 weeks of gestation. Typically, pregnancy is broken down into three 3-month intervals called trimesters. Although changes occur gradually throughout all trimesters, the most significant adjustments are apparent within the first few weeks after conception. After a brief discussion of hormones, this section looks at specific changes in a woman's body as well as the events that occur in the developing fetus during each trimester.

ROLE OF HORMONES

Estrogen and progesterone are two hormones that play crucial roles in preparing the uterine lining for the implantation of an embryo. The primary source of estrogen in a nonpregnant woman is a structure called the **follicle**. Prior to ovulation, the follicle contains a cell called a **secondary oocyte**. The secondary oocyte, more commonly known as the egg, is ovulated each month after puberty. It is this secondary oocyte that may be fertilized by a sperm cell. After ovulation, the follicle collapses inward to form a structure called the **corpus luteum**. The corpus luteum then produces progesterone to maintain the uterine lining for a minimum of 14 days postovulation. In addition, it produces small amounts of estrogen. If fertilization and implantation do not occur, the corpus luteum degenerates and progesterone levels decrease. If fertilization occurs, the corpus luteum continues to produce estrogen and progesterone until the placenta assumes this role during the 3rd month of pregnancy.

In a nonpregnant woman who has a normal menstrual cycle, the innermost endometrial lining of the uterus sloughs off each month as estrogen and progesterone levels decline. Soon after ovulation, however, estrogen and progesterone levels increase under the influence of the corpus luteum. Estrogen, in particular, promotes repair of the endometrium whether a woman becomes pregnant or not. As it restores the lining, estrogen also stimulates blood vessel and lymph vessel formation throughout various body tissues. Most notably, vessels supplying the uterus increase to transport more blood, oxygen, and nutrients to the newly forming cells. As a result, actual blood flow to the uterus increases from 50 mL per minute at 10 weeks of gestation to 500 mL per minute at 38 weeks. If fertilization occurs, estrogen levels remain elevated and stimulate the uterus to grow to up to 20 times its prepregnancy weight. Estrogen also helps maintain a positive maternal nitrogen balance so that body proteins are available for the formation of fetal tissues and associated structures. Lastly, estrogen increases blood volume by causing the collecting ducts and kidney tubules to retain more sodium. As sodium is reabsorbed, water follows. This water then enters blood vessels and thereby increases blood volume. An elevated blood volume can ultimately cause **edema** because the extra weight associated with pregnancy interferes with interstitial fluid movement into lymphatic vessels. See Chapter 2 for more information. Edema is often apparent in the face, hands, legs, and

---

Follicle—a structure in the ovary in which the female gamete develops.
Secondary oocyte—a cell that is released by an ovary each month after puberty. This is the cell that fuses with a sperm cell if fertilization occurs.
Corpus luteum— a structure formed from an ovarian follicle following ovulation; it releases hormones, most notably estrogen and progesterone.
Edema—fluid accumulation in the spaces in between cells.

feet. As blood volume continues to increase (by as much as 50% above normal by the end of pregnancy) to meet the needs of the fetus, **cardiac output** increases. This often results in a more rapid pulse rate at rest and during exercise.

Like estrogen, progesterone levels rise after ovulation and remain elevated for a minimum of 14 days whether a woman becomes pregnant or not. Without progesterone, the endometrial lining sloughs off and cannot support a growing fetus. Progesterone not only maintains the thickened state of the endometrium but also increases its secretions. These secretions nourish the developing embryo as it enters the uterine cavity and prepares to implant. Progesterone, along with estrogen, stimulates breast tissue but prevents lactation until after birth. In addition, it relaxes the smooth muscle lining of the uterus to prevent contraction and dislodging of an implanting embryo. At the same time, progesterone relaxes other smooth muscle tissue in the body, including the muscular layer of the gastrointestinal (GI) tract. This slows **peristalsis**, or the movement of food particles through the GI tract, and enables the small intestine to absorb more nutrients for fetal growth. Unfortunately, a slower rate of peristalsis allows the large intestine to absorb a greater amount of water. This compacts feces and can ultimately cause constipation. Finally, progesterone also causes headaches, blurred vision, tender breasts, and heartburn, all of which complicate an active lifestyle. As pregnancy progresses, progesterone levels drop so that the muscular layer of the uterus can contract when the fetus is finally ready for delivery.

Relaxin is another important hormone that affects joint stability. Early in pregnancy, the corpus luteum releases relaxin to limit the activity and natural movements of the uterus and to soften the cervix in preparation for delivery. The actions of relaxin, however, are not restricted to the uterus. Instead, this hormone relaxes all joints throughout the body, which promotes joint instability throughout pregnancy.

Once the embryo implants about 6 or 7 days after fertilization, the embryonic membranes begin to release a hormone called human chorionic gonadotropin (hCG). As hCG is produced, it enters body fluids and is actually detectable in the blood and urine within

TABLE 3-1   MAJOR HORMONES INVOLVED WITH PREGNANCY

Hormone	Action in the Body
Estrogen	Repairs the endometrial lining of the uterus after the menstrual cycle. Enlarges the breasts during pregnancy and prepares them for lactation. Helps regulate progesterone levels during pregnancy
Progesterone	Maintains the endometrial lining during pregnancy. Limits the natural movements of the uterus early in pregnancy to prevent contractions.
Human chorionic gonadotropin	Produced by the chorion, a membrane that begins forming around the developing embryo by day 12 after fertilization. Maintains the corpus luteum so that the corpus luteum continues to produce progesterone until the placenta fully develops. This is the hormone detected by pregnancy tests.
Relaxin	A hormone released early in pregnancy to limit uterine contractions. Also softens the cervix in preparation for childbirth. Affects joints in the body, making them more flexible and less stable.
Prolactin	Not produced during pregnancy because high levels of estrogen and progesterone limit its production by the anterior pituitary gland. As estrogen and progesterone levels drop after birth, prolactin is released and stimulates milk production in the mammary glands.
Oxytocin	The hormone that stimulates uterine contractions at the time of birth. Also stimulates milk ejection, or letdown.

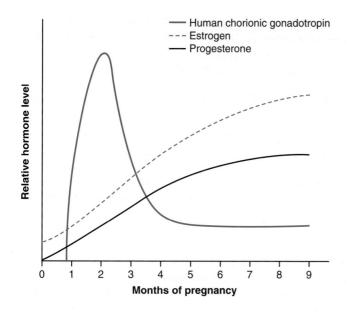

FIGURE 3.1 ■ Relative concentrations of estrogen, progesterone, and hCG during the 9 months of pregnancy.

2 weeks after ovulation. In fact, hCG is the hormone detected by pregnancy kits. Overall, the level of hCG rises dramatically in the early weeks of pregnancy, peaks at about 2 months, and then tapers off. The function of hCG is to ensure that the corpus luteum continues to release both estrogen and progesterone until the placenta assumes this role at the end of the 3rd month of pregnancy. Some of the notable symptoms associated with early pregnancy—nausea, vomiting, and fatigue—are thought to result from the presence of hCG.

Additional hormones play a role either during pregnancy or immediately after birth (Table 3.1). Prolactin, produced by the anterior pituitary gland, is released toward the end of pregnancy as estrogen and progesterone levels drop (Fig. 3.1). Prolactin stimulates the mammary glands to produce milk in preparation for breastfeeding. Oxytocin, released in large quantities by the posterior pituitary gland as delivery approaches, stimulates powerful uterine contractions that assist in expelling a baby during birth. It also stimulates milk letdown, or ejection, in response to a suckling infant.

Since both the pregnant woman and the fetus undergo drastic changes during pregnancy (Table 3.2), exercise professionals working with pregnant clients must understand these changes and evaluate their impact on exercise. The following paragraphs present the changes that occur in both the mother and the fetus during each trimester of pregnancy.

Cardiac output—the amount of blood pumped by the heart per minute; usually measured in liters per minute. CO = SV × HR, where CO is cardiac output, SV is stroke volume, and HR is heart rate.

Peristalsis—alternating rhythmic contractions of the smooth muscle lining of the digestive tract that propel contents along. It must occur at an appropriate rate to allow nutrient absorption.

TABLE 3-2	CHANGES THAT OCCUR IN A PREGNANT WOMAN DURING EACH TRIMESTER
First trimester	Hormone levels fluctuate dramatically promoting nausea. Breasts swell and become tender. Perspiration increases. Fetus enlarges and puts pressure on urinary bladder resulting in increased frequency of urination.
Second trimester	Body adjusts to hormone levels, so nausea subsides. Enlarging fetus promotes back pain and changes the center of balance. Joints become less stable. Reflux develops as uterus and fetus are displaced out of the pelvis. Breasts continue to swell and become tender. Edema develops.
Third trimester	Fetus continues to grow and crowd out maternal organs. Consequently, frequent urination continues and constipation develops. The increasing weight strains the woman's heart and lungs, so fatigue ensues. Braxton-Hicks contractions might occur.

FIRST TRIMESTER

The most dramatic hormonal changes and fluctuations occur during the first 3 months of pregnancy. This often causes a pregnant woman to feel lethargic and nauseous—symptoms collectively known as morning sickness. Because of the extreme fatigue experienced during this time, pregnant women often lack the energy to exercise. However, if they are able to overcome this fatigue, they discover that exercise actually alleviates the discomfort of morning sickness. In addition to nausea, estrogen and progesterone cause tender breasts and increased vaginal secretions and body perspiration. The increased vaginal secretions prepare the vaginal canal for delivery, while increased perspiration eliminates excess heat from the body as metabolism increases. Lastly, the uterus, positioned above the urinary bladder, also begins to grow as the fetus enlarges, so it puts pressure on the urinary bladder and increases the frequency of urination.

The first trimester is the time when fetal organ systems begin to develop. It is important to note that each system has a specific and unique "**critical period**"—a time during which rapid cell division and growth occur within a given organ system (Fig. 3.2). For some organ systems, this period of intense cellular activity is concentrated into 2 or 3 days; for other organ systems, it extends over several months. In either case, an organ system is particularly vulnerable to damage from toxins, nutrient deficiencies, or trauma during its critical period, so extra caution is advised when training during the first trimester. Since the critical period for one system differs from that of another, not all organ systems are susceptible to damage at the same time. Consider development of the neural tube as an example. A neural tube defect typically occurs on day 28 of development if some factor disrupts the process that enables a particular sheet of embryonic tissue to fold into the neural tube (a structure that later forms the central nervous system). Whether the disruption results from a nutrient deficiency or some sort of trauma, the neural tube remains open whenever conditions are not ideal during this time. Unfortunately, the critical period for the central nervous system occurs early in pregnancy—often before a woman is aware that she is pregnant. Consequently, many women participate in harmful behaviors before discovering that they are pregnant and ultimately interfere with the ability of the fetus to thrive.

Weeks

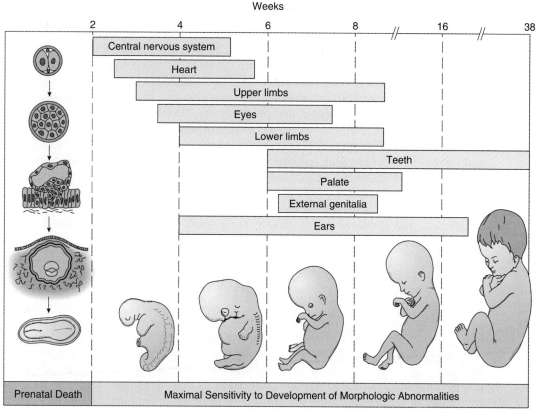

FIGURE 3.2 ■ Critical periods of organ and system development. (Modified from Rubin E., Farber JL. Pathology. 3rd Ed. Philadelphia: Lippincott Williams & Wilkins, 1999 and Pillitteri A. Maternal and Child Nursing. 4th Ed. Philadelphia: Lippincott Williams & Wilkins, 2003.)

By the end of the first trimester, the fetus is about 4 in. long and weighs about 1 oz. The eyes and ears begin to form and small buds that eventually develop into the arms and legs are evident. By the end of 4 weeks, the heart is actually beating. The circulatory, digestive, urinary, skeletal, and nervous systems continue to form as the fetus takes on a humanlike appearance with an unusually large head relative to its body size.

> **Critical period**—a finite time period during which an organ system is growing rapidly. An organ system is particularly vulnerable to harmful conditions such as nutrient deficiencies or exposure to toxins during its critical period. Therefore, pregnant women should avoid harmful behaviors from the moment of conception until delivery to ensure optimal development.

SECOND TRIMESTER

By the start of the second trimester, the placenta is fully functioning. Not only does it produce the major hormones mentioned earlier, but it is also the site of nutrient, oxygen, and waste exchange between the mother and the fetus. At this point, the woman's body has typically adjusted to the elevated hormone levels, so much of the fatigue and nausea subsides. Other discomforts, such as nasal congestion and frequent nosebleeds, might result from high levels of estrogen and progesterone. The abdomen enlarges as the fetus grows causing back pain and an altered center of balance. The instability created by excess weight coupled with joint laxity from the hormone relaxin raises the risk of falling and joint injury. The **cardiac sphincter** remains relaxed, so reflux becomes even more of an issue as the uterus is displaced upward and out of the pelvis. As the weeks pass, the breasts continue to swell in preparation for lactation. To deliver blood more efficiently, blood vessels dilate, which makes the skin look flushed. Additionally, skin pigmentation on the face and abdomen might darken. Long bouts of standing cause edema in the legs—a painful condition that occurs as extra pregnancy weight interferes with the return of interstitial fluid to the blood. This increased pressure then impairs venous valve functioning and causes uncomfortable varicose veins or painful hemorrhoids. Exercise seems to relieve the symptoms of edema and provides other physiological and psychological benefits as well.

During the second trimester, all major organ systems have begun developing, and the fetus grows in size and weight. By the end of 6 months, the fetus averages 14 to 16 in. long and weighs close to 3 lb. By delivery, its weight increases by over seven times. The fetus also develops external genitalia and becomes noticeably active. At this time, the fetus hears its mother's voice and responds to certain stimuli. The brain undergoes its most substantial development during the 5th month as nervous tissue acquires its specialized functions. The fetus swallows, sucks, sleeps, awakes, and begins to open its eyes. Lanugo, a soft hair, develops on the skin surface, and a creamy white vernix develops to protect the skin.

Because of technological advances and rapid fetal growth and development during the second trimester, a baby born by the end of 6 months usually survives if placed in a neonatal intensive care unit.

THIRD TRIMESTER

As the fetus grows in size, it puts more and more pressure on the mother's surrounding organs and structures. Frequent urination and constipation continue. The risk for hemorrhoids and varicose veins persists as more weight is gained. This excess weight strains the woman's heart and lungs and causes greater fatigue and discomfort. Skin continues to darken while the abdomen becomes itchy as the skin stretches. Women often experience false labor contractions called **Braxton-Hicks contractions** as well. If present, these occur at irregular intervals prior to delivery.

In the fetus, organ systems continue to mature with the respiratory system being the last to complete development. Toward the end of the third trimester, the fetus is about 19 to 21 in. long and weighs 6 to 9 lb.

In summary, significant changes occur in a pregnant woman's body as the fetus grows and develops during the 9 months of pregnancy. These changes help meet the increased metabolic demands of the fetus and provide the basic building blocks for fetal growth. As mentioned, blood volume begins increasing during the first trimester and reaches 150% of normal blood volume by 36 weeks. Cardiac output increases during the first 8 months of pregnancy by as much as 50% to ensure adequate supply to all body tissues, including the placenta. This places an extra burden on the maternal heart, which sometimes responds by growing slightly larger than normal. During the last month of pregnancy, cardiac output usually declines by about 10% to 30%, but **stroke volume** remains high to sustain fetal needs. Pulse rate gradually increases until it is about 10 to 15 beats above normal. Blood pressure fluctuates more than usual, especially in response to changes in body position. Because of her increased metabolism, a woman requires more oxygen. Since blood volume and cardiac output increase, she has a greater capacity to deliver oxygen to body cells. In addition, a pregnant woman has a greater **tidal volume** and more efficient **alveoli**—all of which ensure adequate oxygen delivery. Interestingly, respiratory rate increases only slightly (by about two breaths per minute; Fig. 3.3).[1,2]

Blood composition also changes during pregnancy. Blood triglycerides and fatty acids increase to meet increasing energy demands. Blood cholesterol levels also rise because the pregnant woman's body needs it to synthesize estrogen and progesterone.[3] Lastly, proteins become more available in the blood to ensure adequate building blocks for fetal tissue formation.

PRECAUTIONS DURING EXERCISE

Because pregnancy already places tremendous stress on a woman's body, any additional stress added by exercise can be hazardous if the exercise is not monitored and adjusted to ensure safety. Hypothetically, exercise could increase fetal core temperature to a dangerously high level; it could reduce blood flow to the uterus and result in insufficient oxygen delivery; it could cause low–birth-weight babies; or it could increase the risk

---

Cardiac sphincter—also called the lower esophageal sphincter. Regulates the passage of food substances from the esophagus into the stomach. A weakened cardiac sphincter often results in reflux, or the backup of stomach contents into the esophagus. Because stomach contents are acidic, reflux results in burning and possible damage to the esophageal lining.

Braxton-Hicks contractions—irregular uterine contractions that usually begin midway through pregnancy and persist throughout pregnancy. Often occur with increased physical activity. Typically not intense but quite uncomfortable.

Stroke volume—the amount of blood pumped by the left ventricle with one heart beat. Usually expressed in milliliters.

Tidal volume—the amount of air breathed in or out during normal respiration.

Alveoli—tiny air sacs in the lungs through which gases are exchanged. Each lung contains millions of alveoli.

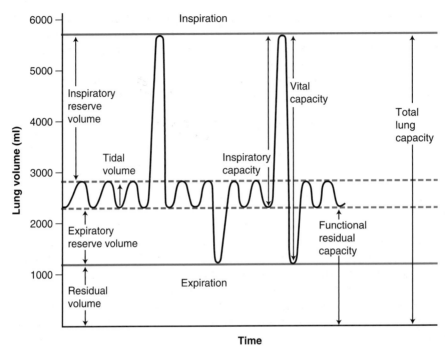

FIGURE 3.3 ■ Respiratory changes during pregnancy. (From Beckmann CRB, Ling FW, Laube DW, et al. Obstetrics and Gynecology. 4th Ed. Baltimore: Lippincott Williams & Wilkins, 2002.)

of musculoskeletal injuries during pregnancy (Table 3.3). This section explores these concerns.

INCREASED CORE BODY TEMPERATURE

Proteins exist in various forms and perform various functions in the body. They form basic body structures; they transport materials in fluids and across cell membranes; they help maintain pH balance and appropriate fluid distribution; and most importantly, they act as enzymes. Because proteins are responsible for most cellular functioning, cells often die if their proteins are damaged or unavailable.

The three-dimensional shape of a protein determines its function. Some proteins are long and filamentous; others fold into globular shapes; others have active sites with a unique configuration that allow the protein to bind to specific substances. The shape is not arbitrary; instead, it is designed to enable a protein to perform a specific job. **Denaturation** is the process that alters protein shape and ultimately interferes with protein function. Inappropriate pH, excessive agitation, exposure to chemicals, and *extreme heat* can all denature proteins. Thus, the major problem with an elevated core temperature is that an extreme temperature denatures proteins and renders them unable to fulfill their intended roles. Since heat is a by-product of normal metabolism, anything that elevates metabolism also increases heat production, which in turn elevates core body temperature. A pregnant exerciser, therefore, must be cautious. During pregnancy, **anabolic processes**

TABLE 3-3 POTENTIAL RISKS OF EXERCISE	
Increased core body temperature	Extreme and prolonged elevated temperature increases risk for neural tube defect because it alters the shape and functioning of body proteins.
Interrupted blood flow to fetus	Working muscles demand increased blood flow. Blood might be diverted from the fetus to supply skeletal muscles with oxygen and nutrients. This might restrict their availability to fetal tissues.
Decreased oxygen delivery to fetus	Maternal cells require more oxygen when stressed with exercise. This could deprive fetal cells of oxygen and interfere with growth and development.
Low–birth-weight	An exercising mother requires extra kilocalories to sustain activity. Nutrients, particularly carbohydrates, might be preferentially given to maternal tissues and promote fetal growth problems.

occur at a faster rate than usual to allow fetal structures to develop. Exercise, of course, also stimulates anabolism and **catabolism** as the body adjusts to new demands. It seems reasonable to assume that the combined effect of both pregnancy and exercise could theoretically increase core body temperature to dangerous levels.

Current evidence suggests that a maternal body temperature exceeding 102.6°F could be deadly to a fetus—particularly during the first trimester. Animal studies indicate that elevated temperature typically does not lead to death, but it impairs growth and development of the central nervous system. In fact, **hyperthermia** is strongly correlated with neural tube defect. Exercise, however, does not seem to increase core temperature to such extremes as long as pregnant exercisers drink plenty of cool water or juice, avoid exercising outdoors in hot or humid conditions, exercise indoors during the hottest part of the day, and exercise for shorter intervals at lower intensities than normal. In addition, they should wear light clothing to facilitate evaporative cooling. Interestingly, the pregnant woman's body "learns" to begin sweating at a progressively lower body temperature as pregnancy proceeds to ensure appropriate heat dissipation as metabolism increases.[1,2,4–7]

BLOOD FLOW TO THE FETUS

Blood flow to the placenta is essential because maternal blood is the source of oxygen and nutrients for the fetus. Some research suggests that damage to a fetus occurs when

Denaturation—a process that alters the three-dimensional shape of a protein. Since shape determines function, a denatured protein is often inert. Denaturation results from extreme heat, agitation, or exposure to strong acids or bases.

Anabolic processes (anabolism)—metabolic processes that build up. A reaction in which two smaller molecules or structures combine to form a larger molecule or structure.

Catabolic processes (catabolism)—a metabolic process that breaks down. A reaction in which a large molecule or structure is broken down into two or more smaller molecules or structures.

Hyperthermia—a condition of higher than normal body temperature.

placental blood flow drops by 50%. Since blood is diverted from deep organs to working muscles during exercise, there is a fear that bouts of exercise deprive the fetus of these essential substances. Currently, research findings are contradictory, so future studies are necessary to determine the actual effects of reduced blood flow to the placenta during exercise. Keep in mind, however, that during pregnancy blood volume, number of red blood cells, and vascular resistance change in such a way that benefits the fetus. The increased blood volume and number of red blood cells coupled with the increased cardiac output and **heart rate** increase the amount of blood delivered to the placenta. Consequently, blood flow likely remains adequate during physical exertion.[1,4,7–9]

OXYGEN DELIVERY TO THE FETUS

Oxygen demand increases during both exercise and fetal development. When a woman is pregnant but at rest, tidal volume and oxygen consumption increase to meet the growing needs of the fetus; however, respiratory frequency is not affected. In the initial stages of mild exercise, respiratory frequency increases up to a certain point to satisfy the greater demand. As intensity reaches moderate to maximal levels, however, respiratory frequency, tidal volume, and oxygen consumption tend to decrease. This drop probably occurs because the growing fetus limits the diaphragm's ability to fully contract. When this happens, the pregnant woman cannot tolerate the greater intensity and must slow down. Although studies are lacking in this area, it appears that pregnant women voluntarily decrease exertion when exercising, which helps counteract the effects of exercise on fetal oxygen supply. As mentioned earlier, blood volume and number of red blood cells increase during pregnancy. Since these values also increase with training, a fit body is better able to deliver oxygenated blood to tissues. The placenta itself also experiences an improved capacity to deliver oxygen and remove wastes from fetal tissues, so more oxygen is transported overall to meet increasing demand.[1,4,5]

LOW–BIRTH-WEIGHT

Current research indicates that pregnant exercisers are more likely to have lower birth weight babies than their less active counterparts. In fact, in one study of 750 low-risk pregnant exercisers, the babies were about 86.5 g (0.1907 lb) lighter than those of a control group. Whether or not this lower weight is harmful, however, is unknown. Basically, researchers concluded that the lower weight resulted from limited fat stores rather than underdeveloped muscle or other tissues. Although once thought to impair a baby's ability to maintain core body temperature, low fat stores actually do not promote low body temperature. Therefore, experts believe that lighter babies suffer no complications as a result of low fat stores. On the contrary, they might be less likely to become obese as they get older.[1,10]

Why do exercisers sometimes have lower births weight babies? It might be because carbohydrate availability to the fetus decreases slightly during and immediately following exercise. This occurs because working muscles have a high demand for carbohydrates, so much of the active mother's carbohydrates are delivered to her muscles rather than to the fetus. Evidence, however, suggests that as long as the mother consumes adequate kilocalories and carbohydrates, there are no harmful effects on the fetus because glucose metabolism changes during pregnancy to favor fetal development. The placenta becomes more efficient at delivering nutrients to the fetus as the pregnancy proceeds, and though the mother is at a higher risk of hypoglycemia during exercise exceeding 45 minutes in duration, the fetus tends to receive adequate nutrition. Of course, frequency, intensity, and type of exercise should also be considered, but as long as energy intake is sufficient, the fetus receives adequate nutrients for development.[4,9,10]

MUSCULOSKELETAL CHANGES

As pregnancy progresses, a woman's body weight increases, her center of gravity shifts, and her joints become less stable under the influence of relaxin. All of this promotes loss of balance, stability, and control over body movements, so fitness professionals must be cautious when designing exercise programs for this population. Heavy weight lifting could cause strains, sprains, and dangerously high blood pressure. Aerobic training that requires frequent changes in direction or excessive lateral movements could promote falling.

Interestingly, actual studies have failed to show increased incidences of musculoskel-etal injuries in physically active pregnant women. Perhaps this is because pregnant women consciously avoid contact sports and activities that require quick movements or high-impact. Overall, fitness professionals must consider the significant musculoskeletal changes that develop in this population and design exercise programs that minimize risk.[4]

BENEFITS OF EXERCISE

Although it is best for a woman to begin an exercise program prior to becoming pregnant, evidence suggests that initiating physical activity after becoming pregnant is still safe for both mother and fetus. The sooner an expectant mother begins exercising, the better the outcome. The following section discusses some of the specific benefits experienced by pregnant exercisers.

HEALTHY WEIGHT GAIN

Before considering weight gain during pregnancy, understand that being overweight, obese, or underweight before conception is associated with greater difficulty in conceiv-ing and an increased risk of complications during pregnancy. Obese women tend to have prolonged gestation, so their babies often weigh more than 9 lb. This results in a more difficult labor and delivery and increases the likelihood of delivery by cesarean. An over-weight pregnant woman has an increased risk of **gestational diabetes**, hypertension,

---

Heart rate—the number of times the heart beats in one minute.

Gestational diabetes—a type of glucose intolerance that develops during pregnancy. Affects approximately 7% of all pregnancies.

and **preeclampsia** with risk increasing linearly as **body mass index** (BMI) increases. This means that the greater the weight, the more complicated the pregnancy. Even more disconcerting than the effects of obesity on birth weight is the higher incidence of congenital defects in babies born to overweight mothers. Obesity doubles the risk of neural tube defect (discussed shortly) and significantly increases the risk of heart abnormalities. Since authorities do not recommend dieting during pregnancy, it is best if a woman achieves and then maintains a healthy weight prior to conceiving.[1,4,11]

Underweight women who become pregnant also have difficulty during pregnancy and delivery. Their babies are often born preterm and are likely to be low–birth-weight. Since birth weight is the most reliable indicator of infant health, low–birth-weight babies are at a disadvantage. They have a higher risk of death and the development of degenerative diseases.

During pregnancy, a healthy weight gain is 25 to 35 lb over the course of 9 months assuming that the woman's prepregnancy weight was within normal limits. Underweight women need to gain a little more, while overweight woman need to gain a little less. Women with multiple fetuses need to gain 35 to 45 lb to meet their demands. The average woman should gain about 3.5 lb during the first trimester and then 1 lb per week thereafter. Any rapid weight gain during a short time should sound an alarm and be addressed by a physician.

As mentioned, birth weight is the greatest predictor of infant health. Since birth weight positively correlates with maternal weight gain, a pregnant woman and her physician should monitor changes in weight throughout pregnancy. Although the exact amounts vary somewhat among different women, the extra weight is usually distributed in the following manner:

- 7.5 lb: average baby's weight
- 7 lb: extra stored protein, fat, and other nutrients
- 4 lb: extra blood
- 4 lb: additional body fluids
- 2 lb: increased breast size
- 2 lb: increased size of uterus and supporting muscles
- 2 lb: amniotic fluid surrounding the fetus
- 1.5 lb: placenta

Overall, studies show that the increased energy expenditure from exercise moderates weight gain and reduces total increase in body fat throughout pregnancy. Pregnant exercisers are still able to achieve doctor recommended weight gain, but the increase is within healthy limits. Although weight loss after delivery is associated more with postpartum exercise than with exercise during pregnancy, women who consistently exercise during pregnancy are more likely to continue exercise after delivery.

IMPROVED CIRCULATION

Continual weight gain during pregnancy negatively affects circulation and promotes edema. Because exercise increases blood volume, cardiac output, and number of blood vessels, it improves circulation and prevents painful and uncomfortable swelling. Furthermore, exercise improves the efficiency of the lymphatic system by promoting return of accumulating interstitial fluid to the blood. In addition, exercise enhances nutrient and oxygen delivery so that they are more available to maternal and fetal tissues. Overall, exercise during pregnancy improves blood composition and circulation, which enhances a woman's tolerance to the anatomical changes that occur.[1,4,6]

REDUCED OVERALL DISCOMFORT AND IMPROVED MOOD

Exercise alleviates some of the discomforts associated with pregnancy including lower back pain, edema in the legs, stiff joints, constipation, bloating, and insomnia. Exercise involving major joints maintains normal functioning and range of motion. In addition, it preserves muscle mass and increases strength—this extra strength then translates into increased energy levels. Lastly, regular activity improves sleep, another factor that positively affects energy level.[2]

Few studies have focused on the psychological effects of physical activity during pregnancy. In the studies available, however, pregnant exercisers express being happier and more content throughout all three trimesters compared to their sedentary counterparts—perhaps because exercise stimulates the release of chemicals that elevate mood. In addition to elevating mood, participation in structured exercise programs also seems to decrease the incidence of depression according to one study that used a popular depression scale to measure psychological disposition.[1,12] Another study indicated that pregnant exercisers who participated in prepared programs improved self-image considerably. This is significant since a negative body image during pregnancy sometimes promotes practices such as strict dieting or even purging—behaviors not compatible with a healthy pregnancy.[13] Unhealthy behaviors such as these have been associated with inadequate weight gain, premature delivery, low–birth-weight, and delayed child development later in life.

IMPROVED CARDIORESPIRATORY AND MUSCULAR FUNCTIONING RESULTS IN EASIER PREGNANCY, LABOR, AND DELIVERY

Cardiovascular exercise profoundly affects cardiorespiratory functioning. In addition to an increase in blood volume and the number of circulating red blood cells, the oxygen-binding capacity of hemoglobin increases during and following exercise. Consequently,

Preeclampsia—a condition that affects both the mother and the fetus. It is characterized by high blood pressure, persistent swelling, and excessive protein in the urine. Preeclampsia is more common during a first pregnancy. Risk is higher for those whose mother or sister had it; those with multiple fetuses; those still in their teens or over the age of 40; those with hypertension prior to pregnancy; and those suffering from kidney disease. The exact cause is unknown.

Body mass index— a measure of weight in relation to height; indicates overall risk for chronic disease; does not measure body fat percentage or indicate body fat distribution.

more oxygen travels to both maternal and fetal cells. Ultimately, this places less stress on the maternal heart and improves stamina during pregnancy.[1,14] In addition, aerobic conditioning improves endurance so much that it eases the cardiorespiratory burden associated with labor and reduces the actual length of labor.[2]

Since resistance exercise that complies with current recommendations strengthens the skeletal muscles involved with childbirth, many women who strength-train during pregnancy claim that they experience less pain and soreness both during and following delivery. Their muscles have adapted to challenges and are consequently better able to handle the stress of childbirth. According to a 2002 study, women who participated in strength training during all three trimesters required less pain medication and had a healthier delivery overall than women who did not. In addition, most exercisers did not have to undergo induced labor or any other type of medical intervention such as a cesarean.[1,14]

DECREASED RISK FOR PREECLAMPSIA

According to the Preeclampsia Foundation, preeclampsia occurs in 5% to 8% of all pregnancies. It is characterized by high blood pressure and protein in the urine and affects both the mother and the fetus. This condition progresses rapidly and is suspected when a pregnant woman experiences sudden weight gain, headache, and unusual swelling. A pregnant woman noticing any of these symptoms should seek medical care immediately. New studies suggest that moderate cardiovascular exercise helps prevent preeclampsia and its harmful effects on pregnancy outcomes. Additionally, exercise effectively reduces blood cholesterol levels throughout pregnancy. A lower blood cholesterol level is associated with a lower risk for gestational diabetes *and* preeclampsia during pregnancy.[10]

RECOMMENDATIONS

Years ago, physicians noticed that women in physically demanding jobs had preterm deliveries and low–birth-weight babies, so they strongly discouraged physical activity during pregnancy. Controlled studies since then have indicated that exercise more than likely *benefits* rather than harms the developing fetus, so exercise is no longer discouraged during pregnancy.[2]

As mentioned earlier, since both pregnancy and exercise stress the body, guidelines must consider the potential adverse affects of this added stress on the fetus.

EXERCISE TESTING

According to the American College of Sports Medicine (ACSM), pregnant women without contraindications (see Table 3.4) should continue exercise throughout the duration of pregnancy. They should undergo maximal exercise testing only if medically necessary and only under physician supervision. Most pregnant women may undergo submaximal exercise testing (<75% heart rate reserve) to predict maximum oxygen uptake for better program design.

TABLE 3-4 CONTRAINDICATIONS TO AEROBIC EXERCISE DURING PREGNANCY ACCORDING TO ACOG

Relative

- Severe anemia
- Unevaluated maternal cardiac arrhythmia
- Chronic bronchitis
- Poorly controlled type I diabetes
- Extreme morbid obesity
- Extreme underweight (BMI < 12)
- History of extremely sedentary lifestyle
- Intrauterine growth restriction in current pregnancy
- Poorly controlled hypertension
- Orthopedic limitations
- Poorly controlled seizure disorder
- Poorly controlled hyperthyroidism
- Heavy smoker

Absolute

- Hemodynamically significant heart disease
- Restrictive lung disease
- Incompetent cervix/cerclage
- Multiple gestation at risk for premature labor
- Persistent second-trimester or third-trimester bleeding
- Placenta previa after 26 weeks gestation
- Premature labor during current pregnancy
- Ruptured membranes
- Preeclempsia/pregnancy-induced hypertension

Source: Exercise during pregnancy and the postpartum period. ACOG Committee Opinion No. 267. American College of Obstetricians and Gynecologists. Obstet Gynecol 2002;99:171–173.

EXERCISE PRESCRIPTION

Available information suggests that both strength training and cardiovascular training are safe and beneficial for women with low risk pregnancies.[15,16] In compliance with existing literature and guidelines from the American College of Obstetricians and Gynecologists (ACOG), the following recommendations are considered safe for generally healthy pregnant women experiencing no complications.[14,17–19]

- Previously sedentary women, or women experiencing any of the contraindications listed in Table 3.4, should receive clearance from a physician prior to beginning an exercise training program. If encouraged by a physician, exercise can be a healthy adjunct to pregnancy.

- ACSM suggests that all pregnant women be screened using the Physical Activity Readiness Medical Examination (PARmed-X for Pregnancy) before participating in exercise.[20]
- Precede all forms of exercise by at least 5 to 10 minutes of a low impact, low-intensity warm-up such as walking or stationary cycling (Fig. 3.4). As for all exercisers, the warm-up prepares the joints and muscles for movement by increasing blood flow and heart rate. Follow each workout with a 5- to 10-minute cooldown to return heart rate and blood flow to normal levels. Perform stretching exercises *following* either the warm-up or the cooldown.
- *Regular* aerobic exercise (at least 3—preferably all—days of the week) provides more benefit than *intermittent* exercise. Fifteen to thirty minutes of moderate intensity (40% to 60% of VO_{2R}) exercise appears safe (for a total of 150 minutes of activity per week). See Table 3.5 for recommended heart rate ranges for pregnant women. Consider using the "talk test" or the rating of perceived exertion scale to monitor intensity since heart rate is already elevated during rest and exertion in this population. To pass the talk test, a woman should be able to carry on a light conversation during exercise. If she becomes short of breath when speaking, she should lower her intensity. If she can recite a 20-minute monologue, she should increase intensity. If using the 6 to 20 Borg rate of perceived exertion scale (see Appendix A), a rating of 12 to 14 is classified as moderate.
- Overall, a pregnant woman should avoid exercise to exhaustion and should stop exercise when fatigued.
- Avoid contact sports and other activities that have a high risk of falling or abdominal trauma. Examples of activities to avoid are soccer, basketball, and horseback riding.
- In general, low-impact exercise, such as stationary cycling (Fig. 3.5) or swimming, is preferred to high-impact activities such as running, jumping, and bouncing. In addition, avoid rapid changes in direction to reduce trauma to the fetus, injury to joints, and risk of falling. Remember—a pregnant woman's center of gravity changes.
- Resistance training is recommended, especially for the abdominal muscles, back muscles, and pelvic floor muscles. Training these muscles makes it easier to support the increasing weight of the growing fetus; helps the pregnant woman push more effectively during the last phase of delivery; maintains posture and reduces lower back pain; and prevents urinary problems after delivery. The hormone relaxin

TABLE 3-5 RECOMMENDED TARGET HEART RATE RANGES FOR PREGNANT WOMEN	
Age (years)	**Heart Rate Range (bpm)**
<20	140–155
20–29	135–150
30–39	130–145
>40	125–140

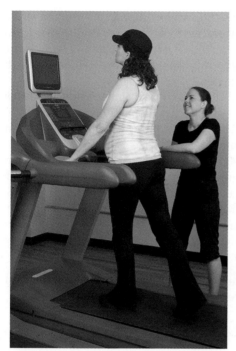

FIGURE 3.4 ■ Precede all forms of exercise with a 5- to 10- minute warm-up that includes a low impact, low-intensity activity such as walking.

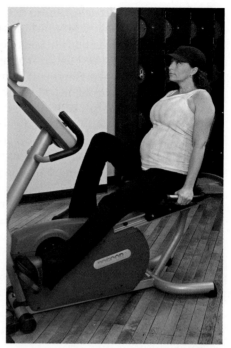

FIGURE 3.5 ■ Low-impact activities such as stationary cycling or swimming are preferred for pregnant exercisers.

affects not only the joints involved with childbirth but also every joint in the body. Therefore, deep flexion or extension of joints is discouraged because of joint instability. Make pregnant exercisers perform all movements slowly and with control to prevent injury. Pay attention to body mechanics and ensure neutral joint alignment. Encourage participants to exhale during the exertion and inhale during the return phase. This prevents lightheadedness and an unsafe increase in blood pressure. Ensure that the participant does not grip any weights or dumbbells too tightly—a tight grip can cause dangerous increases in blood pressure. Strength train all major muscle groups at an intensity that allows for 12 to 15 repetitions. Avoid isometric exercises and the Valsalva maneuver.

■ Avoid full sit-ups throughout pregnancy. After the 3rd month of pregnancy, avoid any exercise performed in the supine position (lying on the back) since this position decreases cardiac output, lowers blood pressure, and potentially decreases oxygen flow to the fetus. In addition, avoid any activity that requires extended motionless standing since motionless standing interferes with the return of deoxygenated blood to the heart and promotes blood pooling.

■ Avoid strenuous exercise during the first trimester. This is when most major organ systems develop, so the fetus is particularly vulnerable at this time.

- Avoid strenuous exercise during hot, humid weather. A pregnant woman already has a high metabolic rate (which means she is producing more heat than normal), and even though her body has adapted to initiate sweating at a lower temperature, excessive heat can be life-threatening to the fetus. Exercising indoors allows for more control over environmental temperature.
- Drink plenty of fluids before, during, and after exercise to maintain normal body temperature. Consume two additional 8-oz glasses of water for every hour of exercise.
- Do not exercise when severely fatigued—especially during the third trimester. This can put undue stress on both mother and fetus.
- Avoid exercise at altitudes above 6,000 ft since this increases the risk of preterm labor and vaginal bleeding. Note: pregnant women do not need to avoid altitudes above 6,000 ft altogether; they just need to avoid physical exertion at this level.
- Energy needs increase *slightly* during pregnancy, so pregnant exercisers should consume enough kilocalories to compensate for the combined demands of pregnancy *and* exercise. Women need approximately 300 extra kilocalories per day to accommodate pregnancy.

A pregnant woman should stop all activity and seek immediate medical attention if she experiences any of the following during exercise:

- Shortness of breath
- Vaginal bleeding
- Dizziness
- Headache
- Chest pain
- Amniotic fluid leakage
- Decreased fetal movement
- Significant calf pain, swelling, or muscle weakness as these are signs of deep venous thrombosis

Additionally, previously sedentary pregnant exercisers might tolerate exercise better at the start of the second trimester because of the severe fatigue, nausea, and vomiting often associated with the first 3 months of pregnancy. They should choose a low-intensity, low-impact activity initially performed just 3 days per week for approximately 15 minutes at a time. This allows their unconditioned bodies to gradually adapt to activity and decreases the risk of injury. Ultimately, the previously sedentary pregnant woman should strive for 30 minutes of moderate activity on most days of the week. Low-impact exercises such as swimming, walking, or water aerobics are the safest and most tolerable, but stationary cycling and other low-impact aerobic training machines are also good choices.

If an active woman becomes pregnant, she can usually continue her regular exercise routine well into her pregnancy. Performance typically declines as the pregnancy progresses, so these women should allow physical comfort to dictate intensity. A few studies have investigated the effects of high-intensity activities on the fetus or baby; most have found no complications or harmful effects other than low–birth-weight. Yet, caution is still advised.

All pregnant women should avoid motionless standing for prolonged periods because it interferes with the return of blood to the heart. It also increases the likelihood of developing **varicose veins**. Strenuous exercise during the third trimester can predispose the pregnant woman to hypoglycemia, possibly because both the fetus and maternal cells increase their intake of glucose and the maternal liver's glycogen stores diminish. Consuming about 30 to 50 g of carbohydrates prior to exercising minimizes the risk of hypoglycemia.

Free weights can be hazardous to a pregnant woman because of joint instability. If possible, use weight machines. They provide built-in protection and limited range-of-motion to decrease the risk of joint injury. After five minutes of warming up, begin resistance training. Most resistance exercises performed in the nonpregnant state are safe during pregnancy as long as the preceding guidelines are followed.

> ### QUICK REFERENCE
> In most cases, a woman who participated in strength training prior to becoming pregnant may continue this activity after becoming pregnant. She must adjust intensity based on comfort level and avoid sets with maximal effort. The goal during pregnancy should be to maintain strength—not make substantial improvements.

> ### QUICK REFERENCE
> A previously sedentary woman who becomes pregnant may participate in strength training with physician approval. The goal should be to prepare the body for the demands of pregnancy and delivery—not to lose weight or make significant improvements in muscle mass and body composition.

Postpartum exercise helps the pregnant woman's body return to prepregnancy conditions; however, it is typical for a woman to feel the physiological effects associated with pregnancy for up to 6 weeks after delivery. Increases in exercise duration, intensity, and frequency should be gradual and based on individual condition. In other words, someone who delivered by Caesarean needs a longer recovery time than someone who delivered naturally. Most experts claim that women who breast-feed their infants need not worry about exercise interfering with the quality of milk. Milk composition and milk volume seem unaffected by increased activity and any subsequent weight loss that often accompanies exercise.

> **Varicose veins**—visible, dilated, lumpy veins near the surface of the skin. Occur when venous valves function improperly and blood pools in a small section of a vein; typically seen in the lower legs.

SAMPLE EXERCISES FOR THE PREGNANT WOMAN

WARM-UP

Warm-up for 5 to 10 minutes on a treadmill. Include limbering movements of the upper extremities, but avoid keeping hands overhead for an extended period of time (this increases blood pressure). Mildly stretch the shoulders, back, chest, biceps, triceps, hip flexors, quadriceps, and hamstrings after the warm-up.

UPPER BODY EXERCISES

Strengthening the upper body helps maintain posture and enables the woman to handle the weight gained during pregnancy. Maintain neutral body alignment throughout each exercise.

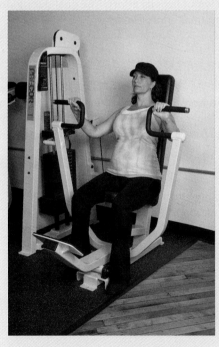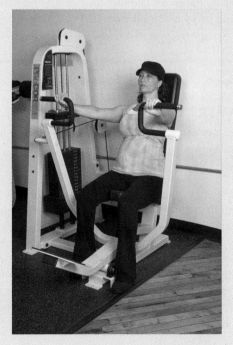

■ **Seated Chest Press (Fig. 3.6)**
Sit on a seated chest press machine and grasp handgrips. Using a light resistance, perform the exercise like any other population: push handgrips forward until arms are straight but not locked. Pause. Return to starting position. Repeat 12 to 15 times. A seated chest press machine is preferable to a lying chest press machine. The chest can also be worked using elastic bands or by doing wall push-ups.

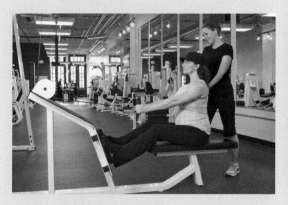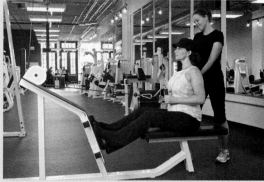

■ **Seated Row (Fig. 3.7)**

Sit in a seated row machine with spine neutral; avoid arching the back and maintain a stable core. After setting the machine to a lightweight, grasp hand grips and pull elbows back. Pause. Return to starting position. Repeat for 12 to 15 repetitions. Ensure that the client is breathing out during the exertion and in during the return phase. This exercise can also be done using elastic bands.

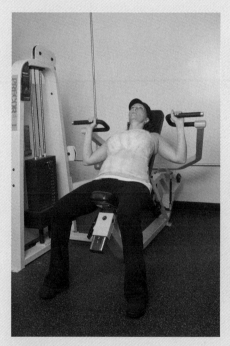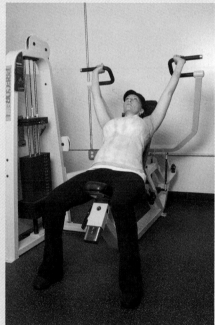

■ **Seated Shoulder Press (Fig. 3.8)**

Sit at a shoulder press machine. Adjust seat so that arms are parallel to ground with hand grips at ear level. Grasp hand grips and push up until arms are fully extended but not locked. Pause. Return to starting position. Repeat for 12 to 15 repetitions. This exercise may be done using resistance equipment, bands, or light dumbbells. Ensure neutral alignment and smooth movements. A more vertical machine is preferable, especially as pregnancy progresses.

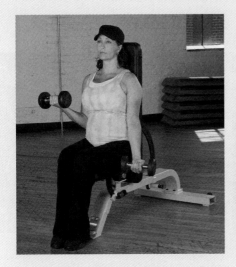
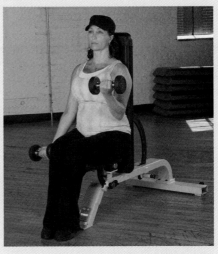

■ Biceps Curl (Fig. 3.9)

Sit on a bench with one light dumbbell in each hand. Flex the right elbow while curling the weight up toward the shoulder. Pause. Return right arm to starting position. Repeat on left side. Alternate right then left for 12 to 15 repetitions each. This exercise can be done with resistance equipment, bands, or light dumbbells. Avoid hyperextension at the elbow, but perform through a full range-of-motion.

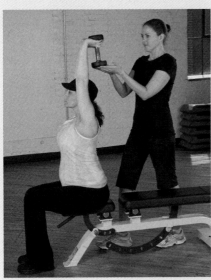
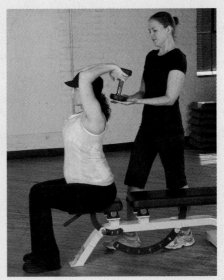

■ Seated Triceps Extension (Fig. 3.10)

Select a dumbbell with a weight that can be held overhead with both hands. Sit on a bench with spine neutral and feet flat on floor (choose a bench with a backrest if possible). Grasp the dumbbell around the weight and raise above head. Lower the weight with control until forearms are parallel to the floor. Pause. Return to starting position. Repeat 12 to 15 times. Avoid hyperextension at the elbow. Resistance equipment targeting the triceps might become difficult to use as the belly enlarges. Alternately, elastic tubing can be used.

LOWER BODY EXERCISES

Strengthening the lower body improves balance, increases support of the pelvic joints, and assists in delivery. Maintain neutral body alignment throughout each exercise.

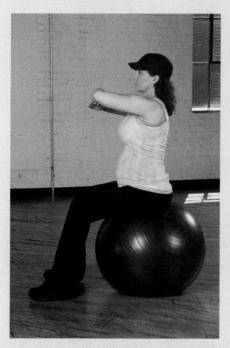 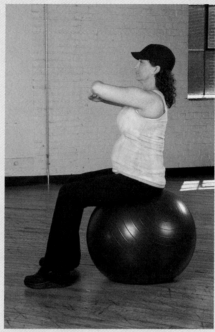

■ Seated Pelvic Tilt (Fig. 3.11)

This exercise increases core strength by targeting the abdominals, buttocks, and pelvic floor muscles. To perform this exercise, stand with knees aligned over toes. Slowly contract the abdominals, buttocks, and pelvic floor muscles (which slightly tilts the pelvis). Relax and repeat for 12 to 15 repetitions. This is a slight movement; avoid rocking. This exercise may also be done in the seated position.

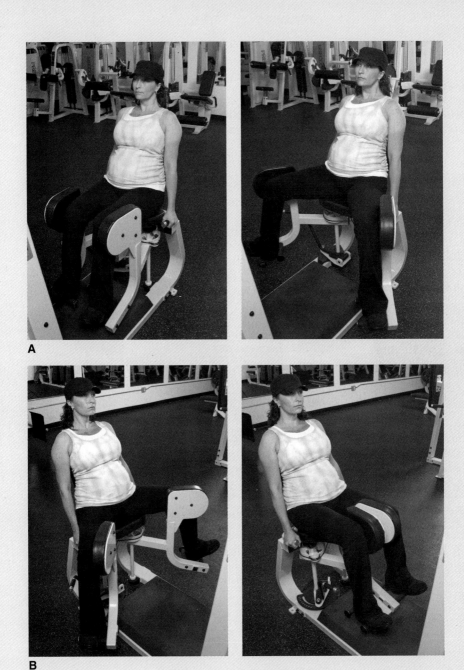

A

B

■ **Thigh Abduction and Adduction. A: Abduction. B: Adduction (Fig. 3.12)**
Thigh abduction (Fig. 3.12A) and adduction (Fig. 3.12B) exercises may also be performed using a piece of weight lifting equipment with light resistance. They can also be done in the side-lying position using body weight as resistance (this is preferred for the previously sedentary pregnant woman). The all-fours position should be avoided during the third trimester. Avoid the supine position after the 3rd month of pregnancy. When using resistance equipment, follow manufacturers instructions. Avoid overstretching the hip joints.

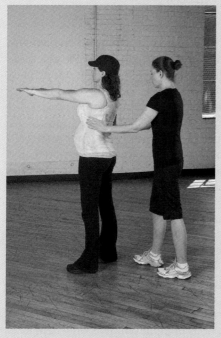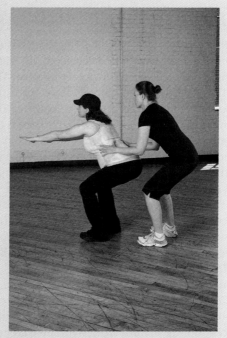

■ Squat (Fig. 3.13)

Have the woman stand with feet slightly wider than shoulder width apart, back neutral. Contract the abdominal muscles and bend the knees until the hips are parallel to the floor. Knees should stay at or behind an imaginary vertical line drawn from the toes straight up to the ceiling. Slowly return to an erect position without locking the knees. Exhale while lowering the hips; inhale when returning to the standing position. For added resistance, hold one dumbbell in each hand or use a body bar and squat. Note: The squat might become difficult during the third trimester (and perhaps toward the end of the second trimester). Lunges in a stationary position are also effective. The leg press is another alternative that effectively trains the buttocks and hamstrings. It should be done with light resistance. Sit with back and head against pad. Place feet hip-width apart on footplate. Make sure that heels are flat. Hips and knees should be at a 90-degree angle. Grasp the handles, keep knees in line with feet, and push with legs.

KEGEL EXERCISES

Kegel exercises strengthen the pelvic floor muscles to prevent uterine prolapse and urinary incontinence. To perform, contract the muscles that form the floor of the pelvic cavity for 5 to 10 seconds. Relax. Repeat for 10 repetitions. Perform only one set at a time; however, multiple sets may be done if they are scattered throughout the day (for up to 100 repetitions per day).

NUTRITIONAL CONSIDERATIONS

People in all stages of life require the same basic nutrients. What differs is the amount necessary to support growth and development. During times of rapid cell division and tissue formation, nutritional needs obviously increase. This is exactly what happens during pregnancy. The pregnant woman's body develops tissues to support a growing fetus and provides the nutrients for fetal tissue development. This means that a pregnant woman's diet must provide sufficient kilocalories and nutrients to support increased metabolism.

Ideally, a woman should strive for optimal physical, mental, and emotional well-being prior to conceiving. This prepares her body for the stresses of pregnancy and helps ensure a positive outcome. Although maternal and fetal blood never mix, maternal and fetal blood vessels have an intimate connection; therefore, a pregnant woman must avoid consuming anything that can negatively affect her fetus. This includes certain over-the-counter and prescription medications, alcohol, nutritional supplements, herbal supplements, and anything else that is potentially dangerous. In fact, a pregnant woman should check with her physician before ingesting any supplements or medications.

Maternal nutrition at the time of conception greatly affects fetal growth and development. Consequently, all women of childbearing age should consume an adequate and balanced diet to prevent malnutrition. Remember that critical periods in fetal development occur during the first trimester. These are periods of rapid cell division where most organs and organ systems begin developing. Since a woman is often unaware that she is pregnant during the first few weeks of pregnancy, she could inadvertently harm her fetus if she is malnourished. The following sections discuss particular nutrients that are of interest prior to and during pregnancy.[21,22]

ENERGY-YIELDING NUTRIENTS: CARBOHYDRATES, PROTEIN, AND FAT

Although pregnant women need to increase energy intake to meet their higher metabolism, experts now recognize that a pregnant woman is not technically "eating for two." During the second trimester, energy needs increase by about 340 kilocalories per day. During the third trimester, they increase by 450 kilocalories per day. Considering the fact that energy needs do not increase during the first trimester, this averages out to an extra 300 kilocalories per day throughout the course of the pregnancy. That is it! This extra energy supports the increased workload of the cardiovascular and respiratory systems; the growth of breast tissue and uterine muscle; and the formation and operation of the placenta and fetal tissues. By consuming **nutrient-dense foods**, foods that have a high nutrient content relative to their total number of kilocalories, a pregnant woman can ensure appropriate nutrition without excess and unnecessary weight gain (Table 3.6).

Carbohydrate intake should average a minimum of 175 g per day (or at least 50% to 65% of total kilocalorie intake) to fuel metabolism, spare dietary and body proteins, and provide glucose to fuel the fetal brain. To meet this need, pregnant women should include whole grain breads and cereals, dark green vegetables, fresh fruits, and low-fat dairy products.

TABLE 3-6 SUMMARY OF THE REQUIREMENTS FOR ENERGY-YIELDING NUTRIENTS

Carbohydrates	50%–65% of total kilocalorie intake; no less than 175 g per day for the average pregnant woman.
Proteins	Pregnant women require 25 g more per day than nonpregnant women. Avoid protein supplements.
Fats	Obtain approximately 13 g of omega-6 fatty acids per day and 1.4 g of omega-3 fatty acids per day.

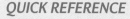

QUICK REFERENCE

Pregnant exercisers have an increased risk for hypoglycemia during exercise, especially during the last several weeks of pregnancy. Adequate carbohydrate intake prevents this.

Pregnant women need about 25 g more protein per day than nonpregnant women. To ensure protein adequacy, expectant mothers should choose lean cuts of meat, poultry, and fish. In addition, milk, other dairy products, legumes, and whole grains contain appreciable amount of protein. Since high protein supplements can damage a developing fetus, women should avoid these during pregnancy.

Fat, the third energy-yielding nutrient, is also a healthy part of a pregnant woman's diet for several reasons. First of all, fat provides a concentrated source of energy that helps meet the slightly higher energy requirements. Secondly, fat is the only source of the two essential fatty acids: linoleic acid (omega-6 fatty acid) and linolenic acid (omega-3 fatty acid). These fatty acids, which perform several crucial functions within the body, must be obtained from food sources because the human body cannot make them on its own. Without them, cell membranes would not form properly; eicosanoids (substances that regulate certain body functions) would be scarce; and the nervous system would not develop appropriately. Currently, recommendations suggest that pregnant women consume 13 g of omega-6 fatty acids and 1.4 g of omega-3 fatty acids per day. More important than the actual intake of each of these fatty acids, however, is the relative proportion of omega-6 fatty acids to omega-3 fatty acids in the diet. Ideally, adults should consume about five times more omega-6 fatty acids than omega-3 fatty acids. Actual intake, however, is close to 20 to 40 times more omega-6 fatty acids than omega-3 fatty acids. To improve this ratio, people should consume fish two times per week or seek other sources including flaxseed, flaxseed oil, or walnuts. Although fatty fish are the best sources of omega-3 fatty acids, they can also contain large amounts of contaminants. A pregnant

Nutrient-dense foods—foods that have a high nutrient content relative to their kilocalorie content.

woman should be aware of this and avoid consuming excessive amounts of fatty fish. Futhermore, she should not ingest fish oil supplements because they potentially contain high levels of contaminants that can severely damage the fetus.

VITAMINS AND MINERALS

Folate, vitamin B_{12}, iron, calcium, and vitamin D are of particular concern during pregnancy (Table 3.7). Over the years, studies have confirmed the importance of folic acid in the prevention of neural tube defect. The neural tube is a structure that develops into the spine (often by day 28 of gestation, before a woman is even aware that she is pregnant), so folic acid intake is important *before* conception as well as during pregnancy. The most common types of neural tube defects are anencephaly and spina bifida.

Anencephaly, a word that literally means "no brain," is an uncommon condition that occurs if the upper end of the neural tube fails to close. This results in severely diminished brain development—or in some cases, the complete absence of a brain. Most cases of anencephaly abort early; others are carried to term, but the baby is either stillborn or dies shortly thereafter.

Spina bifida is a more common condition that occurs when the spinal cord and the vertebral column fail to close completely. The spinal cord, covered by protective membranes called meninges, protrudes, a condition that might be life-threatening. Spina bifida varies in severity and causes a wide range of physical disabilities including different levels of paralysis. In addition, those suffering from spina bifida often experience clubfoot, muscle weakness, mental deficiencies, and kidney disorders.

To prevent neural tube defect, women should consume 600 μg of folate per day, with 400 μg coming from fortified foods or supplements and the additional 200 μg deriving from fruits and vegetables. To ensure adequate intake, all grain products in the United States are fortified with folate, a practice that has improved the outcome in cases of

TABLE 3-7	VITAMINS AND MINERALS IMPORTANT DURING PREGNANCY	
Vitamin/ Mineral	**Importance**	**Amount Required per Day**
Folate	Necessary to prevent neural tube defect. Significant food sources include fortified grains, leafy greens, legumes, seeds, and liver.	600 μg
Vitamin B_{12}	Helps maintain nerve cells. Necessary for the body to use folate. Significant food sources include meat, fish, poultry, eggs, and fortified cereals.	2.6 μg
Iron	Attaches to oxygen in hemoglobin. Significant food sources include red meat, poultry, fish, eggs, dried fruit, and legumes.	27 mg
Calcium	Needed for muscle contraction and nerve impulse propagation. Forms the structure of bones and teeth. Significant food sources include milk, tofu, broccoli, and legumes.	1,000 mg
Vitamin D	Needed for calcium absorption in GI tract. Significant food sources include meat, eggs, and fortified milk, butter, cereals.	5 μg

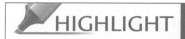

HIGHLIGHT The Intimate Connection Between Mother and Fetus

Maternal blood and fetal blood normally never directly mix; however, the placenta provides an intimate connection between the two. The placenta develops as one of the fetal embryonic membranes grows into the endometrial lining of the mother's uterus. A permeable membrane remains between the two, but many substances easily cross it. For example, oxygen and nutrients from maternal blood diffuse through the placenta to enter fetal blood vessels, while carbon dioxide and other wastes diffuse from fetal blood vessels into maternal blood. This allows the mother to provide the building blocks for fetal development; to provide oxygen for cellular respiration; and to remove metabolic by-products to prevent dangerous accumulation within fetal blood.*

Unfortunately, several potentially hazardous substances take advantage of this intimate connection and must be avoided. These harmful substances include or are associated with alcohol, cigarette smoke, some drugs, listeria monocytogenes, and caffeine.

Alcohol—alcohol consumption is not compatible with a healthy pregnancy. In fact, it directly endangers the fetus. Alcohol easily crosses the placenta to enter fetal circulation. Once within fetal circulation, it wreaks havoc on growth and development—particularly within the central nervous system—because the immature fetal liver cannot catabolize it. Although experts do not yet know the precise amount that causes damage, a pregnant woman who consumes any amount of alcohol increases her baby's risk of heart defects, cleft palate, urinary system problems, abnormal facial features, growth retardation, poor motor skills, hyperactivity, incoordination, and severe central nervous system malfunctioning. Collectively, these impairments are referred to as fetal alcohol syndrome (FAS). Sadly, these symptoms are irreversible once they develop. Encouragingly, FAS is 100% preventable—just avoid alcohol prior to conception and during pregnancy.[17,23,24]

Cigarette smoke—exposure to smoke, even second-hand smoke, drastically decreases oxygen and nutrient availability to a developing fetus because cigarettes contain many harmful substances that reduce blood oxygen levels and constrict the blood vessels that transport oxygen to cells. Therefore, pregnant women should avoid smoking. Pregnant smokers often experience spontaneous abortions, excess vaginal bleeding, placental detachment, preterm births, prolonged and difficult labor, and low weight births. Their babies sometimes suffer sudden infant death syndrome (SIDS), mental retardation,

(continued)

Anencephaly—literally means "no brain." A serious birth defect represented by absence of all or part of the brain and/or skull.

Spina bifida—literally means "an open or severed spine." A serious birth defect that exposes part of the spinal cord thereby making the spinal cord vulnerable to injury.

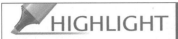

asthma, and heart problems. Although dangerous throughout pregnancy, smoke is particularly harmful during the first 8 weeks of embryonic development as major organ systems form. Ideally, anyone planning to conceive should quit smoking; however, smoking cessation after conception—or even a decrease in the number of cigarettes smoked during pregnancy—significantly benefits the fetus.[15,21]

Drugs—whether they are illegal, prescribed, or over-the-counter, many drugs are dangerous to pregnant women because they can often cross the placenta. At the very least, they can impair fetal growth, promote preterm and low weight births, and cause mild to severe withdrawal symptoms in the fetus. If those side effects are not bad enough, drugs can also cause mental retardation, rapid fetal heart rate, congenital birth defects, irritability, intracranial bleeding, and sepsis. Therefore, pregnant women should seek physician advice when considering drug or medication use.[17,23]

Listeria—Listeria monocytogenes is a bacterium found in some soft cheeses, unpasteurized milk, deli meats, and undercooked meat, poultry, or shellfish. If consumed, it often results in severe vomiting and diarrhea that can leave the sufferer dehydrated and lethargic. It can also cause fever, chills, and muscle aches—symptoms that resemble those of the flu. Unfortunately, it easily crosses the placenta and can cause spontaneous abortion or stillbirth, so pregnant women must limit exposure. During pregnancy, women should avoid soft cheeses such as Brie, Camembert, and Roquefort. Additionally, they should consume deli meats with caution. Reheat deli meats—and hot dogs—until they are steaming so that any existing bacteria are destroyed. Furthermore, thoroughly cook all meat, fish, and poultry and wash fruits and vegetables prior to consumption.[17]

Caffeine—caffeine intake during pregnancy does not appear to increase the risk for birth defects; however, it does cross the placenta and ultimately elevates fetal heart and respiration rate. Some research suggests that caffeine increases the risk for spontaneous abortion, premature birth, low–birth-weight, and withdrawal symptoms in newborns, but the March of Dimes contends that pregnant women—or those trying to conceive—may consume 200 mg of caffeine per day (which is the equivalent of one 12-oz cup of coffee per day) without any side effects. Those who consume more than 200 mg per day are two times more likely to experience a miscarriage than those who consume no caffeine.[17,23,25,26]

*The placenta performs additional functions as well. It synthesizes several hormones such as progesterone, which maintains the uterine lining during pregnancy and is used by the fetal adrenal glands to synthesize estrogen. Estrogen influences fetal organ development, maternal breast development, and changes in the maternal uterus.

unplanned pregnancy. There is no upper limit when folate is derived strictly from dietary sources; however, there is an upper limit of 1,000 μg per day for supplemental folate. Excessive folate can mask the signs of a vitamin B_{12} deficiency, and a deficiency of vitamin B_{12} can have devastating effects on the mother and fetus. Under physician supervision, however, women who have previously delivered a baby with a neural tube defect should take 4,000 μg of folate in supplement form to avoid a recurrence. Most over-the-counter supplements contain 400 μg of folate; whereas, prenatal supplements contain at least 800 μg. Note: Taking folate supplements *after* conception will not benefit the fetus if the woman was deficient prior to conception.

Vitamin B_{12}, found abundantly in animal-based foods such as meat, fish, eggs, and dairy products, plays a significant role in activating the enzyme necessary for folate use in the body. It is also added to many fortified products such as soy milk to prevent the permanent decline in neurological functioning associated with a vitamin B_{12} deficiency. Pregnant women need 2.6 μg of vitamin B_{12} per day, while lactating women need 2.8 μg per day.

Partly because of the expanding blood volume and increase in red blood cells during pregnancy, a pregnant woman's need for iron increases substantially. On average, a pregnant woman needs about 1,000 mg more iron over the course of gestation than her non-pregnant counterpart. Three hundred milligrams are used by the fetus and placenta; 250 mg are lost at delivery; and 450 mg support the increased blood volume. Since most women have difficulty maintaining normal iron levels in the body, many women enter pregnancy below optimal levels. This can be dangerous because a woman with iron deficiency anemia at the start of pregnancy has a three times greater risk for preterm delivery and low–birth-weight upon delivery. Iron deficiency anemia is also associated with cognitive development problems and poor motor function later in life. Although the exact reasons for these impairments are unknown, experts believe it has to do with inadequate oxygen availability and delivery to the fetus. Iron is a necessary component of hemoglobin, a molecule that attaches to and transports oxygen throughout the body. As metabolism increases while fetal tissues grow, the need for oxygen—and subsequently iron—also increases. If the supply of iron is limited, oxygen delivery is diminished. To counteract this, most pregnant women should take a daily prenatal supplement that contains 30 to 60 mg of iron. Note that absorption from a multivitamin-mineral supplement is much lower than from an iron-only supplement. To enhance iron absorption, take an iron supplement on an empty stomach, but be aware that taking it on an empty stomach often causes nausea. Calcium, coffee, and tea actually inhibit iron absorption, so supplements should not be taken along with these liquids. Vitamin C, on the other hand, enhances iron absorption from food sources, so consuming orange juice along with a meal high in iron might be beneficial. Vitamin C, however, has no effect on iron absorption from supplements since the form found in the supplement is already the most highly absorbable form available. Fortunately, iron absorption increases as iron levels decrease, so iron becomes more **bioavailable** during times of greater demand.

Calcium, phosphorus, magnesium, and vitamin D are necessary for the proper development of fetal bones and teeth during pregnancy. Although calcium, phosphorus, *and* magnesium form the actual structure of bone tissue, calcium is required in the greatest quantity. How does the body handle calcium during pregnancy? During pregnancy, calcium absorption in the digestive tract increases significantly because fetal

---

Bioavailability—the degree and rate at which a substance is absorbed into body cells.

demands increase tremendously. At the same time, calcium excretion by the urinary system decreases. Under normal conditions, the body's goal is to maintain blood calcium levels within a very narrow margin to ensure calcium availability for muscle contraction and nerve impulse conduction. During pregnancy, the body has an additional goal of maintaining appropriate amounts for development of the fetal skeleton. If dietary intake is low, the mother's body sacrifices her own bone tissue to ensure that enough calcium is available for the developing fetal skeleton. To meet these needs and to prevent unwanted destruction of maternal bone, experts recommend that a pregnant woman obtain extra calcium by consuming an additional three cups of fat-free or low-fat milk products per day. Only in rare cases is a supplement of 600 mg of calcium per day suggested.

Vitamin D promotes calcium absorption and limits calcium excretion, so it helps to ensure that the building blocks of bone are available. Because vitamin D is fat soluble and can reach toxic levels in the body, supplements are not advised. Instead, a pregnant woman should obtain an adequate amount by consuming dairy products (three cups of vitamin D fortified milk per day, which helps to supply the needed 5 μg per day) and/or ensuring regular exposure to the sun (½ to 2 hours of sun exposure per week, without sunscreen) since UV radiation actually activates provitamin D stored in dermal blood vessels. Keep in mind, however, that unprotected exposure to UV radiation increases the risk for skin cancer.

Vitamin A plays a significant role in cell differentiation, so an adequate intake is crucial during fetal development. A deficiency of vitamin A is rare; however, toxicity is possible if supplements are taken or if topical acne and wrinkle treatments containing retinol or retinoic acid are used. Excesses lead to abnormal ears, missing ear canals, brain malformations, and heart defects in babies. Because of these tragic side effects, women should not consume more than 5,000 IU of vitamin A from supplements.

Pregnant women tend to consume lower-than-recommended amounts of zinc, but zinc supplements are not suggested under most circumstances. Animal studies suggest that a zinc deficiency correlates with limited body growth and the development of malformed body parts, but no clear effect has been demonstrated in humans. Researchers have seen a slightly increased risk of preterm delivery, infections, and long labor in humans when zinc levels are low. As with iron, however, zinc absorption actually increases in response to declining stores. The only time a supplement might be necessary is if a pregnant woman is taking a high-dose iron supplement. Why? Because both iron and zinc compete for the same transporters and iron receives "preferential treatment."

Women on vegetarian diets sometimes wonder whether or not they can supply their fetuses with adequate nutrition. A general rule is that the more inclusive the diet, the more nutrient-sound it is, so vegetarians who consume various foods including dairy products and fish are rarely deficient. Vegans, on the other hand, exclude all animal-based products and are particularly vulnerable to a deficiency of kilocalories, protein, vitamin B_{12}, vitamin D, calcium, zinc, omega-3 fatty acids, and riboflavin. This is because quality sources of most of these nutrients tend to be of animal origin. The conscientious vegan, therefore, must be careful when making food choices. Choosing **complementary protein** sources and selecting fortified vegan products can prevent deficiencies that might impair brain development, growth, and functioning. Excellent vegetarian sources of protein, iron, and zinc include tofu, other soy products, kidney beans, chickpeas, dried pumpkin seeds, sunflower seeds, cashews, ready-to-eat cereals, and oatmeal. Excellent sources of calcium, vitamin D, and riboflavin include fortified soy yogurt, tofu, fortified soy milk, black beans, almonds, spinach, broccoli, and fortified breakfast cereals. Fortified cereals, soy meats, and soy milk are also excellent sources of vitamin B_{12}. Lastly, walnuts, flaxseed oil, canola oil, wheat germ, and soybean oil are good choices for omega-3 fatty acids.

Women of childbearing age as well as women who are already expecting should select healthy foods that contain a vast array of nutrients with an emphasis on calcium, vitamin D, iron, protein, complex carbohydrates, and essential fatty acids. The pregnant woman's diet should contain enough kilocalories to meet her increased metabolism but not enough to cause excessive weight gain. She should also maintain hydration by consuming approximately nine cups of water, diluted juice, or other nonalcoholic and noncaffeinated beverages per day. In certain cases, prenatal vitamins/minerals are recommended to reduce the risk of preterm delivery, low–birth-weight, and congenital abnormalities. Yet, the only supplement that is routinely suggested is iron.

SUMMARY

Existing evidence suggests that exercise during a low-risk pregnancy enhances and improves pregnancy outcomes for the mother without putting undue stress on the fetus. Ideally, a woman should begin exercise prior to becoming pregnant to allow her body time to adapt to the stress of exercise before adding the stress of pregnancy; however, even if a woman was sedentary prior to becoming pregnant, she can still safely reap benefits by starting a low-intensity, low-impact exercise program early in her pregnancy as long *as her physician gives her permission*. Whether fit or not, pregnant women need to adjust intensity based on how they feel during exertion.

Fitness professionals should tailor programs to meet the needs of individual pregnant exercisers based on advice from physicians. Pregnant exercisers report a better self-image, fewer incidences of depression, better weight control, less overall discomfort, and an overall better pregnancy experience than nonexercisers. By adhering to the safety guidelines presented in this chapter, health professionals can ensure that their pregnant clients continue to exercise throughout their pregnancies with minimal risk.

Complementary proteins—two or more dietary proteins whose amino acids complement each other in such a way that the essential amino acids missing in one are supplied by the other. Example: Grains are usually high in methionine and tryptophan but low in isoleucine and lysine. Legumes, on the other hand, are high in isoleucine and lysine but low in methionine and tryptophan. Combined, grains and legumes supply an adequate amount of these four essential amino acids (which are the most commonly deficient amino acids in a vegan diet).

CASE STUDY

A previously sedentary woman wants to begin an exercise program during her first trimester. She is 26 years old, maintains a healthy weight, and has no significant medical history. She is 5′6″ tall, weighs 130 lb, and mentions that she is a vegan.

■ As a fitness professional, describe how you would handle this situation. What type of exercise program would you recommend?

■ What type of nutritional advice would you offer?

■ Calculate her BMI. What is her classification according to the BMI chart?

THINKING CRITICALLY

1. Describe some of the changes that a woman's body undergoes during each trimester. How do these changes impact her ability to exercise?
2. If an active woman came to you to ask how she should modify her exercise program now that she is 2 months pregnant, what would you tell her? Give details.
3. How does exercise help alleviate some of the discomforts of pregnancy?
4. Define "critical period" and explain its significance.
5. Identify the activities and exercises that a pregnant woman should avoid. Why are these dangerous?
6. Explain the importance of hydration for a pregnant exerciser.
7. List and explain several contraindications to exercise for this population.
8. What are some nutritional concerns during pregnancy? How does exercise affect nutrition and exacerbate these concerns?
9. Explain the development of neural tube defect? Give two examples of neural tube defects.
10. What nutrients are of particular concern for a pregnant vegan?

REFERENCES

1. Clapp JF. The effects of maternal exercise on fetal oxygenation and feto-placental growth. Eur J Obstet Gynecol Reprod Biol 2003;110(1):S80–S85.
2. Wang T, Apgar B. Exercise during pregnancy. Am Fam Physician 1998;57(8):1846–1852.
3. Horton MJ. Stay active for healthier cholesterol. Prevention 2005;57(3):129.
4. Artal R, Sherman C. Exercise during pregnancy. Physician Sportsmed 1999;27(8):51–60.
5. Berk, B. Recommending exercise during and after pregnancy: what the evidence says. IJCE 2004; 19(2):18–22.
6. Larsson L Lindqvist PG. Low-impact exercise during pregnancy—a study of safety. Acta Obstetricia Gynecol Scand 2005;84:34–38.
7. McArdle W, Katch F, Katch V. Exercise Physiology. 5th Ed. Philadelphia: Lippincott Williams & Wilkins, 2001:193–194,491–495.

8. Walsh N. Prenatal exercise cuts preeclampsia risk by 34% during first 20 weeks of pregnancy. OB/GYN News March 15, 2002.
9. Wolfe LA, Weissgerber TL. Clinical physiology of exercise in pregnancy: a literature review. J Obstet Gynaecol Can 2003;25(6):473–483.
10. Walling AD. Exercise during pregnancy is associated with thinner babies. Am Fam Physician 2002;65(10):2156.
11. Jeffreys R, Nordahl K. Preconception, prenatal, and postpartum exercise. Healthy Weight J 2002;16(3):36–39.
12. Polman R, Kaiseler M, Borkoles E. Effect of a single bout of exercise on the mood of pregnant women. J Sports Med Phys Fitness 2007;47(1):103–111.
13. Boscaglia N, Skouteris H, Wertheim EH. Changes in body image satisfaction during pregnancy: a comparison of high exercising and low exercising women. Aust N Z J Obstet Gynecol 2003;43(1):41–45.
14. Kramer MS, McDonald SW. Aerobic exercise for women during pregnancy. Cochrane Database Syst Rev 2006;3:Cochrane AN: CD000180.
15. Horton MJ. Basic training. Fit Pregnancy 2003/2004;10(5):74.
16. Weiss A, Harmon K, Rubin A. Practical exercise advice during pregnancy: guidelines for active and inactive women. Physician Sportsmed 2005;33(6):24–30,47–48.
17. American College of Obstetricians and Gynecology (ACOG) Education pamphlet. 2005. Online. Available at: http://www.acog.org/publications/patient_education
18. ACOG guidelines. J Obstet Gynecol 2002;99:171–173.
19. American College of Sports Medicine. ACSM's Guidelines for Exercise Testing and Prescription, 8th Ed. Philadelphia: Lippincott Williams & Wilkins, 2010:183–187.
20. http://uwfitness.uwaterloo.ca/PDF/parmed-xpreg_000.pdf
21. Ladipo O. Nutrition in pregnancy: mineral and vitamin supplements. Presented at Iron and Maternal Mortality in Developing World Conference in Washington, DC. July 6–7, 1998.
22. Whitney E, Rolfes S. Understanding Nutrition, 11th Ed. Belmont: Thomson Wadsworth, 2008:509–545.
23. March of Dimes. www.marchofdimes.com
24. American Pregnancy Association. www.americanpregnancy.org
25. Chiaffarino F, Parazzini F, Chatenoud L, et al. Coffee drinking and risk of preterm birth. Eur J Clin Nutr 2006;60:610–613.
26. Nobuo M, Tinney J, Liu L, et al. Modest maternal caffeine exposure affects developing embryonic cardiovascular function and growth. Am J Physiol Heart Circ Physiol 2008;294(5):H2248.

SUGGESTED READING

Howley ET, Franks BD. Fitness Professionals Handbook. 5th Ed. Champaigne, IL: Human Kinetics, 2007.

4 EXERCISE FOR YOUTH

Research confirms that adults who exercise regularly improve their overall health and reduce their risk for chronic conditions such as cardiovascular disease, diabetes, and stroke. A logical conclusion, therefore, is that regular physical activity can also improve the health status of children and adolescents and possibly prevent the development of chronic conditions.

> ### QUICK REFERENCE
> ACSM designates those under the age of 13 as "children" and those between the ages of 13 and 18 as "adolescents."

Unfortunately, children and adolescents in the United States are less active than recommended. In fact, statistics show that one third of Americans under the age of 18 are physically unfit according to measurements of **maximal oxygen uptake**, or VO_{2max}. Differences exist, however, between males and females. Data from studies comparing boys and girls suggest that boys between the ages of 12 and 19 are in better shape than girls in the same age range. Moreover, boys tend to become fitter as they get older; whereas, girls tend to become less fit as they age. As expected, overweight and obese adolescents are in the worst shape overall and have the greatest risk for developing chronic diseases.[1] Because risk factors tend to persist throughout life, children and adolescents who are at high risk tend to remain at risk as they age.

Overall, only 50% of those between the ages of 12 and 21 participate in regular vigorous physical activity (Fig. 4.1) and a shocking 25% are completely inactive. This is partly because many schools no longer offer daily physical education (PE) classes. Surprisingly, only 33% of students in grades 5 and over have a daily PE class. The rate drops to 20% for most high school students.[2] For some children and adolescents, PE is the only time they are active; thus, decreasing the amount of time permitted for PE predisposes students to a sedentary lifestyle. In addition, all age groups are spending a significant amount of time watching television. The American Academy of Pediatrics estimates that the average child watches 3 to 4 hours of television per day. That leaves little time for physical activity. Unfortunately, children—specifically boys—who accumulate that amount of screen time are two-and-a-half times more likely to be overweight than those who do not. Being overweight as a child sets into motion a viscous cycle of inactivity and the propensity to gain more and more weight.[3]

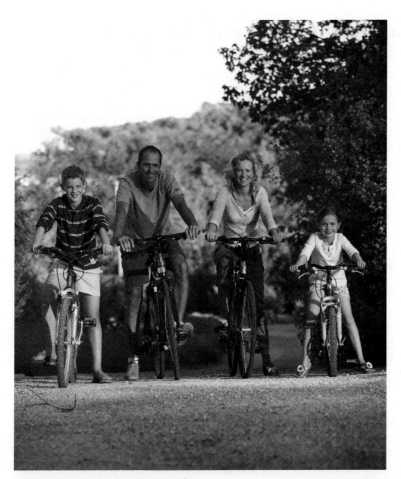

FIGURE 4-1 ■ Family exercising together.

QUICK REFERENCE

According to the American Academy of Pediatrics, boys should take at least 11,000 steps per day and girls should take at least 13,000 steps per day to maintain health. Additionally, total television time should be limited to a maximum of 2 hours per day.

Maximal oxygen uptake—the maximum amount of oxygen the body can take in and use. Improves with endurance training. A high VO_{2max} correlates with a low risk for chronic disease, while a low VO_{2max} correlates with an elevated risk.

ANATOMICAL AND PHYSIOLOGICAL DIFFERENCES BETWEEN ADULTS AND YOUTH

GROWTH AND DEVELOPMENT

The bones, muscles, and joints of children and adolescents are growing and developing at a rapid rate. Long bones grow in length because of the presence of the **epiphyseal plate**. Muscles grow in size as myofibrils form and fill individual muscle fibers. Joints develop stability and flexibility as muscle strength increases and range of motion improves.

> ### QUICK REFERENCE
> Muscle mass in a newborn constitutes 25% of total body weight. Muscle mass in an adult can make up 45% or more of total body weight.

Growth and development are not smooth, continuous processes; instead, body size and proportions change during growth spurts, which occur in response to increasing hormone levels. These growth spurts result in weight gain, height increases, and an altered center of balance that can interfere with biomechanical properties.[4] Ultimately, this can affect performance in physical activity and sports.

NEUROMUSCULAR CONTROL

The nervous system controls the muscular system; therefore, communication between the two is essential for optimal performance. A nerve cell called a motor **neuron** extends from the **central nervous system** to one or more muscle fibers within a given muscle. Although the motor neuron and skeletal muscle fiber do not touch, they are located close to one another at a place called the neuromuscular junction. The space in between the two cells is the synaptic cleft. When an impulse traveling along the motor neuron reaches the terminal portion of the neuron, it stimulates the release of a chemical communicator (called a neurotransmitter) into the synaptic cleft. The chemical communicator, in this case acetylcholine (ACh), binds to receptors on the muscle fiber surface and initiates an impulse along the muscle fiber's cell membrane. Ultimately, the muscle fiber's impulse causes actin and myosin filaments to slide past one another and generate force.

During growth and development, communication between motor neurons and their muscle fibers gradually improves. Neurons begin to branch more, which means they exert better control over muscle fibers. They synthesize neurotransmitters more efficiently, which facilitates interaction with muscle cells. Impulses propagate more rapidly along the neuron as **myelin sheath** develops. Overall, these changes improve neuromuscular functioning as infants, children, and young adolescents mature. In addition, the ability to concentrate, remember, and learn new skills continues to develop as the nervous system matures. This increases attention span and allows growing children to master difficult tasks.

RESPONSE TO EXERCISE

Children and adolescents have a different physiological response to exercise than adults. For instance, they require 20% to 30% more oxygen per unit of body mass when running at a given pace.[5] This means their energy expenditure and VO_{2max} are higher during endurance activities such as running or walking. Their less-efficient respiration is likely due to a shorter respiratory cycle caused by a higher respiratory frequency. The higher respiratory rate also causes a greater **minute volume**.[4,6]

Young boys and girls have similar values for VO_{2max}, and though VO_{2max} tends to remain constant in boys as they age, it steadily declines in girls up until age 16.

Though a child's VO_{2max} improves slightly with training, improvements are minimal. Precisely why these improvements are not as pronounced as they are in adults is still unknown. It might be because of the hormonal fluctuations that occur at puberty.

When compared to adults, children have a lower stroke volume both at rest and during exertion. This probably accounts for the lower overall cardiac output (which is 1 to 3 L per minute lower than that of an adult). Furthermore, heart rate tends to be higher at rest and during exercise in this group; therefore, maximal heart rate cannot be accurately determined by subtracting age from 220 for anyone under the age of 16.[7] In fact, studies show that training heart rate for this group should reach 170 to 180 bpm to achieve even slight improvements in cardiorespiratory functioning.[7]

Lastly, blood pressure at rest and during exertion is lower in children because of their smaller surface area. Average systolic blood pressure while working maximally is approximately 140 mm Hg in a child with a small surface area (1.25 m²); whereas, it is 160 mm Hg in someone with a larger surface area (1.75 m²).[7] Additionally, a child's blood pressure and heart rate return to resting levels following exertion much more quickly than in adults.[7]

Epiphyseal plate—a cartilage layer also known as the growth plate. Found in the ends of long bones like the femur and humerus. Bone continues to grow in length as long as the epiphyseal plate is present. Bone ceases to grow in length when this cartilage layer is replaced by bone.

Neuron—a nerve cell.

Central nervous system—the part of the nervous system consisting of the brain and spinal cord; responsible for coordinating the activities of the entire nervous system and maintaining homeostasis.

Myelin Sheath—a lipid-rich covering found on the axons of many neurons. Increases the speed of impulse propagation along the axon.

Minute volume—the amount of gas moved per minute; the product of tidal volume and respiratory frequency.

REGULATION OF BODY TEMPERATURE

All metabolic processes produce heat; therefore, anything that increases metabolism increases heat production. Ultimately, the body must dissipate heat to prevent dangerous increases in core body temperature. The integumentary system, which includes the epidermis, dermis, hypodermis, and glands, assists in body temperature regulation.

Sweat glands play a crucial role in maintaining body temperature. As the internal body temperature rises, sweat glands become more active. Sweat contains a large amount of water, which carries large amounts of heat with it as it evaporates from the skin surface. Fortunately, the human body contains a significant amount of water, so extreme temperature changes are uncommon and extreme temperature variations are rare.

Children produce more heat per kilogram of body weight during activity than adults; however, they do not sweat as efficiently. They do have more sweat glands than adults, but their glands are underdeveloped and not as active as mature glands. Additionally, their sweating mechanism is not activated until they reach a much higher core body temperature than adults. Overall, these factors make it much more difficult for children to dissipate heat and maintain a normal body temperature during activity.

In addition to evaporative cooling, which occurs as sweat evaporates from the skin surface, radiative cooling allows heat to radiate into the surrounding environment as blood is diverted from deeper vessels to more superficial vessels. Although the epidermis is **avascular**, the dermis contains a rich supply of blood vessels. As internal body temperature rises, these dermal vessels dilate. Blood flow to dilated vessels increases, which means that blood travels from deeper vessels to more superficial vessels. As the blood passes through vessels near the body's surface, heat radiates into the surrounding environment. As body temperature returns to normal, dermal vessels return to their normal state thereby decreasing blood flow as well as radiative cooling. This is called negative feedback; it maintains body temperature at homeostatic levels. Figure 4.2 shows a diagram of this negative feedback loop.

The hypodermis, the deepest layer of the integument, also participates in the maintenance of body temperature. This layer contains **adipose**, which insulates and protects the body from excessive heat loss.

Children are generally more vulnerable to dehydration than adults are. When dehydrated, the body has difficulty eliminating body heat and is therefore prone to heat illness—especially during intermittent activity, the type of activity common in this population. If children are exercising for a prolonged time period, ensure that they consume fluids every 15 to 20 minutes to facilitate efficient heat dissipation and better performance.[4]

OVERWEIGHT AND OBESITY AMONG CHILDREN

Overweight and obesity are serious problems for today's youth.[8,9] According to the Centers for Disease Control, 16% of those between the ages of 6 and 19 are overweight or obese with an additional 15% dangerously close to meeting the criteria for overweight.[10,11]

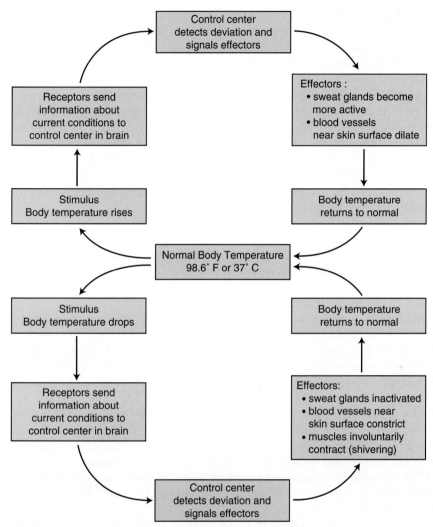

FIGURE 4-2 ■ Homeostasis of body temperature through negative feedback.

Additionally, the obesity rate for children between the ages of 2 and 5 and adolescents between the ages of 12 and 19 is twice as high as it was 30 years ago. It is nearly three times as high for those between the ages of 6 and 11.[10,12] Excess weight tends to be more common in girls than in boys and more prevalent among black, Mexican-American, and

> **Avascular**—lacking blood vessels.
> **Adipose**—a type of connective tissue that stores excess fat.

Hispanic youth than among non-Hispanic whites.[13] Unfortunately, those carrying excess weight have a greater risk for impaired glucose tolerance, insulin resistance, and high blood insulin levels as well. These conditions predispose them to type 2 diabetes, a chronic disease that previously almost exclusively affected adults.[11] The prevalence of type 2 diabetes among younger individuals has increased dramatically over the past three decades—right along with the prevalence of overweight and obesity.[8,14,15] Excess weight at a young age promotes the same consequences as excess weight at an older age—it increases the likelihood of high blood pressure, elevated cholesterol levels, heart disease, and joint disorders. Interestingly, when asked what they consider the most severe consequence of overweight or obesity, children and adolescents list lowered self-esteem, increased social isolation, and difficulties with interpersonal relationships. Not surprisingly, these psychosocial factors are of higher priority to children and teens than the health consequences of excess weight.[2]

Sadly, 70% of overweight adolescents remain overweight or become obese in adulthood. This rate increases to 80% for those who have a parent who is overweight or obese.[2,14] Chapter 7 discusses hypertension, type 2 diabetes, and cardiovascular disease, health problems associated with excess weight in adults.

Children and Body Mass Index

Body mass index is the most commonly used method for categorizing children and adolescents as overweight, at risk of becoming overweight, or normal weight.[16] The BMI for this special population is calculated using the same formula used for adults. It equals body weight in kilograms divided by height in meters squared. Determining the correct weight and height is imperative for ensuring an accurate BMI value. Unfortunately, healthy BMI ranges are not available for children as they are for adults (see Fig. 4.3) because healthy ranges increase as height increases. Additionally, values vary considerably with each month of age and by sex.[9,16] Consequently, the Centers for Disease Control established BMI-for-age growth charts (see Appendix C). After calculating BMI, compare it to the BMI-for-age growth charts. Note that BMI for children and teens is age-specific and sex-specific—unlike it is for adults—because body fat content changes substantially as children age and varies significantly between boys and girls. According to the CDC, those in the less than 5th percentile are underweight; those in the 5th to 85th percentile are at a healthy weight; those in the 85th to 95th percentile are at risk for becoming overweight; while those in the ≥95th percentile are overweight. Those classified as overweight need additional medical assessments to ascertain their risk for chronic disease.

Though easy to use, inexpensive, and informative, body mass index indicates nothing about the percentage or distribution of body fat. Often, body fat distribution is even more reliable for assessing risk for conditions such as heart disease. Children and adolescents who store fat in the abdominal area consistently have higher levels of blood cholesterol, triglycerides, and insulin coupled with lower HDL values (as indicated by a **blood lipid profile**). Additionally, they tend to have a higher blood pressure, which can predispose them to atherosclerosis.[5] This is true for adults as well and emphasizes the importance of using multiple measures for determining health status.

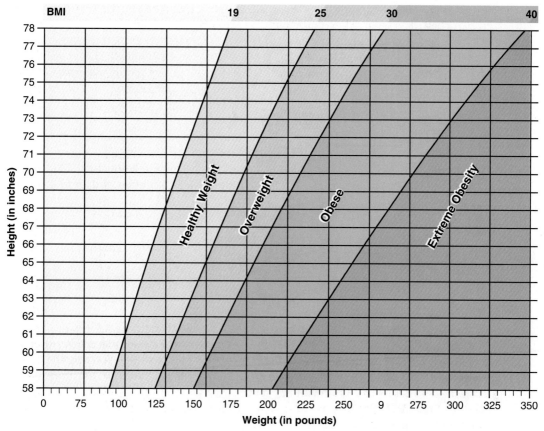

FIGURE 4-3 ■ Body mass index risk stratification for adults. (Asset provided by Anatomical Chart Co.)

Fat Cell Growth

Fat cells, also called **adipocytes**, undergo two processes of growth. **Hypertrophy** occurs when existing adipocytes fill with fat and increase in size. Once they reach a certain capacity, these cells divide to produce two daughter cells. **Hyperplasia** describes this process.

Blood lipid profile—includes a value for total cholesterol, high-density lipoprotein (HDL), triglycerides, and low-density lipoprotein (LDL).

Adipocytes—fat cells that cluster to form adipose tissue.

Hypertrophy—an increase in cross-sectional area of a cell that results in an increase in overall size.

Hyperplasia—an increase in the number of cells.

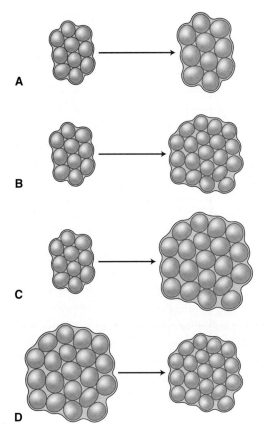

FIGURE 4-4 ■ Growth of fat cells. **A**. Hypertrophy of fat cells during growth and development. **B**. Hyperplasia of fat cells during growth and development. **C**. Hypertrophy and hyperplasia of fat cells with excess energy intake. **D**. Atrophy of fat cells with weight loss.

The resulting daughter cells continue to fill with fat until they reach capacity; then they divide to form two additional daughter cells, each of which can store as much fat as the original cell (Fig. 4.4). In fact, whenever kilocalorie intake exceeds kilocalorie output, the excess energy is stored as adipose. This happens at a rapid rate during growth and development, but it continues into adulthood if energy supplies exceed demand. Unfortunately, the number of fat cells never decreases—even with weight loss. When a person loses weight, fat cells shrink in size, but the total number remains constant. This means that anyone who has ever been overweight has the storage capacity to accommodate more fat than someone who has never been overweight. This is one reason why maintaining weight loss is difficult and requires strict balance between energy intake and energy output. Moreover, excess dietary fat is not the only nutrient stored as fat. Excess kilocalories in the form of carbohydrates, protein, or fat are stored as adipose. Thus, weight gain occurs whenever an individual consumes surplus energy—no matter what the source. Additionally, because fat cells are particularly prone to hypertrophy and hyperplasia during adolescence, achieving and maintaining a healthy weight during this time are crucial in preventing overweight and obesity in adulthood.

> ## QUICK REFERENCE
>
> To maintain weight, make sure that energy in equals energy out.
> To lose weight, make sure that energy in is less than energy out.
> To gain weight, make sure that energy in is greater than energy out.

Factors Contributing to Overweight and Obesity

Both genetics and environmental factors contribute to the prevalence of overweight and obesity in children and adolescents. For example, genes—the units that contain heredi-tary characteristics passed from parent to child—determine the body's metabolic rate. In other words, they influence how the body stores and uses fat for fuel. Since children receive their DNA from their birth parents, they tend to process energy just like them. In fact, research on adopted twins supports a genetic link as indicated by the fact that adopted twins usually have body weights similar to the weights of their biological par-ents, not their adoptive parents. If both birth parents are of normal weight, their children have only a 14% risk of becoming overweight. If one parent is obese, the child has a 40% risk of becoming overweight. And if both parents are obese, the child has an 80% chance of becoming obese.[11,17]

Environmental factors, such as sedentary lifestyle and excess energy consumption, probably have the greatest influence on the prevalence of overweight and obesity among school-aged children. As mentioned, children and teens are not as active today as they were in the past. They spend increasingly more time watching TV and playing on the computer and less time engaging in outdoor activity. Unfortunately, surveys suggest that sedentary youth are much more likely to be obese than their active counterparts.[13]

Now consider excess energy consumption. Children consume large quantities of high kilocalorie, high fat foods[18] and fewer fruits and vegetables.[13] This might be because many parents have less time to prepare meals at home; instead, they visit fast food or sit-down restaurants where portion sizes are often two to three times larger than they were two decades ago.

Increased Risk for High Blood Pressure

The number of adolescents diagnosed with high blood pressure is increasing, and it seems to correlate with inactivity and excess weight.[11,19] One study showed that 60% of those between the ages of 5 and 18 diagnosed with high blood pressure had a BMI greater than the 95th percentile.[11] Another suggested that obese adolescents have a three times greater risk of hypertension than normal weight adolescents.[11,20] At one time, experts believed that hypertension only occurred in children with **comorbidities** such as kidney disease.

Comorbidity—the presence of two or more related medical conditions.

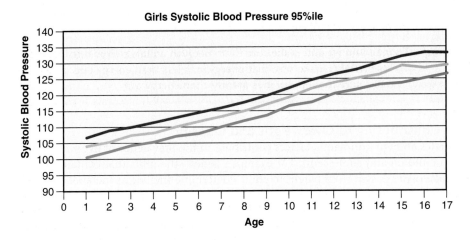

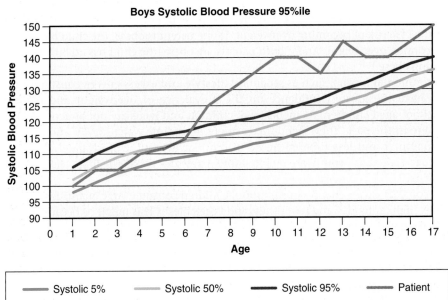

FIGURE 4-5   ■   High blood pressure from childhood through adolescence. (From Bickley LS, Szilagyi P. Bates'
Guide to Physical Examination and History Taking. 8th Ed. Philadelphia: Lippincott Williams & Wilkins, 2003.)

They now realize that many children—especially those who carry excess weight—
experience **primary (or essential) high blood pressure** that occurs in the absence of
comorbidities.

According to the American Heart Association, blood pressure tends to increase as a
child ages (Fig. 4.5), but the extent is influenced by sex and height. Therefore, they recommend thorough evaluation before classifying a child or adolescent as hypertensive.
In many cases, a careful diet and routine exercise effectively control blood pressure in this
particular group.

PRECAUTIONS DURING EXERCISE

Because the bodies of children and adolescents are not fully mature, they must practice care when exercising. Hypothetically, exercise could increase core temperature to a dangerously high level; it could increase the risk for musculoskeletal injuries; it could cause hypothermia in cold climates; or it could lead to fatal heart failure in certain young athletes. This section explores these issues.

INCREASED CORE TEMPERATURE

As mentioned, children and adolescents have difficulty dissipating heat; therefore, they need to practice care when exercising for prolonged periods in extreme heat and humidity. Chapter 3 provides further details on the dangers associated with an elevated body temperature. In general, extreme temperatures denature proteins and subsequently interfere with most body processes since proteins are involved with nearly every body function. Ensuring adequate hydration and encouraging appropriate breaks from activity help minimize the risk.

INCREASED RISK FOR MUSCULOSKELETAL INJURY

Because the bones and muscles of children and adolescents are still growing, excessive physical activity could possibly interfere with their development. The skeletal system is prone to epiphyseal plate damage and intervertebral disc rupture with excessive loads during resistance training.[5] Damage to the epiphyseal plate is problematic because it stimulates ossification. The affected bone then stops growing in length and never reaches full potential. Associated long-term problems depend upon which bone is broken. Imagine the complications resulting from damage to the femur's growth plate. One leg might grow longer than the other—a condition that impairs walking, throws off center of balance, and increases the risk for abnormal spinal curvatures such as scoliosis. Excessive loads accompanied by improper lifting technique can also result in intervertebral disc herniation followed by life-long back problems. Moreover, since muscles are not fully developed, moveable joints throughout the body are not as stable as they should be; this increases the likelihood of joint injuries.

As mentioned, growth usually occurs in spurts, so response and performance can be unpredictable. Additionally, hormone levels (especially testosterone levels) are variable and inconsistent; therefore, the results of strength training might not be as expected.[5]

Primary (essential) high blood pressure—the most common form of hypertension. No known medical cause explains its presence. Secondary high blood pressure is a result of another condition such as kidney disease.

Scoliosis—an abnormal lateral spinal curvature. Rather than appearing straight from an anterior or posterior view, the spine has an "S" shape.

INCREASED RISK FOR HYPOTHERMIA

Because children have a large surface area relative to body mass, they lose large amounts of heat when exercising in water. In fact, children lose heat so rapidly when playing in water that they become prone to hypothermia. Encourage children to exit the water periodically whenever they are in a pool, lake, or river for extended times.[2]

FATAL HEART FAILURE IN SOME YOUNG ATHLETES

Over the past few years, several young high school athletes have died as a result of fatal heart problems even though they passed physical exams prior to competition. These deaths follow vigorous activity and are associated with genetic heart problems such as **hypertrophic cardiomyopathy**. The American Heart Association is calling for more intensive and sensitive tests to identify those with genetic defects, but they also suggest that parents, coaches, nurses, and trainers more earnestly look for signs that suggest serious problems. These include fainting, sudden chest pain, high blood pressure, irregular heart rate, family history of heart disease, and family history of unexplained, sudden death.[2]

BARRIERS TO EXERCISE

As with most populations, lack of time is the number one barrier to exercise, particularly for girls. Students report spending 4 hours or more on some days doing homework. Many have part-time jobs that occupy them on weekends. Others have family obligations that fill their schedules. These responsibilities often interfere with activity.[21]

Self-consciousness about physical attributes and competency in activity tend to be the primary barriers for boys. If boys feel that they are too young, too small, too overweight, or lacking skills for a particular activity, they tend to avoid it.[22,23] Some fear failure and would rather pass up opportunities than risk ridicule by their peers.[22]

Many adolescents prefer to work on computers, talk on cell phones, or watch television rather than participate in activity. In fact, they are "playing" football, "riding" bicycles, or "hitting" tennis balls on a TV or computer screen. Thus, they *choose* to spend time on sedentary, technology-related activities[21,22] and might not even realize how unhealthy that is.

Peer pressure greatly influences this population, so it likely affects involvement in physical activity as well. Teens like to be a part of a group, so if their friends are playing sports, they also play sports. However, if their friends are playing video games or going out to parties, they choose these other activities.[21]

Another barrier to exercise is inaccessibility or cost. Many neighborhoods lack recreation or fitness centers, while school sports programs are often only available for a limited number of students with obvious athletic ability. This forces many adolescents to seek other opportunities for activity. Unfortunately, many do not have transportation to other facilities, so they simply miss out. Even if they have transportation, most teens cannot afford the cost of fitness centers.[21,22]

These are only a few of the barriers to exercise perceived by this special population. Health and fitness professionals need to be aware of these as they design programs that are enjoyable, easy to access, and affordable. Offer some activities that are competitive and others that are not. Challenge clients and help them develop new skills that foster confidence and improve self-esteem.[21–23]

BENEFITS OF EXERCISE

DECREASED RISK FOR OBESITY

Since a sedentary lifestyle is linked to excessive weight gain in children and adolescents,[2,15,23,24] it seems reasonable to assume that regular exercise could reduce the occurrences of overweight and obesity in this population. Although it is still uncertain whether overweight/obesity leads to poor physical performance—or whether poor physical performance leads to overweight/obesity[25]—evidence suggests that inactive youth have a greater amount of body fat than active youth.[2,24,26] Thus, increasing the amount of time young people physically exert themselves will likely decrease the prevalence of obesity. Since overweight during childhood is a strong predictor of overweight and obesity in adulthood, children—even very young children—should be encouraged to increase daily activity.[17,26]

INCREASED MUSCULAR STRENGTH AND BONE DENSITY

Authorities once believed that resistance training in children prior to puberty was pointless because of low prepubescent testosterone levels. Moreover, they considered weight lifting to be too dangerous during growth and development.[7] Recent research, however, suggests that resistance training is not only safe for most children, but also beneficial. In fact, both prepubescent boys and girls who participate in strength training often experience a 15% to 30% increase in muscular strength.[2,27] Though they improve strength (with comparable improvements in endurance[27]), they do not experience a corresponding increase in muscle size.[2] Strength gains are likely a result of improved neuromuscular functioning and better communication between motor neurons and muscle fibers—factors that result in better motor development.[25]

While improving communication between the nervous and muscular systems, exercise also affects the skeletal system.[27] In fact, exercise promotes a higher peak bone mass that reduces the risk of developing osteoporosis later in life. Overall, the long-term effects of resistance training also improve body composition and reduce the risk for injury in other activities.[27]

IMPROVED CARDIORESPIRATORY PERFORMANCE

Studies indicate that regular exercise improves cardiorespiratory endurance and fitness in children and adolescents.[1,28] Though the gains are not as significant as they are in adults, they are still notable.[2,29] Additionally, improved cardiorespiratory fitness in youth is

---

Hypertrophic cardiomyopathy—a genetic disorder characterized by a thickened left ventricular wall. It is the number one cause of death in elite, young athletes and can occur at any time.

associated with lower subcutaneous body fat—particularly in the abdominal area. Since intra-abdominal fat is strongly correlated with cardiovascular disease, this population should strive to incorporate routine aerobic activity into their daily routines.[28,30]

IMPROVED PSYCHOLOGICAL FACTORS

As expected, children and adolescents who participate in regular exercise experience improvements in mood, self-confidence, and self-esteem. They also face less anxiety, stress, and depression than their inactive counterparts.[10,19,31–33] Overall, active children have more energy, are able to participate in more activities with their peers, and tend to have healthier weights—factors that positively influence mental well-being.

DECREASED RISK FOR CHRONIC DISEASE

Inactive children are at an increased risk of developing certain chronic conditions such as type 2 diabetes, **metabolic syndrome**, hypertension, atherosclerosis, and **dyslipidemia**.[19,34,35] Some sources estimate that the incidence of type 2 diabetes alone is 20 times what it was just two decades ago. This is particularly apparent in minority populations. Additionally, sedentary children and adolescents develop insulin resistance and impaired glucose tolerance—early predictors of diabetes and metabolic syndrome.[34,36] Metabolic syndrome, once considered an adult condition, is becoming more common in adolescents.[37] It consists of a cluster of risk factors that significantly increase the risk for heart disease, stroke, and diabetes. The National Cholesterol Education Program states that metabolic syndrome is diagnosed whenever three or more of the following factors are present: excess weight stored in the abdominal area; an elevated blood triglyceride level; a low HDL level; hypertension; and a high fasting blood glucose level. See Chapter 6 for more details on the diagnosis of metabolic syndrome. Studies confirm that participation in routine exercise decreases the risk of developing metabolic syndrome in children and adolescents.[37]

Hypertension is becoming much more common among today's youth—particularly in adolescents.[38] Since physical activity is associated with a lower blood pressure across all age groups,[38,39] it might help prevent the development of chronic high blood pressure. If blood pressure is normal, blood vessels tend to be healthier; therefore, atherosclerosis is less likely to develop (see Chapter 7 for details on atherosclerosis). Because the fatty streaks that precede atherosclerosis begin appearing as early as age 10, and because atherosclerosis increases the risk for a cardiac event, most authorities agree that preventive steps need to begin early in life. Increasing physical activity in children and adolescents is one step toward decreasing risk later in life.[19,34,35,39,40]

Dyslipidemia, or abnormal blood levels of cholesterol, LDL, HDL, and triglycerides, is dangerous because it increases the risk for cardiovascular disease. Studies of children with dyslipidemia indicate that a healthy diet coupled with regular physical activity normalizes blood lipid levels. Since this particular population adheres to an increased activity level better than they adhere to improved dietary intake, fitness professionals should focus primarily on exercise.[37]

Overall, the risk for chronic conditions in overweight or obese youth can be minimized by weight loss. Physical activity increases energy expenditure, enhances weight loss, and likely improves blood glucose levels and insulin sensitivity—factors that protect against the development of type 2 diabetes, metabolic syndrome, hypertension, and dyslipidemia.

RECOMMENDATIONS FOR EXERCISE

Because of the anatomical and physiological differences between youth and adults, exercise guidelines for the younger population differ from those for adults.

EXERCISE TESTING

According to Skinner, exercise testing in children, as in adults, is done to determine fitness level; to indicate the prognosis for a child suffering from a chronic condition; to reveal the need for further assessment when exercise response is poor; to determine the effectiveness of a given exercise program by providing baseline data to which future measurements can be compared; and to confirm the safety of exercise in cases where safety is questioned.[4] In most cases, basic adult exercise testing guidelines apply to healthy children and adolescents, but response to exercise differs.[7] For instance, immediately following exercise, a child has a lower absolute oxygen uptake, cardiac output, stroke volume, blood pressure, tidal volume, and minute ventilation than an adult. Additionally, a child experiences a higher relative oxygen uptake, heart rate, and respiratory rate than an adult.

According to ACSM, exercise testing is generally not needed for children and adolescents provided they are healthy and have no special health concerns. When exercise testing is warranted, however, familiarize the child with the testing protocol ahead of time. This alleviates fears and helps ensure accurate measures.[7] The treadmill test is the most appropriate means of exercise testing for young children because of its simplicity and because it accommodates various body sizes (Fig. 4.6). Many fitness professionals use the Bruce treadmill protocol, modified to 2-minute work stages. The cycle ergometer is also useful, but because it is designed for an adult body, it might not "fit" a child's body size if the child is less than 50 in. tall. Additionally, the cycle ergometer usually requires maintenance of a particular cadence—something that is sometimes difficult for young children to sustain. See *ACSM's Guidelines for Exercise Testing and Prescription*, 8th Ed., for explanations of different types of tests.[7]

> *QUICK REFERENCE*
> Fitness professionals can use the FITNESSGRAM test battery to assess the components of fitness in youth if testing is to occur outside the clinical setting.[6,7,41]

Metabolic Syndrome—also known as insulin resistance syndrome or syndrome X. Increases the risk for cardiovascular disease, stroke, and diabetes.

Dyslipidemia—a disorder of blood lipids. Includes elevated blood cholesterol levels, high LDL levels, low HDL levels, and increased triglycerides. This condition increases the risk for cardiovascular disease.

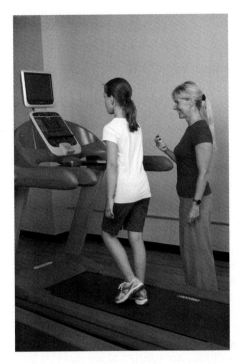

FIGURE 4-6 ■ Child undergoing fitness testing on a treadmill.

During exercise testing, keep in mind that resting heart rate is higher in children than in adults. It gradually decreases as children age, even though maximal heart rate does not change. Peak heart rates during the treadmill test or cycle ergometer are typically 185 to 225 bpm but can vary. Cardiovascular and muscular endurance improve gradually with age, so young children often cannot last as long as adults during exercise testing.[7] A small attention span, lack of enjoyment, and inexperience might make testing difficult.

QUICK REFERENCE
The common formula used to determine maximal heart rate in an adult (220 – age) is not appropriate for those under the age of 16.[7]

Most physical education classes in schools use simple field tests to assess the fitness status of students. For cardiorespiratory fitness, they perform the 1-mi walk-run; for muscular fitness, they use the curl-up test and the pull-up or push-up test; for flexibility, they use the sit and reach test; and for body composition, they take skin fold measurements. Additionally, they calculate BMI as an indicator for overweight or obesity.

EXERCISE PRESCRIPTION

General Guidelines

- Include about 5 minutes of light activity such as walking, jumping jacks, and stretching prior to increasing intensity to prepare the body for activity. Additionally, include a 5-minute cool-down at the end of activity to return the body to a resting state. This age group needs to learn the importance of warm-up and cool-down sessions.
- Groups such as the American Heart Association and ACSM suggest that all children over the age of two receive 60 minutes of moderate-to-vigorous intensity physical activity each day. ACSM specifically recommends 30 minutes of moderate activity (activity that moderately increases breathing, heart rate, and sweating) plus 30 minutes of vigorous activity (activity that substantially increases breathing, heart rate, and sweating) *at least* 3 to 4 days per week. The activity should be enjoyable and varied but does not necessarily have to be continuous. In fact, children under the age of 12 tend to perform better with intermittent activities that change from vigorous intensity to moderate intensity back to vigorous intensity, so encourage it.[7,14,19,40,42]
- Table 4.1 lists recommendations from the National Association for Sport and Physical Education (NASPE). Overall, NASPE suggests that parents discourage prolonged periods of inactivity in young children. Unless they are sleeping, do not allow them to be sedentary for more than 1 to 2 hours at a time. Create a schedule that incorporates activity into daily routines, and plan enjoyable "exercise sessions" that engage children. Discourage idle television watching and limit access to no more than 2 hours per day. Most importantly, adults should be positive role models for children and show enthusiasm and commitment to regular exercise themselves so that children mimic this healthy lifestyle behavior.
- To ensure compliance, make the activities fun, nonthreatening, unembarrassing, and developmentally appropriate. Offer words of encouragement and support. Elicit family support.

TABLE 4-1 GUIDELINES FROM THE NATIONAL ASSOCIATION FOR SPORT AND PHYSICAL EDUCATION	
Age	**Minimum Daily Activity**
Infants	No minimum; encourage activity that develops motor skills.
Toddlers	1.5 hours; encourage 30 minutes of structured activity plus 60 minutes of unstructured activity.
Preschoolers	2 hours; encourage 60 minutes of structured activity plus 60 minutes of unstructured activity.
School-age children	≥1 hour; encourage bouts of activity lasting 15 minutes or more.

TABLE 4-2	GUIDELINES FOR RESISTANCE TRAINING
Age (years)	**Recommendations**
7 or younger	Introduce child to basic exercises with little or no weight; develop the concept of a training session; teach exercise techniques; progress from body weight calisthenics, partner exercise, and lightly resisted exercises; keep volume low.
8–10	Gradually increase the number of exercises; practice exercise technique in all lifts; start gradual progressive loading of exercises; keep exercise simple; gradually increase training volume; carefully monitor toleration to the exercise stress.
11–13	Teach all basic exercise techniques; continue progressive loading of each exercise; emphasize exercise techniques; introduce more advanced exercise with little or no resistance
14–15	Progress to more-advanced youth programs in resistance exercise; add sport-specific components; emphasize exercise techniques; increase volume.
16 or older	Move child to entry-level adult programs after all background knowledge has been mastered and a basic level of training experience has been gained.

Note: If a child of any age begins a program without previous experience, start the child at previous levels and move to more advanced levels as exercise toleration, skill, amount of training time, and understanding permit.
Source: From Kraemer WJ, Fleck SJ. Strength Training for Young Athletes. Champaign, IL: Human Kinetics, 1993.

- The consensus for resistance training is that "closely supervised resistance training using … relatively high repetitions and low resistance significantly improves muscular strength with no adverse effect on bone, muscle, or connective tissue."[5] See Table 4.2 for recommendations based on age.
- Encourage children to drink one to two 8-oz glasses of water before activity and provide them with water during activity to prevent dehydration.

QUICK REFERENCE
Encourage daily active play rather than structured exercise for young children ages 2 to 6 years old.

Tips for Cardiovascular Exercise[7]
- As mentioned, children and adolescents should participate in 30 minutes of moderate activity and 30 minutes of vigorous activity on at least 3 to 4 days per week.[7] Overweight children, however, might not initially be able to accumulate 60 minutes of daily activity. Start them out slowly and gradually increase duration and frequency until they meet minimum recommendations.
- Exercise in a cool environment. Children and adolescents have immature thermoregulatory systems, so they can become overheated quickly. Encourage them to drink adequate water to help reduce risk of overheating.

Tips for Resistance Exercise[7]

- In general, adult guidelines apply to children.
- Remember that most equipment is designed to "fit" the bodies of adults. Adjustments are likely needed when working with children.
- Closely monitor any resistance training program to ensure neutral body alignment and execution. Emphasize gradual progressive overload and develop a program that improves motor skills along with fitness level.
- Use light resistance with a greater number of repetitions. Have the child perform 8 to 15 repetitions to moderate fatigue and do not increase intensity until the child is able to perform the specified number of repetitions with proper form. Reduce the resistance if a minimum of eight repetitions cannot be executed with neutral body alignment. Avoid maximal training until physical maturity is reached.

QUICK REFERENCE

According to the Centers for Disease Control, physical activity programs for children and adolescents are most effective when they

- Emphasize activities that are enjoyable and not monotonous
- Include both competitive and noncompetitive activities to meet the needs of different age groups and ability levels
- Foster skills and abilities that develop confidence
- Promote interaction and coordination between the school and the community

SAMPLE EXERCISES

Most children and adolescents can safely perform the same exercises suggested for adults. Obviously, modifications are necessary to accommodate size, coordination, development, and maturity. For cardiovascular improvements, encourage activities such as swimming, bicycling, and roller blading. For bone health, encourage weight bearing activities such as running and jumping rope. To improve muscular strength, have children lift or move objects—or perform activities that require the support of their own body weight. For more structured programs, encourage them to do crunches, push-ups, pull-ups, lunges, heel raises, biceps curls with light free weights, triceps kick backs, lateral shoulder raises, and any other exercises they enjoy and are capable of executing properly. Watch body alignment and ensure a full range of motion.

> ## *QUICK REFERENCE*
> Circle running is a fun way to warm-up or workout. Have participants march in a very large circle. Call out a description that can only apply to some of the children. For example, call for everyone who has a birthday in January and have those children exit the circle and run around the circle in a specified direction one full time. Once they have finished, they take their places in the circle again. Alternatively, have children march in a circle, call out a description, and have those who fulfill the description run into the middle of the circle and dance for 30 seconds. Then they take their places in the circle again.

WARM-UP

A fun workout for youth of all ages is a circuit program. Begin with a warm-up that includes limbering movements and some basic dynamic stretching. Children tend to enjoy upbeat, age-appropriate music, so pump-up-the-volume and encourage dancing or basic cheerleading moves to get the workout started. Young participants like their instructors to demonstrate movements for them, so join in on the fun. Alternatively, warm up with basic marching, jogging, jumping, hopping, skipping, grapevines, knee lifts, or any other familiar movements.

EXERCISES

Arrange the circuit ahead of time and adjust the number of stations based on the number of participants. Children prefer to work in pairs, so set up eight stations for 16 children. Alternate an upper body station with a lower body station so that energy level will be high at each station. Demonstrate the activity at each circuit before expecting the participants to perform. Place a sign with a short exercise description at each station to prompt their memories. Allow 45 to 60 seconds at each station with a 20- to 30-second active rest in between.

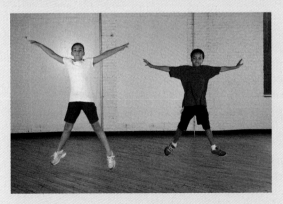

■ Station 1: Star Jumps (Fig. 4.7)
Jump high off the floor while abducting and then adducting shoulders and hips.

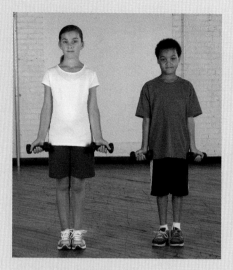 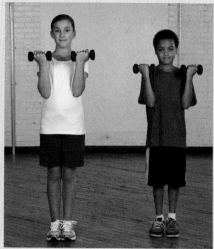

■ **Station 2: Bicep Curls (Fig. 4.8)**
Use lightweight dumbbells. Keep elbows in but not pinned to sides. Control the movement. Flex both elbows to lift weights slowly. Return to start.

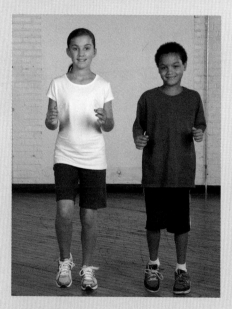 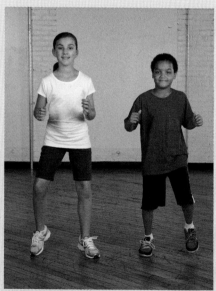

■ **Station 3: Football Feet (Fig. 4.9)**
Teach this by having children march at a normal speed. Begin increasing speed until they are moving their feet as fast as they can. They will be landing on the balls of their feet, not the entire foot. Start with feet shoulder width apart; move them out; move them in; move them back to center; repeat.

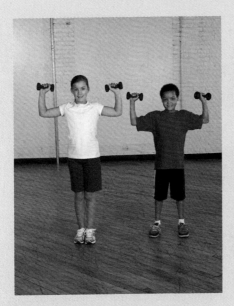
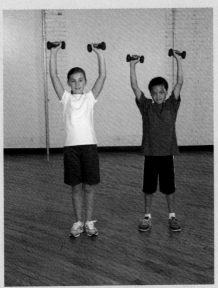

■ Station 4: Shoulder Press (Fig. 4.10)

Use lightweight dumbbells. Start with dumbbells at ear-height, arms parallel to floor. Push up. Return to start. Control the movement.

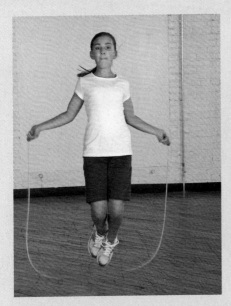
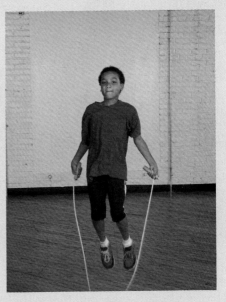

■ Station 5: Jump Rope (Fig. 4.11)

This may be done with or without a jump rope. Jump rope in place until time is called.

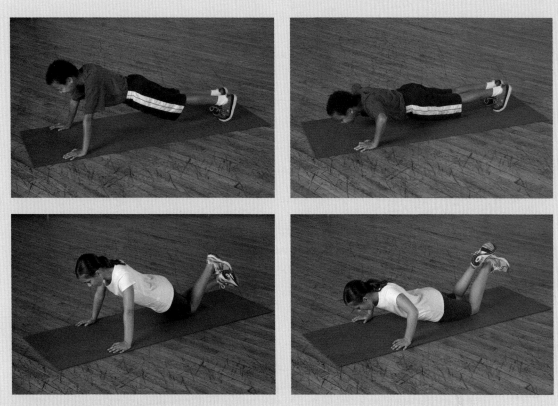

■ Station 6: Push-Ups (Fig. 4.12)
Demonstrate both full body and knee push-ups. Ensure a neutral spine.

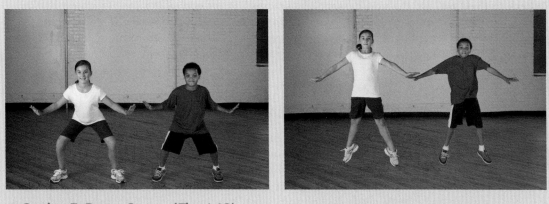

■ Station 7: Power Squats (Fig. 4.13)
Begin with feet shoulder width apart. Squat down. Push up and jump from this position. Repeat.

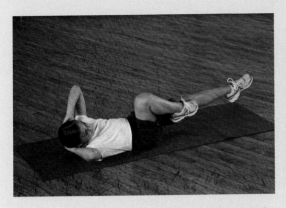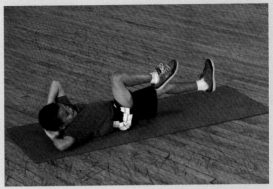

■ **Station 8: Bicycles (Fig. 4.14)**
Lie on floor, hands behind head. Bend knees and lift feet. Lift head, neck, and shoulders off ground. Alternate right shoulder to left knee and then left shoulder to right knee. Continue riding the bicycle until time is called.

> *QUICK REFERENCE*
>
> Most children love participating in group activities, so relays are fun and effective for encouraging participation. Set up mats at one end of a room, or simply use tape to mark off a certain distance on the floor. Assign children to groups of 3 or 4 and have the members of each group line up at one end of the room. At the sound of a whistle, have the first person in each line run to the mat or to the tape at the other end of the room and perform a specified exercise (such as 10 jumping jacks or 5 push-ups). When finished, they should run back to their line, tap the next person, and sit down at the end of the line. That next person should run to the other end of the room, perform the exercise, and return. Continue until all group members are sitting. Instead of simply running to the other end of the room, have children skip, hop, dribble a ball, lunge, or do any other moves specified by the instructor.

NUTRITIONAL CONSIDERATIONS

Nutritional needs for this particular population vary depending upon age because the rate of growth and development, and subsequently basal metabolic rate, gradually slows as **infants**, **toddlers**, **children**, and **adolescents** get older. The fastest rate of growth occurs during the first 12 months of life during which an infant's weight triples. By age 2, growth and energy needs decline somewhat, but they are still high throughout adolescence as bones and muscles increase in density and mass. During adolescence, growth occurs in spurts until physical maturity is reached.[43]

QUICK REFERENCE

Log into www.mypyramid.gov to input a child's age, gender, and activity level and determine an appropriate, healthy diet for that child. It is fun and it is free!

INFANTS, TODDLERS, AND PRESCHOOLERS

Energy Needs

Up until the age of 5, children actually self-regulate food intake to meet energy requirements.[44] Though daily intakes vary significantly, the average energy consumption for toddlers and **preschoolers** over a week tends to be quite close to what their bodies need. Unfortunately, this inborn ability to adjust energy intake does not enable this age group to select a nutritionally sound diet, so parents need to provide healthy options to ensure adequate nutrition. Additionally, this self-regulating mechanism for energy intake actually falters when parents force kids to eat when they are not hungry. This can then predispose them to long-term eating issues. Caregivers are important role models for lifelong healthy eating because eating habits and food preferences begin developing between the ages of 2 and 5. Thus, caregivers need to establish healthy habits early to prevent eating problems later in life.

QUICK REFERENCE

Parents should routinely expose toddlers and preschoolers to various healthy food options. Furthermore, they should not restrict foods, use food as a reward for good behavior,[43,45,46] or force children to be members of the "clean plate club."

How many kilocalories are appropriate for this age group? To calculate the energy needs of those between the ages of 13 and 35 months, use the following formula: (89 × weight in kg) − 100 + 20. For estimated energy requirements of children older than age 1, see Table 4.3. For more specific guidelines based on age, gender, weight, and height, see the Food and Nutrition Board (Institute of Medicine) at www.iom.edu/Object.File/Master/21/372/0.pdf. Table 4.4 has additional tips concerning nutritional eating for toddlers.

Infants—the age group between birth and 12 months old.
Toddlers—the age group between years 1 and 2.
Children—the age group between years 3 and 11. ACSM designates those under the age of 13 as children.
Adolescents—the age group between years 11 and 21. ACSM designates those between the ages of 13 and 18 as adolescents.
Preschoolers—the age group between years 3 and 5.

TABLE 4-3 ESTIMATED ENERGY REQUIREMENTS FOR BOYS AND GIRLS ACCORDING TO THE DIETARY REFERENCE INTAKE

Age	Energy Needs (kcal/day)
Boys	
1–3	1,046
4–8	1,742
9–13	2,279
14–18	3,152
Girls	
1–3	992
4–8	1,642
9–13	2,071
14–18	2,368

Source: Adapted from the USDA's Dietary Reference Intakes, available from the National Academy of Sciences Institute of Medicine, Food and Nutrition Board; www.usda.gov.

TABLE 4-4 TIPS FOR TODDLERS

- Offer toddlers various food choices, colors, textures, and flavors
- Provide small quantities of food since a toddler's stomach is small
- Include various snacks. Toddlers typically obtain 25% of their total daily kilocalorie intake from snacks
- If a toddler has a small appetite, be careful with liquids—they are filling
- Limit salt intake
- Toddlers need fat in their diets for proper nervous system development; make sure they get the healthy monounsaturated fats and limit saturated and trans fats

Vitamins and Minerals

A varied diet that meets minimum energy requirements is usually rich in vitamins and minerals. Therefore, toddlers should consume plenty of milk, lean meats, iron-fortified cereal, whole grain breads, fruits, and vegetables.[19] Appetite often diminishes by age 1, so it is not always consistent from one meal to the next. This is not unhealthy as long as a child's average energy consumption meets minimum requirements.

Iron deserves special attention because it is often deficient in this particular age group. In fact, iron-deficiency anemia is quite common among infants and toddlers as they switch from iron-fortified infant formulas and foods to "adult foods" and cow's milk (cow's milk is notoriously low in iron). To ensure normal growth and development, make

| TABLE 4-5 | RECOMMENDED VITAMIN AND MINERAL INTAKES FOR VARIOUS AGE GROUPS |

Recommended Vitamins

	Thiamin (mg/day)	Riboflavin (mg/day)	Niacin (mg/day)	Biotin (μg/day)	Folate (μg/day)	Vitamin C (mg/day)	Vitamin A (μg/day)	Vitamin D (μg/day)
Boys								
1–3	0.5	0.5	6	8	150	15	300	5
4–8	0.6	0.6	8	12	200	25	400	5
9–13	0.9	0.9	12	20	300	45	600	5
14–18	1.2	1.3	16	25	400	75	900	5
Girls								
1–3	0.5	0.5	6	8	150	15	300	5
4–8	0.6	0.6	8	12	200	25	400	5
9–13	0.9	0.9	12	20	300	45	600	5
14–18	1.0	1.0	14	25	400	65	700	5

Minerals

	Sodium (mg/day)	Chloride (mg/day)	Potassium (mg/day)	Calcium (mg/day)	Phosphorus (mg/day)	Iron (mg/day)	Zinc (mg/day)	Fluoride (mg/day)
Boys								
1–3	1,000	1,500	3,000	500	460	7	3	0.7
4–8	1,200	1,900	3,800	800	500	10	5	1.0
9–13	1,500	2,300	4,500	1,300	1,250	8	8	2
14–18	1,500	2,300	4,700	1,300	1,250	11	11	3
Girls								
1–3	1,000	1,500	3,000	500	460	7	3	0.7
4–8	1,200	1,900	3,800	800	500	10	5	1.0
9–13	1,500	2,300	4,500	1,300	1,250	8	8	2.0
14–18	1,500	2,300	4,700	1,300	1,250	15	9	3.0

Source: Adapted from the USDA's Dietary Reference Intakes, available from the National Academy of Sciences Institute of Medicine, Food and Nutrition Board; www.usda.gov.

sure that children receive 7 to 10 mg of iron per day by including iron-rich foods during each meal. Table 4.5 provides specific suggestions about other vitamins and minerals.[45]

SCHOOL-AGE CHILDREN

During childhood and preadolescence, children continue to grow, but they grow at a slightly slower pace than when they were younger. Various foods and adequate energy intake are still important to ensure nutrient availability for the rapidly approaching growth spurts associated with puberty. Fluctuations in appetite and weight typically correspond to growth spurts, so expect children to eat more and put on extra weight just

TABLE 4-6 FIBER RECOMMENDATIONS FOR CHILDREN	
Age (years)	AI (g/day)
1–3	19
4–8	25
9–13 (boys)	31
9–13 (girls)	26
14–18 (boys)	38
14–18 (girls)	26

Source: Adapted from the USDA's Dietary Reference Intakes, available from the National Academy of Sciences Institute of Medicine, Food and Nutrition Board; www.usda.gov.

prior to a growth spurt. This is normal, so do not severely restrict kilocalories when this occurs. Expect weight to normalize as height increases. Children in this age group, however, must learn to balance activity with dietary intake to maintain a healthy weight. It is during this time that children are prone to developing body image issues and unhealthy dietary practices, so be on the alert.

Energy Needs

Total daily energy needs vary based on age, size, and activity level. Kilocalorie intake tends to increase as size increases, but the actual need per kilogram of body weight slowly declines.[45] This is partly because growth and development slow, but it also occurs because activity levels decrease with age. This is true for both boys and girls, but it is much more pronounced in girls. To ensure energy balance, encourage increased activity and discourage sedentary activities. See Table 4.3 for energy recommendations for different ages.

Carbohydrates, Proteins, and Fats

The RDA for carbohydrates is 130 g per day, the same as it is for adults. This is because recommendations are based on the brain's requirement for glucose, which stabilizes after age 1. Active children might require a greater carbohydrate intake to meet the demands of increased activity. Table 4.6 shows dietary fiber recommendations for different age groups.

Protein needs vary and actually decline slightly with age. The RDA suggests 1.05 g/kg/day for those between the ages of 1 and 3; 0.95 g/kg/day for those between the ages of 4 and 13; and 0.85 g/kg/day for those between the ages of 14 and 18.

There is no RDA for total fat; however, children between the ages of 1 and 3 should consume 30% to 40% of their total daily kilocalories in the form of fat. Those between the ages of 4 and 18 should obtain 25% to 35% of their total daily kilocalorie intake in the form of fat. Severely restricting fat in the diet results in deficiencies of the fat-soluble vitamins and essential fatty acids (linoleic and linolenic fatty acids; Table 4.7).

Vitamins and Minerals

According to the International Food Information Council and the American Heart Association, children need various carbohydrate-rich grains, vegetables, and fruits to obtain

TABLE 4-7 RECOMMENDED INTAKES FOR LINOLEIC AND LINOLENIC FATTY ACIDS		
	Linoleic acid (g/day)	Linolenic acid (g/day)
Boys		
1–3 years	7	0.7
4–8 years	10	0.9
9–13 years	12	1.2
14–18 years	16	1.6
Girls		
1–3 years	7	0.7
4–8 years	10	0.9
9–13 years	10	1.0
14–18 years	11	1.1

Source: Adapted from the USDA's Dietary Reference Intakes, available from the National Academy of Sciences Institute of Medicine, Food and Nutrition Board; www.usda.gov.

adequate amounts of vitamins, minerals, and fiber for optimal health (Table 4.5). They also require dairy products, lean meats, and fish to support growth and development.[19,47]

ADOLESCENTS

Compared to children, adolescents are much more interested in and involved with their food choices. They are also greatly influenced by peer pressure. They want to fit in, so they often conform to the eating behaviors of their friends. Thus, they might begin eating large quantities of junk food, or they might begin practicing restrictive dieting. These are two opposite extremes, but they are both unhealthy.

Energy Needs

Energy requirements during adolescence increase because of growth spurts, which occur in response to the changing hormone levels associated with puberty. Growth spurts in girls begin at age 10, peak at age 12, and taper off by age 15. In boys, they begin at age 12, peak at age 14, and last until age 19. Expect energy needs to increase just before each growth spurt.[47]

Overall, the exact needs of adolescents vary depending upon gender, body composition, and activity level. Boys tend to require more energy because they develop greater muscle mass and are more active than girls. Girls, on the other hand, need to consciously increase their daily activity level to avoid becoming overweight or obese.

QUICK REFERENCE

Before puberty, the body composition of boys and girls tends to be quite similar. After puberty, however, girls develop more fat, whereas boys develop more muscle and bone mass.[45]

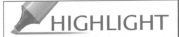

HIGHLIGHT   Steroid Abuse by Children and Adolescents

Steroids and other performance-enhancing drugs have been in the news for years now, so most Americans know that they are used to promote muscle size and strength. Their use is common in the world of body building, but they are becoming much more popular among certain other athletes as well. Although it is legal for physicians to prescribe steroids to patients with osteoporosis, breast cancer, severe muscle wasting, and other medical conditions, the Anabolic Steroid Control Act of 1990 banned the use of *nonprescription* steroids. It is now illegal to possess steroids without a prescription or to distribute steroids without a medical license.[5]

Steroid use causes several side effects. Users have an increased risk for early heart attack, stroke, liver cancer, and kidney failure. They experience an increased incidence of psychiatric issues such as severe rage and aggression.[48] They also have an increased risk of contracting HIV, hepatitis B, hepatitis C, and other bloodborne illnesses because many steroids users share needles.[5,48] Steroid use has a masculinizing effect on female users and often results in decreased breast size, loss of body fat, deepened voice, increased body hair, and loss of hair on the head.[48] It has a feminizing effect on male users and causes shrinkage of the testes, breast development (sometimes accompanied by milk production), and male-pattern baldness.[5,48] Many of the adverse effects are irreversible and likely occur because

of the abnormally high dosages usually taken by users. Illegal users often take amounts 10 to 100 times higher than those used for medical purposes.[48] In addition to the side effects already mentioned, steroids stimulate ossification of the epiphyseal plates on long bones. Therefore, young users typically stop growing prematurely and are shorter than expected.

Because so many athletes—who are role models for children and adolescents—admit to using steroids, teens are now experimenting with these performance enhancers. According to the National Institute on Drug Abuse, 2.7% of those in grades 8 to 10 and 2.9% of those in 12th grade have tried steroids at least once in their lives. This usage rate is on the rise and is much higher than it was just 8 years ago. Why do teens use steroids? Adolescents list improved appearance and the subsequent boost in self-confidence as their primary reasons for using steroids. A secondary reason is for better performance in sports.

To prevent adolescents from using steroids, parents, coaches, and trainers should discuss the dangers associated with steroid use and provide suggestions on how they can refuse offers from friends and teammates. Give them alternatives to steroids such as safe and effective strength training guidelines and proper nutrition. Studies show that steroid use decreases by as much as 50% when parents and teachers are actively involved with adolescents.[48]

Vitamins and Minerals

Adolescents should consume a varied diet that includes whole grains, vegetables, fruits, low-fat dairy products, lean meats, and poultry to meet their increasing needs. Calcium, vitamin D, and iron are of utmost concern.[47]

Calcium is an integral component of bone tissue. A deficiency stunts growth in younger children, interferes with the achievement of peak bone mass in adolescents, and predisposes the bones to osteoporosis during adulthood.[45] Unfortunately, 90% of girls and 70% of boys between the ages of 12 and 19 do not receive enough calcium to support bone health. Adolescents should, therefore, consciously increase daily calcium intake. Milk, other dairy products, small fish with bones, calcium-fortified tofu, broccoli, and legumes are good sources of this nutrient. Vitamin D is necessary for calcium absorption because it stimulates the synthesis of calcium channels along the lining of the small intestinal wall. Without vitamin D, the small intestine is unable to transport dietary calcium into the body. The body can manufacture sufficient vitamin D, provided the skin is exposed to sunlight for 15 to 30 minutes 2 to 3 days per week. It is not, however, found naturally in very many foods. Some good sources include vitamin D–fortified milk, margarine, butter, and cereals. Additionally, egg yolks, beef, liver, and fatty fish also contain vitamin D. A deficiency of vitamin D leads to a condition of soft, rubbery bones called rickets in children and osteomalacia in adults.

Requirements for iron increase during adolescence. Iron is an essential component of hemoglobin, the molecule in red blood cells that binds with oxygen as oxygen is transported to body cells (see Chapter 7 for further information about the importance of oxygen). Adolescent boys need extra iron to support muscle growth, and their needs increase right before a growth spurt. More specifically, they need 2.9 mg per day more than the RDA during a growth spurt. Adolescent girls need an additional 1.1 mg per day above the RDA prior to a growth spurt. Girls who begin their monthly cycle prior to age 14, however, require an additional 2.5 mg per day above the RDA to make up for iron losses during menstruation. Good sources of iron include red meats, fish, poultry, eggs, legumes, and dried fruit. Low iron intake that results in anemia leads to weakness, fatigue, headache, impaired immunity, and diminished cognitive functioning.

SUPPLEMENTS

Overall, the American Academy of Pediatrics (AAP) suggests that children and adolescents obtain proper nutrition through dietary intake rather than through supplements. Still, over 30% take multivitamins/multiminerals. Those between the ages of 4 and 8 have the highest usage rate: nearly 50% in this age group take a daily supplement. The nutrients that are most commonly ingested include retinol, vitamin C, vitamin D, calcium, and iron. Supplemental calcium, vitamin D, and iron are probably safe because the typical American diet is low in these nutrients.[49] In fact, rickets, which results from a deficiency of vitamin D, is still a concern in the United States today; therefore, the AAP encourages supplemental vitamin D. They suggest that breastfed infants or infants who consume less than 500 mL of vitamin D–fortified formula or milk take a supplement containing 200 IU of vitamin D.[3]

Additionally, experts recommend supplemental fluoride in areas where public drinking water does not contain adequate amounts of fluoride. Children diagnosed with specific deficiencies might require additional supplements, but this must be determined by a physician.

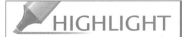
HIGHLIGHT   Eating Disorders

Eating disorders involve unusual eating behaviors that often endanger mental and physical health. They affect both men and women—and boys and girls—but they are most common among adolescent girls and young women. Still, nearly 10% of sufferers are male.[50] Eating disorders are more than just an obsession with food or weight loss. In fact, multiple sociological, cultural, psychological, and physiological factors contribute to their development. Those who have eating disorders have a love/hate relationship with food. They struggle with negative feelings about their bodies and are extremely critical of themselves and their own capabilities. Sufferers usually hide their eating habits from family and friends, which suggests that they know their behavior is not "normal." Consequently, eating disorders are usually difficult to catch in the early stages. The earlier they are caught, however, the better the prognosis.

According to the National Eating Disorders Association, approximately 10 million Americans suffer from some sort of disordered eating.[51] Examples of these disorders include anorexia nervosa, bulimia nervosa, binge eating disorder, and muscle dysmorphia.

Anorexia nervosa is characterized by self-starvation and the inability to maintain a minimally healthy weight. In fact, a major criterion for diagnosis is a body weight that is less than 85% of what is considered healthy.[50] There are two recognized subtypes of anorexia. The "restrictive" anorexic usually limits food intake but rarely engages in purging. The "binge eating/purging" anorexic restricts food intake but regularly engages in episodes of binging and purging (through vomiting, laxative abuse,

or excessive exercise). Anorexics tend to have a highly distorted body image—they can be 5'8" tall and weigh a mere 90 lb, but when they look in a mirror, they see a fat person looking back at them. Interestingly, anorexics often look at normal weight people and think that normal weight people look fine. They rarely admit that they have a problem, yet they often wear baggy clothes and eat in private to keep family and friends from discovering their behavior. Anorexics have an intense, deep fear of gaining weight. As levels of body fat drop, they often develop amenorrhea. Amenorrhea is diagnosed when a young woman does not begin menstruation by age 16 or if she stops having her monthly cycle for 3 to 6 consecutive months. Amenorrhea is dangerous because it results in low blood levels of estrogen, a hormone needed for bone building. Bone loss from amenorrhea can be significant and often promotes the early development of osteoporosis. Other complications associated with anorexia nervosa include protein deficiencies, malnutrition, slowed growth and development, muscle wasting, heart atrophy, drop in blood pressure, and electrolyte imbalance. Sufferers actually lose brain tissue, develop anemia, and have impaired immunity. Digestive problems often arise, blood lipid levels become unhealthy, and the skin dries out.[45,51]

Bulimia nervosa, which is much more common than anorexia nervosa, is characterized by "repeated episodes of binge eating usually followed by self-induced vomiting, misuse of laxatives or diuretics, fasting, or excessive exercise."[45] Bulimics are typically within 10 lb of a normal, healthy body weight, so it is difficult to diagnose. But their opinions about themselves are ruled by their weight and overall

(continued)

HIGHLIGHT Eating Disorders *(continued)*

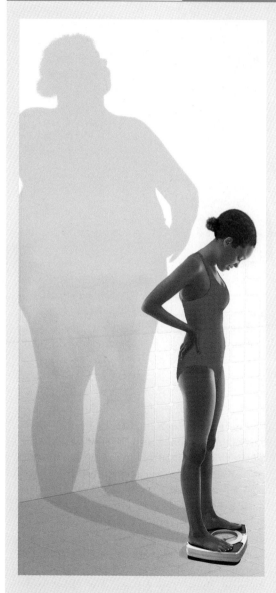

appearance. During a binge, bulimics feel out of control and ingest an inordinate amount of food, sometimes thousands and thousands of kilocalories over the course of one to two hours. They are secretive about these binges, so they usually eat alone at night when everyone else is asleep. Or they might eat at buffets where no one knows them. After a binge, they feel guilty and try to compensate by purging themselves of the excess kilocalories. Vomiting is a common means of eliminating kilocalories, but bulimics also abuse laxatives or try to exercise until they burn off all of the excess energy they consumed. Criteria for the diagnosis of bulimia include the uncontrolled intake of vast quantities of food in a short time coupled with repeated attempts to compensate for the binge. As with anorexia nervosa, bulimia nervosa is categorized into two subtypes. The "purging" type is when a bulimic routinely vomits or abuses laxative, diuretics, or enemas following a binge. The "nonpurging" type is when a bulimic does not routinely vomit or abuse laxatives, diuretics, or enemas; instead, they fast or exercise excessively to compensate for excess intake.[50]

Though not recognized by the American Psychiatric Association as an actual eating disorder, binge eating disorder occurs when people consume vast quantities of food but do not follow it with purging. Binge eaters tend to eat for emotional reasons—even when they are not hungry. They feel shame, embarrassment, and disgust following the binging episode, but they do not usually try to compensate. Therefore, they tend to be overweight or obese.

Muscle dysmorphia, another obsessive compulsive disorder that centers around body image, occurs when an individual has a preoccupation with developing muscle mass. It normally affects men and has symptoms that parallel those of anorexia nervosa. Sufferers

(continued)

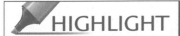 **HIGHLIGHT** Eating Disorders (*continued*)

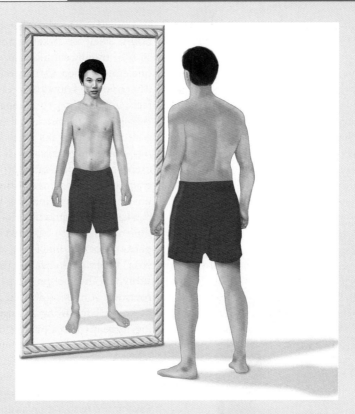

have a distorted body image and feel that their muscles are small and underdeveloped—even though they are actually well developed and large. They feel compelled to lift weights every-day—sometimes more than once per day—to put on muscle mass. This is dangerous because their bodies are often stressed so much that they develop serious pain and injuries. Nevertheless, they work through the pain to try to continue to bulk up. Sufferers often agonize during their hours away from the gym because they intensely fear muscle atrophy. They frequently consume unhealthy diets that are dangerously insufficient in kilocalories,

low in fat, and high in protein. Because their carbohydrate intake is so low, they feel hungry all the time. In an effort to reach their unreal-istic expectations, they sometimes abuse sup-plements—or seek out steroids. For those with muscle dysmorphia, strength training becomes an obsession; therefore, they have little time in their lives for anything else.[52]

Eating disorders are relatively common among children and adolescents. Why? Because these age groups are faced with puberty, changing bodies, and peer pressure. Sometimes concern over weight develops into an obsession with weight loss that can interfere

(*continued*)

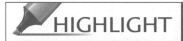 **HIGHLIGHT**   Eating Disorders (*continued*)

with normal activities, relationships, and health. Young people who participate in gymnastics, wrestling, ballet, or other forms of dance seem to have a greater risk of developing eating disorders because excelling at these sports often requires leanness. Young girls who have mothers or sisters who are obsessed with weight and restrictive eating are also vulnerable to developing the same behaviors. Additionally, eating disorders are common in children who have families who abuse alcohol and/or drugs. In these cases, children strive for some sort of control in their lives; since they cannot control their family situation, they control their own body weight.

The media is frequently blamed for the increased prevalence of eating disorders. Television, magazines, movies, and sports programs often show thin females and muscular males as being popular, while overweight people are outcasts. This might promote an obsession with weight in predisposed girls and boys who try to live up to these unrealistic expectations. Sadly, this is starting to affect younger and younger children. In fact, surveys show that 42% of first to third grade girls express a desire to be thinner than they are, and 81% of 10 year olds have an intense fear of becoming fat.

Prevention is the key to dealing with eating disorders. Teaching children to accept and appreciate various body shapes and weights—and encouraging them to focus on characteristics not associated with weight—helps in the fight against dysfunctional eating. Parents, family members, teachers, coaches, and friends should help children develop a healthy relationship with food. Explain the importance of diet and activity without focusing on physical improvements. Give them the tools to make sound food choices. Empower them to take charge of their lives by helping them become as healthy as they can be!

SUMMARY

Existing evidence suggests that physical activity and proper nutrition enhance growth and development during childhood and adolescence. Therefore, it is important to challenge the heart, muscles, and bones early in life while simultaneously providing the building blocks (in the form of food) to allow the body to adapt to imposed demands. This encourages optimal functioning of each body system. Additionally, regular exercise and adequate energy intake reduce the risk for chronic disease later in life. Since research suggests that several chronic conditions—such as atherosclerosis and heart disease—actually begin to develop early in life, establishing healthy lifestyle behaviors at a young age promotes health and might even slow age-related deterioration.

Though children and adolescents respond differently to exercise than adults, they still reap many of the same benefits. Trainers, coaches, and anyone else involved with designing programs for this age group should tailor programs to meet individual needs. They should realize how influential they are in establishing lifestyle behaviors—particularly in those under the age of 10—and try to "create" active children. Active children then grow into active teenagers who develop into active adults. Not only do active youth experience health improvements as they age; they also report a better self-image, improved moods, better weight maintenance, and increased self-efficacy than sedentary youth. By adhering to the guidelines presented in this chapter, health professionals can ensure that their younger clients safely begin exercise programs and continue them throughout life with minimal risk.

CASE STUDY

A 15-year-old girl would like to begin an exercise program to lose weight. She is 5'9" tall and weighs 160 lb. She has recently started a weight-loss diet and is currently consuming 1,000 kcal per day. She has never been active before, but she sees her classmates playing sports and cheerleading and would like to become more active. She read in a popular magazine that dairy products and carbohydrates are high in fat and kilocalories, so she has completely cut out all milk products and breads from her diet. In fact, she consumes little more than fruits, vegetables, and protein shakes each day.

■ Discuss how you would approach this situation.

■ Give specific exercise and nutrition recommendations for this client.

THINKING CRITICALLY

1. Discuss why today's youth is so inactive.
2. What are some of the barriers to exercise for this population? Explain how to overcome these barriers.
3. Describe several anatomical and physiological differences between children and adults. How do these affect exercise performance?
4. Explain how children and adolescents enhance muscular strength during training without significantly increasing muscle mass.
5. Why is there an increased prevalence of overweight and obesity among youth?
6. Describe three precautions for exercise in this particular population.
7. List several benefits of exercise for children and adolescents. What are some guidelines for various age groups?
8. Under what circumstances is exercise testing recommended for children and adolescents? What are some problems when trying to use 'adult tests' to determine status of children?
9. Explain some of the special nutritional considerations for adolescents.
10. Do you think steroid use is a problem for adolescents? Why are these drugs appealing to this age group? What are some of the negative side effects?

REFERENCES

1. Pate R, Wang C, Dowda M, et al. Cardiorespiratory fitness levels among U.S. youth 12–19 years of age. Findings from the 1999–2002 National Health and Nutrition Examination Survey. Arch Pediatr Adolesc Med 2006;160:1005–1012.
2. Nieman D. The Exercise-Health Connection. In: Chapter 19: Children and Youth. Human Kinetics, 1998.
3. American Academy of Pediatrics. www.aap.org
4. Skinner J. Exercise Testing and Exercise Prescription for Special Cases. Baltimore: Lippincott Williams & Wilkins, 2005.
5. McArdle W, Katch F, Katch V. Exercise Physiology. 5th Ed. Baltimore: Lippencott Williams & Wilkins, 2001.
6. Columbia University School of Nursing. www.ccnmtl.columbia.edu
7. American College of Sports Medicine. ACSM's Guidelines for Exercise Testing and Prescription. 8th Ed. Philadelphia: Lippincott Williams & Wilkins, 2010:207–211.
8. Black M, Young-Hyman D. Introduction to the special issue: pediatric overweight. J Pediatr Psychol 2007;32(1):1–5.
9. National Association for Sport and Physical Education. www.aahperd.org
10. Centers for Disease Control. www.cdc.gov
11. Hagarty M, Schmidt C, Bernaix L, et al. Adolescent obesity: current trends in identification and management. J Am Acad Nurse Pract 2004;16(11):481–489.
12. National Association of Children's Hospitals and Related Institutions. www.childrenshospitals.net
13. Shields M. Overweight and obesity among children and youth. Health Rep 2006;17(3):27–42.
14. United States Department of Health and Human Services. www.surgeongeneral.gov
15. Welch G. The growing problems of overweight American youths. Am Fitness 2005;23(5):54–59.
16. Paxton R, Valois R, Drane W. Correlates of body mass index, weight goals, and weight-management practices among adolescents. J Sch Health 2004;74(4):136–143.
17. Maffeis C. Aetiology of overweight and obesity in children and adolescents. Eur J Pediatrics 2000;159:35–44.
18. Anavian J, Brenner D, Speiser P. Profiles of obese children presenting for metabolic evaluation. J Pediatr Endocrinol Metab 2001;14(8):1145–1150.
19. American Heart Association. Dietary recommendations for children and adolescents. Circulation 2005;112:2061–2075.
20. Sorof J, Daniels S. Obesity hypertension in children: a problem of epidemic proportions. Hypertension 2002;40(4):441–447.
21. Dwyer J, Allison K, Goldenberg E, et al. Adolescent girls' perceived barriers to participation in physical activity. Adolescence 2006;41(161):75–90.
22. Allison K, Dwyer J, Goldenberg E, et al. Male adolescents' reasons for participating in physical activity, barriers to participation, and suggestions for increasing participation. Adolescence 2005;40(157):155–171.
23. Trost S, Kerr L, Ward D, et al. Physical activity and determinants of physical activity in obese and non-obese children. Int J Obes Relat Disord 2001;25(6):822–829.
24. McCambridge T, Bernhardt, Brenner J, et al. Active healthy living: prevention of childhood obesity through increased physical activity. Pediatrics 2006;117(5):1834–1832.
25. Graf C, Koch B, Kretschmann-Kandel E, et al. Correlation between BMI, leisure habits, and motor abilities in childhood (CHILT-project). Int J Obes 2004;28:22–26.
26. Reilly J, McDowell Z. Physical activity interventions in the prevention and treatment of paediatric obesity: systemic review and critical appraisal. Proc Nutr Soc 2003;62(3):611–609.
27. Faigenbaum A, Milliken L, Loud R, et al. Comparison of 1 and 2 days per week of strength training in children. Res Q Exerc Sport 2002;73(4):416–414.
28. Lee S, Arslanian S. Cardiorespiratory fitness and abdominal adiposity in youth. Eur J Clin Nutr 2007;61(4):561–566.
29. Payne G, Morrow J. Exercise and VO_{2max} in children: a meta-analysis. Res Q Exerc Sport. 1993;64(3):305–303.
30. Chatrath R, Shenoy R, Serratto M, Thoele D. Physical fitness of urban American children. Pediatr Cardiol 2002;23:608–612.
31. Annesi J. Relationship between self-efficacy and changes in rated tension and depression for 9- to 12-yr.-old children enrolled in a 12-wk. after-school physical activity program. Percept Mot Skills 2004;99(1):191.
32. Valois R, Zullig K, Huebner E, et al. Physical activity behaviors and perceived life satisfaction among public high school adolescents. J Sch Health 2004; 4(2):59–65.
33. Williamson D, Dewey A, Steinberg H. Mood change through physical exercise in nine- to ten-year-old children. Percept Mot Skills 2001;93(1):311.

34. Cruz M, Shaibi M, Weigensberg M, et al. Pediatric obesity and insulin resistance: chronic disease risk and implications for treatment and prevention beyond body weight modification. Annu Rev Nutr 2005;25:435–469.

35. Peterson K, Silverstein J, Kaufman F, et al. Management of type 2 diabetes in youth: an update. Am Fam Physician 2007;76(5):658–664.

36. Scott L. Insulin resistance syndrome in children. Pediatr Nurs 2006;32(2):119.

37. Hardin D, Hebert J, Bayden T, et al. Treatment of childhood syndrome X. Pediatrics 1997;100(2):E5.

38. Luma G, Spiotta R. Hypertension in Children and Adolescents. Am Fam Physician 2006;73(9):1558–1568.

39. Cavallini M, Wendt J, Rice D. Combating obesity in the beginning: incorporating wellness and exercise principles in teacher education programs. J Phys Educ Recreation Dance 2007;78(8):38–41.

40. American Heart Association. www.aha.org

41. Institute for Aerobics Research. The Prudential FITNESSGRAM Test Administration Manual. Dalas, TX: Institute for Aerobics Research, 1994.

42. United States Department of Agriculture. www.usda.gov

43. Brown J. Nutrition Through the Life Cycle. Belmont, CA: Thomsom/Wadsworth, 2005.

44. Horodynski M, Stommel M. Nutrition education aimed at toddlers: an intervention study. Pediatr Nurs 2005;31(5):364–370.

45. Whitney E, Rolfes S. Understanding Nutrition. 11th Ed. Belmont, CA: Thomson/Wadsworth, 2008.

46. Toddlers at the table. Scholastic Parent Child 2007;15(4):52.

47. International Food Information Council. www.ific.org

48. National Institutes of Health. National Institute on Drug Abuse. www.nida.nih.gov

49. Picciano M, Dwyer J, Radimer K, et al. Dietary supplement use among infants, children, and adolescents in the United States, 1999–2002. Arch Pediatr Adolesc Med 2007;161(10):978–985.

50. Academy for Eating Disorders. www.aedweb.org

51. National Eating Disorders Association. www.eatingdisorders.org

52. Eating Disorder Recovery Center. www.addictions.net

SUGGESTED READINGS

Kleinman, R. Pediatric Nutrition Handbook, 5th Ed. Elk Grove Village, IL: American Academy of Pediatrics Committee on Nutrition, 2004.

Robert-McComb, J., Norman, R., and Zumwalt, M. The Active Female. Health Issues Throughout the Lifespan. Totowa, NJ: Human Press. 2008.

EXERCISE FOR SENIOR ADULTS

5

The population of individuals aged 65 and older is the fastest growing segment in the United States today. According to the Administration on Aging, this group represented 12.4% of the population in 2006. That means that one out of every eight Americans was a senior citizen! Advances in medical technology have given 65-year-olds an average life expectancy of an additional 18.5 years, so experts expect this group to comprise 20% of the total population by the year 2030. Obviously, science has managed to prolong life; now health professionals need to help seniors improve and maintain functional capacity so that quality of life remains high and health costs remain low.

The process of aging has become synonymous with anatomical and physiological deterioration. Since the body's organ systems must cooperate to maintain **homeostasis**, a decline in one system often interferes with the performance of another. Over time, this combined functional loss can interfere with all aspects of life—including physical abilities, mental well-being, emotional stability, relationships, and productivity. It is important to ask whether or not all of these changes are truly a part of the "normal" aging process. Or can individuals intervene by making lifestyle choices that slow age-associated functional decline? Furthermore, is it ever too late to begin making positive lifestyle changes?

Studies demonstrate that individuals who are active and eat nutritious foods from childhood through adulthood not only live *longer* but are also *healthier* than their sedentary, poorly nourished counterparts. Since poor diet and inactivity are two of the most modifiable threats to health, it makes sense that efforts should focus on modifying these and other lifestyle behaviors to improve the health of this nation. Consequently, the U.S. Department of Health and Human Services (HHS) established the Healthy People 2010 challenge that seeks to improve both quantity and quality of life for all Americans. In addition, every 5 years, the HHS and the U.S. Department of Agriculture jointly publish Dietary Guidelines to promote overall well-being for U.S. citizens. The 2005 Dietary Guidelines encourage healthy eating habits and increased activity for all age groups. They specifically suggest that older adults "participate in regular physical activity to reduce [the] functional declines associated with aging and to achieve the other benefits of

> **Homeostasis**—the ability of the body to maintain a relatively constant internal environment despite an ever-changing external environment. Homeostasis is crucial for optimal functioning of body cells. Examples of conditions maintained by homeostatic mechanisms include body temperature, blood pH, blood glucose level, blood calcium concentration, and stomach pH.

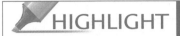 **HIGHLIGHT**   Healthy People 2010

The HHS established the Healthy People 2010 challenge to emphasize 28 areas related to the health of all Americans. The goal of Healthy People 2010 is to motivate individuals, communities, and professionals to take specific steps to eliminate health disparities and to promote health for everyone. At the writing of this book, HHS was in the process of establishing new goals for the Healthy People 2020 campaign which is designed to continue to improve health status, reduce risk, increase awareness, and deliver health services to the people of this nation.

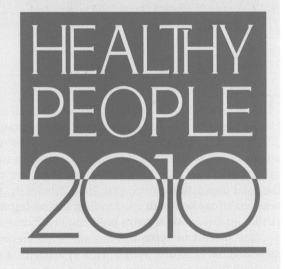

physical activity identified for all adults" such as improved well-being, maintenance of healthy weight, and reduced risk for **chronic diseases**. Interestingly, research demonstrates that benefits accrue even if individuals do not become active until late in life.

Overall, the results of countless studies suggest that physical activity provides benefits to people of all ages, even previously sedentary elderly individuals. Some studies even suggest that frail elderly patients living in nursing homes can achieve phenomenal improvements in **activities of daily living** (ADLs) by incorporating low-level exercise into their daily routines. But what are the guidelines for this population? How much is enough? How much is too much?

Over the past two decades, researchers have investigated the benefits and risks of various types, duration, and intensities of exercise for both active and previously inactive seniors. The results are overwhelming! A full appreciation of these benefits requires a basic understanding of the aging process and its impact on each body system, material that is presented in the next section. See Chapter 2 for a thorough review of the structures and functions of each body system.

ANATOMICAL AND PHYSIOLOGICAL CHANGES WITH AGE

Gerontology is the branch of science that investigates the aging process and tries to identify and control the variables that lead to functional decline. Overall, deterioration of body systems results as body cells lose their ability to function. Some experts suggest that genes dictate the rate of cellular aging and ultimately establish the length of normal cellular functioning. Other experts believe that naturally occurring metabolic reactions

---

TABLE 5-1 LIFESTYLE BEHAVIORS THAT INFLUENCE HEALTH AND BIOLOGICAL AGE

- Adequate water intake
- Eating well-balanced meals regularly
- Sleeping regularly and adequately
- Engaging in routine physical activity
- Avoiding tobacco use
- Limiting or eliminating alcohol intake
- Maintaining a healthy body weight
- Decreasing stress level

---

irreversibly alter and inhibit the ability of cells to perform normal activities. Still others suggest that exposure to environmental hazards has the greatest impact; they suggest that longevity decreases as exposure to environmental toxins increases. More than likely, a combination of all three of these factors sets into motion a sequence of events that eventually destroys body cells. The loss of cells then results in tissue deterioration; damaged tissues interfere with organ function; and malfunctioning organs ultimately weaken organ systems. As organ systems fail, homeostasis falters. Ultimately, chronic homeostatic imbalances lead to death of the organism. Thus, aging leads to death because of its cumulative effects on organ systems.

The *rate* of aging, however, is not the same for everyone. This is obvious when there are notable differences in functional capacity between two people who have the exact same **chronological age**. For example, some 65 to 70 year olds are frail and live in nursing homes, while others live independently, easily perform ADLs, and exercise daily. The observation that some people just do not seem as old as others of the same chronological age led researchers to question whether or not chronological age is a valid indicator of health, especially in those who eat well and are regularly active. Thus was born the idea of **biological age**, which suggests that lifestyle behaviors dramatically influence some aspects of aging.

People with positive lifestyle behaviors (Table 5.1) appear to be healthier than those with negative lifestyle behaviors. Fortunately for personal trainers and other health

---

Chronic diseases—conditions that develop and persist over the long term. Examples of chronic conditions common in the elderly include heart disease, cancer, type 2 diabetes, and osteoporosis.

Activities of daily living (ADLs)—activities that focus on personal care and maintenance; ADLs include eating, drinking, bathing, dressing, getting into and out of a chair, and using the toilet.

Gerontology—the branch of science that studies the causes of aging.

Chronological age—a person's age in years beginning with the date of birth.

Biological age—a concept that suggests that certain aspects of aging are under an individual's control; sometimes referred to as physiological age. Biological age looks at the level of performance of various body organs to determine their functionality. Chronological age and biological age are not necessarily the same.

professionals, studies suggest that next to smoking cessation, physical activity is *the* most influential factor in preventing or slowing many of the changes associated with aging.

AGING OF THE ORGAN SYSTEMS

Throughout life, body cells undergo **apoptosis**. This is essential for optimal functioning since older cells must be removed to make way for newer cells. When the loss of cells outpaces their replacement, however, problems result.

Humans have eleven different body systems which are composed of specialized organs that allow them to function. Since many of these organs deteriorate with advancing age, physical activity level typically declines. Therefore, to safely and effectively develop exercise programs for senior adults, fitness professionals must understand these age-related changes as well as their impact on exercise ability.

Integumentary System

The integumentary system, which includes the epidermis, dermis, hypodermis, sweat glands, oil glands, hair, nails, and nerves, acts as a protective barrier against the external environment, regulates internal body temperature, produces vitamin D, and allows for sensations. As body cells age over time, the ability to perform each of these functions slowly diminishes.

Age-related changes in the integumentary system are probably much more obvious than those associated with other body systems. After all, the skin is clearly visible all the time. Although most of these changes naturally occur with the passage of time, the *rate* at which they occur dramatically increases with excessive exposure to UV radiation. The term used to describe this advanced rate of aging is photoaging. Most of the effects of photoaging are superficial and do not interfere with activity level; however, some impair the ability to handle the stress of activity. These changes must be addressed when designing exercise programs for senior exercisers.

With age, the epidermis thins as cell activity declines. As the cell cycle slows, epidermal cells grow larger and produce a somewhat irregular keratin that results in scaly skin. The dermis also thins as the synthesis of collagen and elastin decreases. The collagen that remains begins to clump, which makes the skin prone to wrinkling. With reduced elastin, the skin is less capable of recoiling after being stretched. Observe this by gently pinching the skin on the back of an elderly person's hand. Notice how long it takes for the skin to return to normal. Now do this to a young person's hand. The skin springs back into place immediately. Moreover, subcutaneous fat in certain areas decreases, which further promotes wrinkling.

Because it thins, the integument is no longer the impenetrable barrier it once was. Pathogens can, therefore, enter the epidermis more easily and cause damage. In most instances, however, Langerhans cells destroy pathogens that actually penetrate the epidermis. Unfortunately, Langerhans cells are also destroyed by UV radiation, so as their numbers decline, risk for infection increases. Ultimately, aging skin is prone to injury, slow to repair, and susceptible to recurring skin infections. Therefore, seniors must minimize exposure to microbes and other toxins in the environment.

The number and activity of **melanocytes** also diminish with age, so skin cells become more vulnerable to UV radiation. To protect themselves, seniors should avoid excessive exposure to sunlight. Because UV radiation is necessary for the body to activate a vitamin D precursor stored in dermal blood vessels, seniors who avoid sunlight can become deficient in vitamin D. A low vitamin D level impairs calcium absorption, a condition that promotes bone loss. Minimal exposure to sunlight coupled with the fact that many seniors avoid dairy products because of lactose intolerance makes them prone to osteoporosis. Osteoporotic bone easily breaks with minimal impact, so sufferers must be careful when exercising.

With age, the number of nerve receptors in the integument declines, so sensitivity to **cutaneous stimulation** diminishes. Older people are, therefore, less responsive to pain, pressure, heat, and cold. This means that seniors might hurt themselves without even knowing it—something that could be particularly dangerous during exercise.

QUICK REFERENCE

An 85 year old has only 1/3 of the number of sensory receptors as a 20 year old.

The ability to regulate body temperature also diminishes with age. This occurs as the number of sweat glands drops, as sweat gland activity decreases, and as the number of capillaries declines, all of which interfere with the ability to evaporate sweat and radiate heat. Thus, a senior's risk for overheating during exertion is high. Additionally, seniors have difficulty retaining heat when exposed to cold environments. Because they lose deep blood vessels, their bodies cannot divert blood to deeper tissues in the cold. This, coupled with the loss of subcutaneous fat, makes it difficult for seniors to maintain a normal body temperature when temperatures drop.

QUICK REFERENCE

The loss of collagen and elastin in the dermis causes the dermis to thin. A thinning dermis coupled with a loss of subcutaneous fat on the face promotes wrinkling as the more superficial epidermis sags inward.

Apoptosis—cell death; this is a natural part of normal development, maintenance, and tissue renewal within an organism; also called programmed cell death. It should not be confused with necrosis, the pathological process that destroys otherwise healthy cells. Apoptosis appears to be intrinsically programmed; it eliminates unneeded cells and allows for "sculpting" of organs.

Melanocytes—cells that produce melanin, a pigment that protects cellular DNA from mutations caused by exposure to UV radiation.

Cutaneous sensation—the ability to sense stimuli to the skin; stimuli include light touch, pressure, pain, warmth, and cold.

Skeletal System

The skeletal system is the structural framework that supports the body. It provides attachment points for muscles and tendons, protects internal organs, acts as a lever system that assists in movement as muscles act across joints, stores and releases minerals, and houses red bone marrow, the tissue in which blood cells are synthesized.

Aging has a dramatic effect on the skeletal system. During childhood and adolescence, osteoblast activity outpaces osteoclast activity so that longer, stronger, and denser bones are formed. In early adulthood, the activity of the bone-builders slows slightly until osteoblast activity equals osteoclast activity. By middle age, osteoclast activity outpaces osteoblast activity, so there tends to be a net loss of bone tissue. As the amount of bone tissue diminishes, the risk for fracture increases (Fig. 5.1). In some instances, bones become so fragile that even a slight bump completely fractures the bone. This is common with bones of the wrist, ankle, or hip. To make matters worse, bone repair in the elderly is exceedingly slow because osteoblast activity decreases with age.

Approximately 70% of the population develops **lactose intolerance** with age. Lactose intolerance occurs when a person produces insufficient lactase, the enzyme required to break down the primary carbohydrate in dairy products. Production usually drops by 90–95%. Without lactase, most of the ingested milk product remains in the small intestine. When lactose remains in the gastrointestinal (GI) tract,

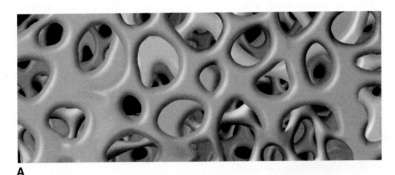

A

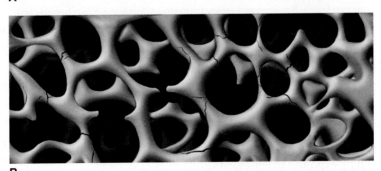

B

FIGURE 5.1 ■ Healthy spongy bone (**A**) and spongy bone with severe bone loss (**B**). (Asset provided by Anatomical Chart Co.)

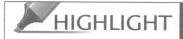
HIGHLIGHT   Osteoporosis

Osteoporosis is a condition of porous bones that can develop with inadequate nutrient intake and minimal activity. Nutrients provide the building blocks for bone remodeling, while exercise stimulates osteoblasts to deposit new bone matrix over older bone tissue. Without nutritional building blocks and mechanical stimulation, bone tissue breaks down faster than it is deposited. This disturbs the overall structure and health of bone. In men, bone loss tends to be steady and slow; however, in women, postmenopausal bone loss is rapid and proportional to the decline in estrogen. Within 5 to 10 years after menopause, women lose spongy and compact bone at a rate three to four times that of men or premenopausal women. Interestingly, by the age of 70, the rate of bone loss in men and women is approximately the same.

Osteoporosis is dangerous because osteoporotic bone is more likely to fracture during a fall. The most common sites of fracture include the vertebrae, hip, wrist, and leg. Since fractures tend to immobilize elderly people, a "simple" fracture can actually cause other body systems to deteriorate as the injured senior loses range of motion, muscle mass, and cardiovascular endurance during recovery. Spongy bone succumbs to the effects of osteoporosis more rapidly and significantly than compact bone, but both deteriorate as the disease progresses. See Chapter 8 for more information on osteoporosis prevention and treatment.

it pulls water from body cells into the **lumen** of the small intestine. The accumulation of extra water in the small intestinal lumen causes cramping and bloating. In addition, **intestinal flora** digest lactose and produce gas and acid as by-products. This promotes flatulence. Although lactose-intolerant individuals do not have to completely avoid dairy products, many sufferers greatly minimize their intake of milk and other milk derivatives. Since dairy products are the major dietary sources of calcium and

Lactose intolerance—the inability to digest lactose, a simple carbohydrate found in dairy products. Results from insufficient lactase, the enzyme that breaks down lactose. Lactose intolerance is not the same as a milk allergy in which a person reacts to the protein found in milk. During an allergic reaction, milk protein evokes an overactive immune response, which can result in death.

Lumen—a passageway, in this case through the digestive tract. Food and its by-products pass through the lumen, which opens to the external environment at both ends.

Intestinal flora—consists of microorganisms found in healthy digestive tracts. The presence of these microorganisms benefits both the microbes and the individual (or host). Bacteria make up the majority of the intestinal flora. They prevent the growth of harmful microbes, produce a small amount of usable vitamins, and metabolize remaining energy nutrients.

vitamin D, a lactose-intolerant elderly person can quickly become deficient and subsequently lose bone mass. Remember: the maintenance of blood calcium is critical, so if a dietary source is lacking, the body catabolizes bone to replenish it. This promotes the development of **osteoporosis**.

Overall, aging bone tends to lose mass and become brittle. By the age of 45, women start to lose approximately 8% of their bone mass every decade. In men, the loss begins at a later age and occurs at a slower rate. At the age of 60, men typically lose 3% of their bone mass every decade. The difference between men and women is largely due to two factors: (i) men typically develop an overall greater bone density than women during their peak bone building years and (ii) women lose bone mass more rapidly with age because of a dramatic drop in estrogen levels postmenopause. Men experience a less-dramatic drop in testosterone production much later in life (see Chapter 2 for the roles of estrogen and testosterone in bone health). Furthermore, bones begin to become brittle as the body loses its ability to produce collagen, a protein essential to bone structure. Brittle bone tissue easily breaks upon impact.

Both men and women typically lose height after the age of 30 at an average rate of 1/16 of an inch per year. A decrease in vertebral bone mass coupled with intervertebral disc deterioration accounts for this loss.

Joints exist wherever two bones meet, so this section presents some of the age-related changes in joints thought to impair a person's ability to participate in activity. Joints are classified as immoveable, slightly moveable, and freely moveable based on the range of motion (ROM) permitted at the joint. This section focuses on the slightly and freely moveable joints since they have the greatest influence on exercise.

The age-related decline in joints is usually noticeable by age 40, sometimes sooner. With age, total water content in the body diminishes, so water is pulled out of cartilage. The effect of this can be devastating. Consider the intervertebral discs, pads of fibrocartilage found in between the vertebrae of the spine. These pads permit spine flexibility and protect against friction. As they lose water, the discs compress, a condition that dramatically decreases spine flexibility. Ultimately, the entire spine stiffens, which interferes with normal daily activities.

Synovial joint function is also affected, often by age 30. Remember that articular cartilage is located on the surfaces of all articulating bones. These hyaline cartilage pads provide shock absorption during impact and minimize friction between bone surfaces. With age, articular cartilage wears away, so bones begin rubbing against one another during movements. Collagen fibers in ligaments also shorten and change orientation; this makes the ligaments less flexible and joint movements more restricted. Capillary supply to the synovial membrane drops as well, so less synovial fluid is made. This decrease in synovial fluid and the simultaneous accumulation of debris and microbes within the synovial cavity reduce overall mobility.

Sprains, bursitis, and arthritis are joint conditions common among the elderly. A *sprain* occurs when the cartilage, ligaments, or tendons associated with a joint are overstretched. Although these supporting tissues are flexible, they are not elastic, so they cannot recoil; therefore, once overstretched, they remain overstretched. Compare a ligament to a piece of taffy. Like taffy, a ligament is strong and resists stretching—up to a certain point. Once stretched beyond its capacity, it never returns to its original length.

Furthermore, if a pulling force is excessive, the ligament, like a piece of taffy, rips. Unfortunately, spraining a joint makes the joint prone to future injury, so caution is necessary in future activities. Symptoms of sprains include swelling, pain, and reduced range of motion in the short term. Most sprains respond well to rest, ice, compression, and elevation, but more serious sprains require medical attention. Active seniors seem to sprain ankles and wrists more frequently than younger people. This is likely because of impaired balance, diminished muscle mass, and shorter and tighter ligaments.

Bursitis refers to inflammation of the bursa sacs associated with joints. Often the result of overuse, bursitis is a chronic condition treated with rest, ice, compression, elevation, and sometimes steroid injections. Bursitis of the shoulder, elbow, or heel is common. Seniors with bursitis should avoid overusing the affected joint since use causes extreme tenderness, pain, and immobility.

More than 100 different forms of *arthritis* exist. Simply stated, "arthritis" means inflammation of the joints. The most common type of arthritis is osteoarthritis (Fig. 5.2A), which affects over 20 million people in the United States alone. Osteoarthritis, also known as "wear and tear" arthritis or "degenerative arthritis," occurs with the passing of time as joints are repeatedly used. Osteoarthritis affects the small joints of the hands, feet, and spine as well as weight-bearing joints such as the hips and knees. In this form of arthritis, the articular cartilage thins as it loses collagen fibers. In extreme cases, the articular cartilage completely wears away. The exact causes are unknown, but it seems to run in families. In addition, factors such as obesity, diabetes, and joint trauma increase the likelihood of developing osteoarthritis.

Rheumatoid arthritis (Fig. 5.2B) is an **autoimmune disease** that affects nearly two million people in the United States. It is three times more common in women than in men, and although it can develop at any age, its onset is typically between the ages of 40 and 60. In rheumatoid arthritis, the immune system attacks the synovial membrane at joints. As the synovial membrane degenerates, it produces a grainy synovial fluid, which actually interferes with joint movements. Imagine the damage to the articular surfaces of two bones that have a grainy fluid between them—the result would be much like rubbing sandpaper on the cartilage. The symptoms of rheumatoid arthritis come and go. More specifically, rheumatoid arthritis has an *active phase* during which the body relapses and experiences inflammation, pain, limited range of motion, and fatigue, and an *inactive phase* during which the body is in remission. Rheumatoid arthritis often affects small joints bilaterally such as those of the hands and wrists. This makes ADLs difficult—if not impossible—to perform. If inflammation is chronic, bone *and* cartilage deteriorate. Movement is limited, which can promote muscle atrophy, joint deformity, and complete loss of function.

As presented in a later section, exercise slows down joint deterioration and preserves functioning; whereas, immobility and inactivity hasten the effects of aging on this system.

Osteoporosis—a condition of porous bones; makes bone vulnerable to fracture.
Autoimmune disease—a disease that occurs when the body's immune system attacks its own cells. The precise symptoms depend upon which body cells are recognized as foreign.

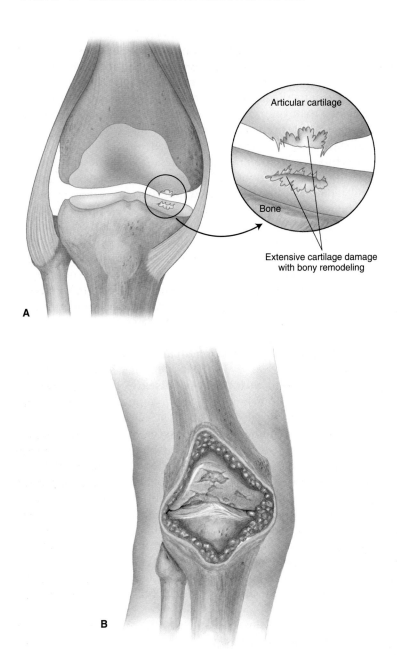

Articular cartilage

Bone

Extensive cartilage damage
with bony remodeling

A

B

FIGURE 5.2 ■ Osteoarthritis (**A**) and subsequent joint inflammation (**B**). (Modified from Werner R, Benjamin BE. A Massage Therapist's Guide to Pathology. 2nd Ed. Baltimore: Lippincott Williams & Wilkins, 2009 and an asset provided by Anatomical Chart Co.)

Muscular System

The major functions of skeletal muscle are to maintain posture, stabilize joints, move the body, and regulate body temperature. With age, all of these functions deteriorate to some extent.

Muscle fibers experience the detrimental effects of aging by the age of 30. The numbers of blood vessels, myoglobin, and mitochondria diminish, which affects the ability of slow fibers to function. Consequently, endurance suffers. The number of myofibrils drops and glycosomes disappear, which interferes with fast fiber function. This also causes a loss of muscle strength and size. Aging has the greatest effect on fast and intermediate fibers—their numbers drop significantly—so the relative proportion of slow fibers increases. As muscle mass diminishes, the relative amount of connective tissue increases, so muscles become stringier, less elastic, and less capable of contraction. All of these changes characterize **sarcopenia**, the gradual loss of muscle mass that develops as muscle proteins are broken down and not replaced. By age 80, muscle strength is half of what it used to be. Part of this decline is attributed to poor neuromuscular communication, an issue that is addressed in a later section of this chapter.

Exercise is really the only means of drastically slowing sarcopenia and preserving muscle mass. Even frail elderly people dramatically improve muscle function when they begin moderate-intensity exercise programs.

Nervous and Endocrine Systems: The Regulatory Systems

The nervous system and endocrine system regulate all other body systems. The nervous system is faster-acting and controls body activities through nerve impulse propagation. The endocrine system is somewhat slower-acting and exerts its influence with **hormones**.

The nervous system enables people to perceive and react to changes in the internal and external environment throughout a lifetime. Interestingly, individuals are born with 100 billion neurons—the maximum number of neurons they will ever have. With age, the total number of neurons drops significantly, but because of the redundancy in the central nervous system, functional decline is rarely detectable until late in life. By age 36, the average person loses 1.6 billion neurons, a loss that primarily occurs in the gray matter of the cerebral cortex. As a result, brain size decreases by an estimated 10% over an average lifetime with a greater loss of gray matter than white matter. Ultimately, this loss impairs memory, hearing, balance, vision, smell, and taste acuity.

In addition to the actual loss of neurons, the capabilities of remaining neurons diminish as the total number of dendrites drops and neurotransmitter levels decrease.

Sarcopenia—age-associated loss of muscle mass.

Hormones—usually steroid or protein molecules that elicit an effect on target cells; target cells have receptors that bind specifically with a given hormone. Hormones then alter the cell's metabolic processes by altering enzyme activity or the rate of transport of specific substances into a cell.

Neurotransmitters allow neurons to communicate with their effectors, so a loss of neurotransmitters interferes with the actions of effectors. In addition, the rate of impulse propagation along axons decreases by 5% to 10%, so reflexes and reaction times also slow. Existing neurons accumulate abnormal intracellular deposits that also interfere with functioning. Additionally, blood flow to the central nervous system drops as atherosclerosis develops in the blood vessels supplying nervous tissue. This increases the risk of stroke as insufficient oxygen and nutrients are delivered to nerve cells. A diminished fight or flight response also causes unexpected transient drops in blood pressure. This predisposes a senior to fainting spells that might result in the fracture of fragile bones. Moreover, special sensory receptors in the inner ear deteriorate, so seniors tend to lose balance and become unstable on their feet. This increases the risk for falling. Lastly, elderly individuals often develop insomnia and spend as little as two to three hours sleeping at night. This affects their ability to exercise since they feel tired and sluggish during daytime hours.

The endocrine system assists the nervous system in regulating body activities. It includes various glands that release hormones. As people age, fibrous connective tissue or fat often replace glandular tissue. Not only does this cause most endocrine organs to shrink in size, but it also interferes with hormone production and release. In many cases, hormone levels drop significantly; in others, levels exceed normal amounts. Treatment under the supervision of a physician, therefore, might involve either supplementing deficient hormones or blocking the action of excessive hormones.

The thymus gland shrinks dramatically with age. Since the thymus releases hormones necessary for the growth and maturation of certain immune cells, a drop in thymus hormones significantly decreases the number of immune cells available to fight pathogens. The result is a less effective immune response to invaders. With age, the pituitary gland produces less human growth hormone (hGH), which decreases strength of both bone and skeletal muscle. The relative concentration of antidiuretic hormone (ADH) increases with age. This stimulates the kidneys to retain water, which might cause high blood pressure. The thyroid gland produces and releases less calcitonin, which means that even when blood calcium levels are high, osteoblasts are not stimulated to build bone tissue. The parathyroid glands are most active in males at age 50; then their activity declines. In women, the parathyroid glands become increasingly active after the age of 40. Since parathyroid hormone essentially causes bone tissue to break down, a woman's more active parathyroid glands make her more prone to osteoporosis as she gets older. Although the pancreas usually continues to produce normal amounts of **insulin** and **glucagon**, aging body cells become less responsive to these hormones. As a result, seniors often have difficulty in regulating blood glucose levels. This promotes **insulin resistance,** which is characterized by rising blood glucose levels and predisposes a person to type 2 diabetes.

Melatonin is a hormone released by the pineal gland, a small endocrine organ attached to the brain. This hormone helps establish normal sleeping patterns. Typically, blood levels increase in low light and decrease in bright light. With age, melatonin release is less responsive to changes in light, so it tends to occur more evenly throughout the day. Consequently, sleeping patterns become irregular.

Cardiovascular and Respiratory Systems

The cardiovascular and respiratory systems work together to deliver oxygen to and remove carbon dioxide from body cells. The cardiovascular system consists of the heart, blood vessels, and blood. The respiratory system includes the nasal cavity, pharynx, larynx, trachea, bronchi and its numerous branches, and the alveoli.

Aging affects all three components of the cardiovascular system, but differentiating between the changes that result from "normal" aging versus those that result from the development of disease is difficult.

Blood Vessels. People are born with clear, smooth blood vessels, but fatty streaks typically develop by age ten. Over time, the blood vessel lining is damaged—perhaps from high blood pressure, cigarette smoking, or infection. This damage increases blood vessel permeability and elicits inflammation. Blood flow to the inflamed area increases. This brings additional white blood cells and basic building materials to the site to assist in damage control and repair. Simultaneously, fibrous connective tissue accumulates and calcifies in the area, thus forming raised lesions that begin a cycle of growth and regression that can last for decades. The lesions also trap circulating LDL molecules, which are then oxidized by free radicals. LDL and its cholesterol then become a part of the developing plaque. Eventually, the lesions stiffen and permanently narrow affected arteries. In the meantime, platelets migrate to the area, cover damaged tissue, and form a clot to prevent excessive bleeding. This narrows the lumen even more. In some cases, abnormal blood clotting triggers life-threatening events such as **thrombosis** or **embolism**. The severity ultimately depends upon which particular vessels are occluded. Arteries are much more prone to dangerous plaque buildup than veins because veins have relatively large

---

Insulin—a hormone released by the pancreas when blood glucose levels increase after a meal. Insulin binds with receptors on muscle, liver, and fat cells and permits the movement of glucose into these cells.

Glucagon—a hormone released by the pancreas when blood glucose levels drop in between meals. Glucagon stimulates the liver to release its glycogen to replenish blood glucose levels. It also stimulates the production of glucose from noncarbohydrate sources.

Insulin resistance—a condition where normal amounts of insulin fail to move adequate glucose into liver, muscle, or fat cells. Insulin is present, but receptors do not respond to it. As a result, the pancreas releases even more insulin, but the insulin remains ineffective. Consequently, blood glucose and insulin levels continue to rise.

Thrombosis—formation of a clot inside a blood vessel. If the clot forms and completely blocks a coronary artery, heart tissue is deprived of oxygen and dies. The clot itself is a thrombus. A thrombus usually affects arteries but might also occur in veins.

Embolism—occurs when an object, called an embolus, migrates from one part of the body and causes blockage of a blood vessel in another part of the body. An embolus usually forms in a vein. It can be a blood clot, air bubble, or fat. Symptoms might not be present; it depends on what vessel the embolus ultimately obstructs.

lumens and are not easily obstructed. Some of the most serious cases of blockage involve the coronary arteries, which supply oxygen to the heart tissue itself. In many cases, narrowing of these arteries goes unnoticed until a major coronary event occurs. Unfortunately, nearly 60% of men over the age of 60 and women over the age of 80 have at least one narrowed coronary artery.

Elastic arteries begin to lose the elastic fibers that enable them to accommodate surges of blood ejected during each heartbeat. Collagen fibers, calcium, and fat further stiffen these arteries and interfere with functioning. The loss of elasticity accompanied by vessel hardening is especially dangerous during times of strenuous exercise—affected blood vessels simply cannot withstand the added stress. In addition, small arterioles are less able to contract in the cold and dilate in the heat, so temperature regulation is impaired.

Aging also affects venous valves. Veins, which are low-pressure vessels, contain valves that prevent blood backflow and encourage movement toward the heart. Over time, valves weaken and no longer close completely—a condition that promotes blood pooling in affected segments of veins. This is especially noticeable in the superficial veins of the lower extremities. The resulting **varicose veins** are not only unsightly, but they can often be painful and itchy as well.

The total number of capillaries in the body tends to diminish with time as well. This interferes with overall oxygen and nutrient delivery to tissues. Much of this loss is associated with decreased activity, so continuing regular exercise can preserve these vessels.

Heart. With age, the elasticity of the heart wall decreases and heart valves thicken and become more rigid. The valves are up to 25% thicker at the age of 80 than they are at the age of 30. Any damaged cardiac tissue is replaced with adipose and fibrous connective tissue, tissues that impair the heart's ability to contract. Though the size of the heart might remain the same, it can increase or decrease. In most cases, the heart **atrophies**. **Hypertrophy** is typically an indication of cardiovascular disease (although the hearts of athletes tend to be larger than expected because of the training effects of routine physical activity). Although the heart enlarges in those with cardiovascular disease, cardiac output (CO) actually declines by as much as 25% over time. Interestingly, recent research suggests that CO *at rest* actually remains the same in seniors who are not suffering from cardiovascular disease; however, CO *during exercise* drops as a person ages.

Systolic blood pressure also increases with age partly because of narrowed vessels and loss of elasticity in arteries. At the same time, blood volume and total red blood cell count drop, so oxygen delivery is impaired. As a result, the heart must work even harder to supply the body with blood at rest—imagine the workload during strenuous activity.

Most of the age-related decline that occurs in the respiratory system seems to be directly proportional to a person's exposure to environmental pollutants. Those chronically exposed to poor air quality are more likely to develop respiratory problems such as emphysema, chronic bronchitis, and lung cancer than those who live in cleaner environments. Even under perfect environmental conditions, however, the coughing reflex slows as a person ages, **macrophages** in lung tissue become less effective, mucus thickens, and the number of cilia diminishes. Cumulatively, these factors interfere with respiratory system functioning.

With age, breathing requires more effort for many reasons. First, lung tissue loses elasticity as collagen fibers replace many elastic fibers. This somewhat reduces the lungs' ability to inflate and deflate. The number of **alveoli** tends to remain constant at about 300 million per lung, but alveolar walls thin and lose surface area. Hence, they are less capable of exchanging gases. Additionally, the walls of the **bronchioles** thin as they lose smooth muscle; this makes it more difficult for them to remain open. Consequently, the amount of air inhaled and exhaled per minute drops by nearly 50% between the ages of 20 and 80. The structure and functioning of the rib cage also change. In particular, the cartilage between the sternum and ribs stiffens as inflammation develops in the rib cage. This interferes with normal breathing.

In healthy people who have had minimal exposure to environmental pollutants, the effects of aging on the respiratory system are only apparent during vigorous activity. In other words, the functional decline is hardly noticeable during normal ADLs. On the other hand, seniors who have been chronically exposed to environmental pollutants experience a dramatic decline in respiratory functioning. Many seniors between the ages of 50 to 70 experience some degree of lung tissue damage because of the cumulative effects of smoking or exposure to other irritants.

Overall, a decline in respiratory functioning can significantly affect all body systems since most body cells require oxygen. Without adequate oxygen, cells, tissues, and organs ultimately cease functioning.

Lymphatic/Immune System

Without the lymphatic system, the cardiovascular system would stop working and the immune system would be seriously impaired, yet few people are aware of its importance. Unfortunately, aging has a detrimental effect on both the lymphatic and immune systems (Table 5.2).

Varicose veins—develop because of weakened venous valves. Blood pools in areas where weak valves cannot prevent backflow.

Atrophy—partial or complete loss of tissue; a decrease in size.

Hypertrophy—an increase in size because of increased cross-sectional area of a cell or organ.

Macrophage—a type of white blood cell that engulfs and digests cellular debris and pathogens; it also enhances the activity of other white blood cells.

Alveoli—microscopic air sacs with thin walls located in the lungs. The site of gas exchange in the lungs. Each lung contains millions of alveoli.

Bronchioles—the branches of the respiratory passageways that terminate in alveoli. The trachea branches into right and left primary bronchi; each primary bronchus branches into right and left secondary bronchi, which branch into tertiary bronchi, which continue to branch up to 25 times. As the walls of the respiratory passageways thin, bronchioles form and terminate into alveoli.

TABLE 5-2 EFFECTS OF AGING ON IMMUNITY
■ Increased risk of infection
■ Diminished ability to fight infection
■ Slower wound healing
■ Increased risk of developing autoimmune disorders
■ Higher rate of tumor growth and cancer development
■ Diminished effectiveness of vaccines

Organs of the lymphatic system begin changing during adolescence. After puberty, the thymus gland begins to shrink as fat and fibrous connective tissue replace most of its glandular tissue. Consequently, T cells mature at a slower rate and enter body fluids in lower numbers. The decreased availability of helper T cells not only affects the activity of cytotoxic T cells, but it also interferes with antibody production since helper T cells are required for adequate B cell proliferation and activity. Moreover, after the age of 70, people are more likely to produce auto-antibodies, antibodies that actually attack body cells. The signs and symptoms of an autoimmune disorder reflect the type of cell under attack. Examples of autoimmune diseases common in the elderly include rheumatoid arthritis, multiple sclerosis, and Graves disease.

Existing cytotoxic T cells also become less responsive to antigens, while macrophage activity slows—factors that together predispose seniors to frequent infection. Moreover, as immune surveillance wanes, tumor cells survive and proliferate, which increases the risk for cancer development. Overall, resistance diminishes by up to 50% in aging adults.

Aging not only affects specific resistance, but it also affects several aspects of nonspecific resistance. For example, surveys indicate that over 20% of adults over the age of 65 do not develop fevers even though they have severe bacterial infections. Since mild to moderate fever is actually protective, these individuals risk longer-lasting and possibly progressive symptoms of infection. Inflammation occurs frequently as arthritis, bursitis, and other inflammatory diseases develop. Wounds take longer to heal in the elderly because of atherosclerosis—a condition that limits blood flow to affected areas (Fig. 5.3). If blood flow is restricted, white blood cells and materials for repair do not arrive where needed. Blood flow, particularly blood flow to the feet, is also restricted in elderly people who have diabetes. Since the risk for diabetes increases with age, seniors must be aware of these potential complications. As blood flow decreases and sensations diminish, the risk for broken skin increases which in turn increases the risk of infection. Although a reduced blood flow inhibits spread of the infection, it also limits the effectiveness of the immune system.

To complicate the physiological age-related decline in immunity, psychosocial factors also affect a senior's resistance to disease. Surveys show that depression often accompanies aging as aging individuals lose loved ones. The surviving spouse is sometimes isolated from family and friends, a condition that increases stress level and correlates

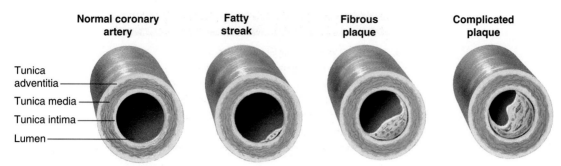

FIGURE 5.3 ■ Development of atherosclerosis. (Asset provided by Anatomical Chart Co.)

positively with impaired resistance. Addressing stress and including regular social activities might help minimize this decline in immune function.

Seniors—especially active seniors who interact with others in a fitness center or other social setting—need to get regular immunizations even though aging interferes somewhat with immunization effectiveness. The elderly account for over 80% of the deaths related to influenza, so a yearly flu shot is imperative.

> ## QUICK REFERENCE
> Medical professionals suggest that older adults receive the influenza vaccination in the form of a shot rather than in the form of a nasal spray since immune system functioning declines with age. The flu shot consists of dead viruses, whereas the nasal spray contains weakened, but live viruses that could cause symptoms in those with weakened immune systems.

Digestive System

The major function of the digestive system is to convert food into small components that can be absorbed into vessels of the cardiovascular or lymphatic system while it passes undigested material out as feces. Although aging only slightly affects the digestive system, the changes that occur are noteworthy.

Most obvious is the effect that aging has on teeth. Healthy teeth promote adequate nutrition, whereas unhealthy teeth indirectly cause major nutrient deficiencies. Why? Those with tooth deterioration or diseased gums tend to avoid nutrient-dense foods such as vegetables, fruits, grains, and meats because these foods are difficult to chew. Instead, they rely on softer products that ease ingestion, digestion, and absorption but are also kilocalorie dense and often nutrient poor. Numerous factors contribute to tooth and gum problems. As people age, tooth enamel thins after years of brushing and grinding, so the teeth become more sensitive to hot and cold. This limits the types of foods that seniors are willing to consume. Additionally, by age 35, the risk for tooth loss and periodontal disease increases. When people lose teeth, they often resort to dentures, which can make eating even more difficult. Consequently, many seniors simply skip meals.

TABLE 5-3 AGE-RELATED CHANGES IN THE GI TRACT

- Rate of cell growth in the GI tract decreases
- Linings of mouth, esophagus, and anus thin
- Peristalsis slows
- Constipation becomes more probable
- Likelihood of developing hemorrhoids increases
- Reflux develops

Medications can also affect the digestive system, and since older adults frequently take one or more medications, they often contend with various side effects. Dry mouth, mouth sores, and tooth decay are just three of the more common side effects experienced by seniors. Each of these causes eating to be painful; therefore, sufferers often limit food intake.

Less obvious are the effects of aging on the GI tract lining (Table 5.3). With years of exposure to abrasion, enzymes, and acid, the linings of the mouth, esophagus, and anus thin. The rate of new cell growth slows significantly, so nutrients are not efficiently absorbed. Digestive secretions also decrease as cells age. That means that substances necessary for nutrient processing are not available. For example, stomach cells produce less **HCl, pepsin,** and **intrinsic factor,** components needed for protein catabolism and vitamin B_{12} absorption. In addition, smooth muscle tone along the entire tract is lost, so peristalsis slows and substances remain in the GI tract lumen longer than necessary. This decreased motility, which encourages excess water absorption in the large intestine, coupled with a drop in mucus production by colon cells, promotes constipation. Constipation, in turn, increases the risk for hemorrhoids since sufferers often strain while eliminating. Loss of smooth muscle tone also interferes with sphincter functioning. Though any sphincter can be affected, the lower esophageal sphincter is frequently weakened, which promotes acid reflux. The resulting burning sensation in the chest near the heart, referred to as heartburn, is sometimes confused with a heart attack.

As the lining of the small intestine wears thin, absorption of vitamins A, D, and K and the mineral zinc decreases. Insufficient vitamin A impairs vision and promotes skin lesions; low levels of vitamin D weaken bones; a deficiency of vitamin K interferes with blood clotting; and insufficient zinc slows wound healing (which is already a problem in the senior population).

The risk and severity of lactose intolerance increase with age. Statistics suggest that 70% of the over-40 population experiences some degree of lactose intolerance because their lactase is 90% to 95% less active than when they were younger. Consequently, sufferers often avoid dairy products and are therefore at risk for calcium, vitamin D, and riboflavin deficiencies.

The risk of colon and stomach cancer increase with age, so the digestive functions of these two organs are also impaired. In addition, olfactory neurons become less sensitive to smell, while taste buds become less sensitive to tastes—changes that make eating less

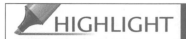

HIGHLIGHT   Lactose Intolerance

Lactose intolerance results from a deficiency of lactase, the enzyme needed to digest the monosaccharide found in milk products. Lactose intolerance has its onset at birth because it usually results from a genetic predisposition to produce insufficient lactase. Lactose intolerance, however, can also result from any disease, surgery, or drug that destroys the intestinal lining or interferes with lactase production or action. Additionally, research finds that the likelihood of developing lactose intolerance increases with age.

The problem with undigested lactose is that it remains in the intestines and attracts water from intestinal cells. Excess water in the intestinal lumen promotes diarrhea. Additionally, the "helpful" bacteria that reside in the intestines ferment lactose and produce gas as a by-product. All of this promotes the cramping, bloating, diarrhea, and gas associated with lactose intolerance. The symptoms can persist for 12 to 48 hours because it takes that long for chyme to pass through the intestines.

Lactose-intolerant individuals who consume fairly small "doses" of lactose might experience no symptoms at all and therefore be unaware of their deficiency. Others who consume larger "doses" of lactose might experience severe symptoms and therefore avoid all foods that provoke a reaction. Strict avoidance of lactose-containing foods usually leads to insufficient calcium and vitamin D intake—nutrients necessary for healthy bones. This can encourage significant bone loss. Fortunately, those who are lactose intolerant typically manage their condition by making careful dietary selections. Rarely do sufferers have to avoid milk products altogether. Instead, they can gradually determine their own tolerable upper intake level. Additional tips include the following:

■ Consume dairy products in moderation
■ Eat other types of food along with milk products
■ Take enzyme tablets with meals
■ Consume foods enriched with enzymes
■ Consume fermented products such as yogurt or acidophilus milk, which contain bacteria that digest lactose
■ Read food labels since many products, such as breads, cereals, salad dressings, and prescription drugs, contain lactose.

Because the symptoms of lactose intolerance resemble the symptoms of several other more serious conditions, those who suspect lactose intolerance should seek diagnosis by a physician.

HCl—hydrochloric acid; produced by cells in the stomach. Denatures proteins in the stomach.
Pepsin—a protein-digesting enzyme secreted by stomach cells.
Intrinsic factor—a substance secreted by stomach cells; necessary for vitamin B_{12} absorption.

desirable. Although age also affects the accessory organs of digestion, these changes have little effect on digestion and absorption.

Overall, age-related changes in the digestive system interfere with food consumption, a factor that affects energy level and ultimately limits exercise ability. Thus, personal trainers should consider these factors when working with the senior population.

Urinary System

The urinary system filters blood to form urine and transports and stores urine prior to elimination. Overall, the goal is to maintain fluid and electrolyte balance while eliminating wastes. As with other body systems, the urinary system is affected by aging. In general, aging kidneys become less adept at removing nitrogenous wastes and toxins from blood. This means that waste products accumulate in body fluids. Superficially, fibrous connective tissue forms around the kidneys as kidney size diminishes. Kidney tissue actually begins to deteriorate at the age of 20, but the loss in size is usually not noticeable until the age of 40. By age 80, the kidneys are approximately half their former size!

As the kidneys age, nephrons are lost. In fact, between the ages of 40 and 70, the kidneys lose 30% to 40% of all nephrons as glomeruli atrophy. The consequence is a drop in glomerular filtration rate (GFR) that begins at age 40. By age 75, GFR is half the rate it was at age 25. It falls from approximately 125 mL per minute to only 60 mL per minute. Granted, drugs such as nonsteroidal antiinflammatory drugs and ACE inhibitors contribute to this decline in GFR, but aging alone affects it as well. Any remaining glomeruli become leakier, so proteins, which are not normally filtered, enter the tubules and become a part of urine. About 33% of the elderly population, therefore, has proteinuria. By age 20, the rate of blood flow to the kidneys begins to diminish by about 1% per year. Simultaneously, renal blood vessels lose their ability to dilate and constrict, and renin release decreases.

The reabsorption of water, sodium, glucose, and other useful substances also drops as the renal tubules thicken and become fattier. The inability to reabsorb water increases the frequency of urination as more water passes into the urinary bladder. The secretion of certain drugs including aspirin and nonsteroidal antiinflammatories slows, so they can linger in the blood and become more potent as people age.

Age-related changes also occur in the urinary bladder, ureters, and urethra. As the urinary bladder loses elasticity, it holds less than half its normal volume. Voiding is often incomplete, so urine can remain in the urinary bladder after elimination and result in a persistent urge to void. Unfortunately, seniors become less perceptive of this urge while the sphincters regulating urination also weaken with time. Combined, these factors can result in embarrassing incidences of leakage or perhaps even complete incontinence. In fact, some degree of incontinence affects nearly 20% of women over the age 65 and nearly 50% of men over the age of 65.

Reproductive System

The basic functions of the male and female reproductive systems are to produce gametes and hormones. The focus here is on the effects of aging on hormone production since the hormones produced by the reproductive systems affect both muscle and bone health.

Male Reproductive System. Unlike women, men do not experience a sudden change in reproductive system functioning. The most significant change occurs as testes tissue is lost. Testosterone levels, however, remain fairly stable. Since testosterone promotes healthy bone and muscle, both bone tissue and muscle tissue remain relatively strong. As the tubes within the testes lose elasticity, the rate of sperm production slows somewhat, but men remain fertile until late in life. Some of the surface cells on the seminal vesicles and prostate gland die, but these glands continue to produce normal amounts of fluid. A number of changes can occur in the prostate gland. In addition to experiencing an elevated risk for prostate cancer, about 50% of men develop an enlarged prostate gland as fibrous tissue replaces glandular tissue. This condition is called benign prostatic hypertrophy (BPH); it can significantly interfere with urination and ejaculation. Some men experience a loss of sex drive or impaired sexual response, but this is typically due to a preexisting condition such as high blood pressure, illness, or medication, not decreased testosterone levels.

Female Reproductive System. Many of the age-related changes in the female body are caused by changes in estrogen levels.

In addition to maintaining female secondary sex characteristics, the different types of estrogen contribute to tissue elasticity and strength. This is apparent when considering aging skin—the skin weakens and wrinkles as estrogen levels drop. In addition, low estrogen levels inflame the gums; loosen teeth; and cause throat dryness, hoarseness, and subtle changes in voice pitch. Low estrogen also correlates with serious conditions such as heart disease and stroke. For instance, cardiovascular disease is responsible for 30% to 50% of deaths in postmenopausal women. With estrogen supplements, however, the incidences of heart attack and stroke decrease by 25% to 50%, while the number of deaths due to heart attack and stroke drops by 50%. Researchers believe that estrogen therapy is beneficial because estrogen lowers blood pressure, dilates arterial walls, improves CO, and reduces the risk of blood clots. It might even decrease total cholesterol level and improve the overall blood lipid profile.[1] In addition, estrogen slows bone loss by inhibiting **osteoclast** activity. Since estrogen is necessary to preserve bone tissue, a decrease in bone mass typically results as estrogen levels decline with age. This increases the risk of developing osteoporosis, particularly in postmenopausal women. Osteoporosis is dangerous because it makes bone vulnerable to fracture during a fall. After menopause, women lose up to 3% of their bone mass per year for the first five years. This rate slows to about 1% to 2% per year thereafter. Since nearly 300,000 osteoporotic women go to the hospital annually for broken bones (with 20% dying within one month after a fall), this is a serious problem. Estrogen replacement therapy can prevent the calcium depletion that often follows menopause, as can weight-bearing exercise and appropriate calcium intake.

Not well understood is the link between low estrogen levels and declining immune function. It appears that immune cells are less effective against pathogens as estrogen drops, so postmenopausal women seem to be more susceptible to infection and disease.

Osteoclast—bone cells that break down bone tissue.

Among its many functions, progesterone assists estrogen in maintaining bone health. Rather than inhibiting bone-destroying cells, however, progesterone stimulates bone-building cells. In addition, progesterone promotes the release of fat, normalizes blood glucose levels, and helps eliminate excess body fluid. Since progesterone is primarily produced by the ovaries, its levels drop as the ovaries age. The adrenal glands continue to produce small amounts of progesterone, but levels never reach premenopausal levels.

Age-related changes in ovary structure and hormone levels also affect the monthly cycle. The monthly cycle begins at puberty and typically continues at regular intervals up until the age of 40 to 50, at which time the average woman undergoes menopause. Menopause occurs as the number of follicles in the ovaries drops, as the remaining follicles become less sensitive to the effects of **pituitary hormones** (FSH and LH), and as ovulation becomes irregular and then ceases. Muscles in the pelvic area lose tone, and ligaments that support the reproductive organs stretch, so the uterus, urinary bladder, and vagina might **prolapse**. Prolapse can cause stress incontinence, an embarrassing condition of urine leakage. To complicate matters, the urinary bladder itself, along with the sphincters that regulate urine flow, weaken—this increases the frequency and urgency of urination. Lastly, yeast infections become more likely because the environment in the vaginal canal changes. Since glandular secretions decrease, this area becomes less acidic and more favorable to microorganisms.

Nearly 50% of menopausal women experience symptoms that interfere with normal activities. **Hot flashes** are common and last from 30 seconds to 10 minutes each. Migraine headaches, fatigue, mood swings, difficulty sleeping and concentrating, sore joints, increased muscle tension, incontinence (particularly upon sneezing or coughing), and GI tract distress are additional complications. Of course, some of these symptoms suggest other disorders such as hypothyroidism, diabetes, or clinical depression, so perimenopausal women experiencing these should seek guidance from a physician.

PRECAUTIONS DURING EXERCISE

All exercisers should practice safe techniques since there are inherent risks in any physical activity. In general, well-conditioned seniors who have been active for most of their lives can continue participating in activities to which they are accustomed. Frequency, intensity, and duration likely need adjusting, but the active person can typically continue a relatively normal exercise regimen well into old age. Previously sedentary exercisers, however, must be more careful because their organ systems typically decline at a faster rate than the organ systems of active people. In either case, special concerns for older exercisers include their impaired body temperature regulation, limited joint movement, decreased lean tissue, loss of balance, and loss of cardiorespiratory functioning (Table 5.4).

INABILITY TO REGULATE BODY TEMPERATURE

Metabolism is the sum of all chemical reactions that occur in the body. It includes processes that build as well as processes that break down. A natural by-product of metabolism is heat; therefore, anything that increases metabolic rate also increases heat production. The liver, kidneys, and skeletal muscle are the most metabolically active organs in the

TABLE 5-4 EFFECTS OF AGING ON BODY SYSTEM FUNCTIONING	
Variable	**Change**
Resting heart rate	Remains the same
Maximal heart rate	Decreases
Maximal CO	Decreases
Resting and exercise blood pressure	Increases
VO_{2max}	Decreases
Residual volume	Increases
Reaction time	Decreases
Muscular strength	Decreases
Flexibility	Decreases
Bone mass	Decreases
Fat-free body mass	Decreases
Percent body fat	Increases
Glucose tolerance	Decreases
Recovery time	Increases

Adapted from ACSM

body. Since muscle contraction increases during activity, skeletal muscle is a major contributor to the body heat generated during exercise. Consequently, active individuals must be able to efficiently eliminate heat to prevent dangerous increases in body temperature.

As mentioned earlier, the ability to regulate body temperature diminishes with age. **Evaporative cooling**, which occurs as sweat vaporizes from the skin surface, is less effective because the number of sweat glands decreases. Furthermore, all remaining sweat glands are less active and thereby produce less sweat overall. Additionally, **radiative cooling** is not as efficient because the total number of capillaries in the body decreases

---

Pituitary hormones—include follicle-stimulating hormone (FSH) and luteinizing hormone (LH). These hormones influence follicle growth rate, progesterone production, and ovulation.

Prolapse—occurs when an organ or structure slips out of its usual position; typically because of weakened support muscles or overstretched ligaments; often involves the uterus or urinary bladder.

Hot flash—a sensation of extreme heat in the face, neck, and upper body that lasts for up to 10 minutes at a time; often accompanied by severe sweating and chills.

Evaporative cooling—occurs at the skin surface as sweat changes from a liquid to a gas. A large amount of heat is carried into the atmosphere during vaporization.

Radiative cooling—the primary means of body heat loss; occurs as blood vessels in the dermis dilate. This transports blood from deeper tissues to the skin surface. Infrared heat rays escape from warm blood to the cooler environment.

with age. Combined, these factors promote heat retention during activity and a subsequent rise in internal body temperature. A senior exerciser must, therefore, lower intensity, exercise in a relatively cool environment, and continuously rehydrate.

Seniors who exercise in cold environments are also at risk. When the body is subjected to cold temperatures, blood vessels in the extremities constrict, while blood vessels in deeper tissues dilate. This diverts blood from the body surface for two primary purposes. First, it reduces the amount of heat lost through radiation. Second, it ensures that major organs like the brain, heart, and kidneys continue to receive adequate blood. Both of these actions are critical for maintaining life. As people age, they lose blood vessels throughout the body, including those that supply deep tissues. This means that seniors cannot as effectively divert blood to deeper tissues when temperature drops. This, coupled with the loss of subcutaneous fat, makes it difficult for seniors to retain heat in cold environments.

LOSS OF ROM

The flexibility permitted by a given joint is specific to that joint, so limited ROM at one joint does not necessarily affect ROM at another joint; however, as increasingly more joints become less mobile, regular ADLs become difficult. If movement is restricted for too long, muscles atrophy, joints deform, and functional ability diminishes.[2,3]

Although time takes its toll on joints, joints tend to age slowly. The spine loses flexibility and eventually stiffens. The cartilage at the ends of long bones wears away. And synovial fluid production decreases. This restricts movement and makes bone vulnerable during impact. Additionally, collagen fibers in ligaments shorten and change orientation, factors that further limit joint flexibility. These changes, coupled with loss of balance and muscle strength, increase the risk for sprained ankles, sprained wrists, bursitis, and arthritis—injuries common among seniors. To minimize risk to clients, fitness professionals should design exercise routines that involve simple yet challenging activities. They should avoid overusing joints as this can worsen inflammatory conditions. Although exercise sometimes improves symptoms of inflammation in the long term, it can exacerbate symptoms in the short term—particularly during flare-ups. Make adjustments based on individual client needs while striving to prevent further decline.[2,3]

QUICK REFERENCE

The typical sedentary individual shows a 20% to 30% decline in overall flexibility by the age of 70.

DECREASE IN LEAN TISSUE

Age-related sarcopenia generally begins at the age of 45; it results in a 1% decrease in muscle mass per year. Accompanying this loss of muscle mass is a loss in strength—

particularly in the back and leg muscles. This substantially weakens joints since muscle tone is the greatest contributor to joint stability. In addition, the number of neurons innervating skeletal muscles decreases, while recruitment ability diminishes. Both of these factors further decrease muscle strength. Between the ages of 60 and 70, average seniors lose 15% of their strength; this accelerates to a loss of nearly 30% between the ages of 70 and 80. Even a minor loss in strength begins a vicious cycle: seniors lose strength and cannot easily perform normal activities; therefore, they avoid difficult activities; this leads to further losses in strength. Before they know it, they are unable to perform even the simplest tasks such as walking around the house, doing laundry, or putting away groceries. Continued muscle loss promotes gait disturbances, muscle imbalance, immobility, and an increased risk of falling.[4]

Sarcopenia can occur in anyone, no matter how fit that person is. Physically inactive people, however, experience the most dramatic and rapid losses in both muscle mass and strength. The best means of preventing sarcopenia is to incorporate resistance exercises into a consistent exercise program.

Muscle is not the only lean tissue at risk. Bone tissue not subjected to mechanical stress also wastes away. As mentioned earlier, bone undergoes a continual process called remodeling where old bone tissue is replaced with new bone tissue. As people age, there tends to be a net loss of bone tissue during remodeling. As bone mass declines, bones weaken and become prone to fractures. Since fractures in the elderly heal slowly and poorly, a broken bone often means an extended stay in bed, which can result in further bone and muscle loss.

LOSS OF BALANCE

Loss of balance is dangerous because it increases the likelihood of falling. Falling is hazardous because it often results in bone breakage, joint dislocation, and acute ligament and tendon damage.

Balance issues develop because of changes in the musculoskeletal and neuromuscular systems. Muscle tone diminishes, joints weaken, range of motion (ROM) decreases, and overall stability wanes. Seniors are prone to fainting spells because of transient drops in blood pressure that result from a diminished fight or flight response. Special sensory receptors in the inner ear responsible for equilibrium and balance also deteriorate, so seniors tend to become unstable on their feet. Combined, these factors promote balance problems in the senior exerciser and must be considered when developing exercise program for older clients.

LOSS OF CARDIORESPIRATORY FUNCTIONING

The age-related decline in both cardiovascular and respiratory functioning can greatly affect exercise capacity, particularly in previously sedentary individuals. With age, the heart's ability to circulate blood diminishes as both heart size and volume capacity drop. A decrease in sympathetic nerve activity to the heart results in a lower maximal heart rate,

TABLE 5-5 COMMON BARRIERS AND MOTIVATORS TO EXERCISE IN THE SENIOR ADULT	
Barriers to Exercise	**Motivators to Exercise**
Time constraints	Independence to perform ADLs
Fear of injury	Improved stamina
Lack of skills and abilities	Improved appearance
Poor health	Maintenance of joint mobility
Limited transportation	Improved sleep
Anticipated discomfort	Maintenance of muscle and bone mass
Limited income	

weaker contractions, and a decreased **ejection fraction**. Reduced elasticity of major blood vessels tends to elevate blood pressure. Simultaneously, the alveoli in the lungs become less capable of gas exchange, while lung tissue itself loses elasticity. Overall, **maximal oxygen uptake**, or VO_{2max}, declines at a rate of 3% to 8% per decade after the second decade of life.[5] Factors other than age, however, account for 84% of that decline. The primary contributor is loss of lean muscle mass, so if people maintain lean muscle mass, the rate of decline slows dramatically. This offers a great deal of promise to the elderly.

Overall, elderly exercisers need to be careful when participating in exercise. With impairments in both the cardiovascular system and the respiratory system, capacity diminishes. Fitness professionals, however, can still provide challenging workouts with minimal risks.

BARRIERS TO EXERCISE

Several barriers prevent older adults from participating in daily activity. Some seniors are simply unaware that exercise is safe and effective for their age group. Others have a fear of the unknown that prevents them from joining a fitness center or seeking out exercise advice even though they know they should. Health and fitness professionals need to be aware of and address these concerns if they want to persuade seniors to adopt healthier lifestyles.[6] Table 5.5 shows additional barriers as well as motivators for exercise.

BENEFITS OF EXERCISE

Despite the fact that exercise provides benefits to all age groups, few seniors engage in regular physical activity. According to data from the HHS, only 31% of individuals aged 65 to 74 participate in 20 minutes of moderate physical activity on three or more days per week. Sixteen percent are slightly more active; they engage in 30 minutes of moderate activity on 5 or more days per week. Unfortunately, only 23% of those 75 years or older continue moderate activity for 20 minutes on 3 or more days per week.

TABLE 5-6 COMMON RISK FACTORS FOR CHRONIC DISEASE
■ Cigarette smoking
■ Hypertension
■ High total cholesterol
■ Obesity
■ Sedentary lifestyle
■ Diet high in saturated fats
■ Diet low in whole grains, fruits, and vegetables

As mentioned earlier, senior adults perceive several barriers to exercise and often intentionally avoid it because of associated risks. Empowering this group with knowledge about the *benefits* of exercise is essential in trying to overcome the barriers.

Although older clients present challenges to the fitness professional, they reap considerable benefits from regular exercise. In fact, several studies show that the improvements seen in older exercisers match those seen in younger exercisers, so it is never too late to become active. Over time, as these benefits accrue, the senior exerciser maintains—and probably even improves—functional capacity. Ideally, it is best for individuals to participate in regular exercise throughout life; however, research demonstrates that initiating an exercise program at any age provides substantial benefits with minimal risks. The sooner a person begins exercising, the better the outcome. The following section discusses some of the specific benefits experienced by senior exercisers.

REDUCED RISK FOR CHRONIC DISEASE AND BETTER MANAGEMENT OF EXISTING HEALTH CONDITIONS

Chronic diseases, responsible for most deaths in the United States today, are typically caused by various factors known as **risk factors** (Table 5.6).[7] People seldom have only one risk factor for a given disease; instead, risk factors tend to cluster. The more risk factors a person has, the greater the chance of developing the disease.

Ejection fraction—the amount of blood pumped out of the left ventricle during each heart beat. A higher ejection fraction suggests a healthier heart. A normal ejection fraction is 50% to 70%.

Maximal oxygen uptake—also known as VO_{2max}. The maximum amount of oxygen the body takes in and utilizes. VO_{2max} is linearly related to energy expenditure, so it provides an indirect measure of a person's maximal aerobic capacity.

Risk factor—a behavior or condition that increases the likelihood of developing a disease. Risk factors do not necessarily cause disease, but they are positively correlated with development.

The number one preventable risk factor for chronic disease is cigarette smoking. Thus, smoking cessation would have a greater affect on health and longevity than any other behavior change. After smoking cessation, increased physical activity likely has the greatest potential to improve health and reduce the risk for chronic disease. Increased activity independently improves risk profile, but a more active lifestyle also reduces the effects of several other risk factors. For instance, regular activity promotes a healthy weight, better long-term control of blood pressure, an increased HDL level, and decreased LDL and total cholesterol levels. All of these also improve heart, lung, and blood vessel health, which reduces chronic disease risk.

Consistent physical activity also helps manage *preexisting conditions* such as cardiovascular disease, diabetes, hypertension, and high blood cholesterol levels.[8] Regular aerobic activities improve heart health by slowing resting heart rate and increasing stroke volume and ejection fraction—factors that reduce the heart's workload. As little as two hours of moderate exercise per week lowers systolic blood pressure, resting heart rate, and body weight, while it increases grip strength and peak exercise capacity.[9] Even seniors suffering from **peripheral artery disease** experience a reduced risk of cardiovascular-related deaths.[10] The MacArthur Study of Successful Aging concurs—it found that subjects facing various chronic conditions experienced protective effects from increased activity.

TABLE 5-7 SYMPTOMS OF CORONARY ARTERY DISEASE

- Chest pain (angina)
- Shortness of breath
- General weakness and fatigue
- Palpitations of the heart
- Lightheadedness

Through its effects on the **blood lipid profile**, exercise helps maintain healthy blood vessels and reduces the risk for atherosclerosis. Atherosclerosis, or the buildup of plaque on arterial wall linings, is life threatening when it affects the coronary arteries that supply the heart. As these arteries narrow, oxygen and nutrient delivery to cardiac tissue decreases. If deprived of oxygen for too long, heart cells eventually die. Since heart cells are unable to repair themselves, they are replaced by fibrous tissue, which cannot contract. Table 5.7 shows the symptoms of coronary artery disease. By improving overall artery health, exercise also reduces the risk for hypertension, heart attack, and stroke.

Exercise also prevents excessive weight gain, a factor associated with the development of type 2 diabetes. In a healthy person, blood glucose levels rise and fall gradually after a meal because of insulin activity. Insulin, a hormone produced by the pancreas when blood glucose levels rise, essentially binds to receptors on **target cells** to allow glucose to enter. If insulin does not bind with its receptor, glucose cannot enter cells, so it accumulates in the blood. This presents two major problems. First, cells can literally starve to death even when blood glucose levels are high since the cells cannot access this glucose. Second, excess glucose in the blood makes blood more viscous, a factor that can damage small blood vessels in the eyes, kidneys, heart, and nerves.

Two types of diabetes exist. Type 1 diabetes occurs when pancreatic cells are unable to produce insulin. Type 1 diabetics, therefore, require an external insulin source so that body cells can access blood glucose to make ATP. Type 2 diabetes is more common than Type 1 diabetes. It frequently develops in overweight or obese people who often continue to produce adequate insulin. The problem is that their insulin receptors cannot bind it. Experts are not sure why this happens, but some think that excess fat alters the shape of insulin receptors, which makes them unable to recognize insulin. If insulin cannot bind to its receptor, body cells are deprived of glucose and blood glucose levels remain elevated.

Peripheral artery disease—a condition that primarily affects peripheral circulation in the legs and feet, causing pain and tingling in the extremities during activity. Results from the accumulation of fatty deposits that block arteries and interfere with blood circulation. Studies show it can be managed and likely prevented with exercise.

Blood lipid profile—blood tests that indicate a person's risk for cardiovascular disease.

Target cells—cells throughout the body that have receptors for a given hormone

Fortunately, Type 2 diabetics can often manage their condition through diet and exercise. These lifestyle changes promote weight management and minimize insulin resistance. With weight loss, insulin receptors usually return to their normal shape, which enables normal functioning.

According to the American Diabetes Association, over 65% of people with diabetes die from heart disease or stroke at a younger age than the general population. Since seniors are already at an increased risk for death from heart disease and stroke, diabetic seniors have serious health concerns.

IMPROVED FUNCTIONAL CAPACITY

Just like younger exercisers, senior exercisers experience improvements in cardiovascular endurance, muscular strength, muscular endurance, and flexibility—factors that *enhance functional capacity* and *decrease the risk for falls*. Maintaining functional capacity improves the ability to perform basic ADLs (Table 5.8) as well as more challenging activities. The more ADLs seniors independently perform, the more active they can be. In other words, exercise preserves functional capacity in the aged and helps maintain independence regardless of existing health problems. In fact, a 14-year study of 74-year-old women found that women who were consistently active had the best functional capacity, while women who were consistently sedentary had the worst functional status.[11–14]

Since seniors have an increased risk for falls because of diminished muscle mass, weakened joints, and loss of balance, exercise should be considered a primary fall-reduction strategy. Not only does it increase muscular strength and joint stability, but it also improves balance.

As mentioned earlier, the average person begins losing muscle mass at the age of 30. Initially, the rate of loss is slow, but it increases progressively with time and ultimately reaches nearly 40% over the course of a lifetime. Strength losses accompany mass losses—both of which interfere with physical performance and increase risk for injury during normal daily activities. Numerous studies show that resistance training slows atrophy and increases muscle mass in frail elderly individuals. In fact, frail elderly subjects who participated in a 10-week resistance-training program had a 189% increase in knee extension strength and an 87% increase in hip extension strength. This is remarkable given that the

TABLE 5-8   ACTIVITIES OF DAILY LIVING

- Feeding oneself
- Bathing oneself
- Dressing
- Grooming
- Independent use of the toilet
- Moving from a chair to the bed
- Working
- Homemaking

group of subjects lived in an institution and participated minimally in additional activities. Surprisingly, musculoskeletal injuries were rare during the duration of this study; only one participant discontinued the prescribed exercise because of musculoskeletal problems.[4,15,16]

Muscle function also improves because of better communication between the muscular and nervous systems. Neurons control muscle fibers, so the more motor units stimulated during a muscle contraction, the stronger the force. Physical training enhances recruitment ability, a factor that often accounts for strength increases during the initial two to three weeks of training in all exercisers.

Consistent aerobic training improves coordination between the cardiovascular and respiratory systems. When physically challenged, these organ systems become more efficient at transporting gases to and from tissues, so demands placed on them become easier. The resulting adaptations allow the physically fit person to participate in activities for a longer duration and at a higher intensity. This is often surprising to seniors who claim that they avoided exercise for years because of frequent and unexplained fatigue! Furthermore, studies indicate that lung function and lung capacity improve as much with moderate activities like walking as they do with more strenuous activities like jogging.[17,18]

FLEXIBILITY AND BALANCE

Use it or lose it—how true this is! People lose flexibility as they grow older, become more sedentary, and fail to move their joints through a full range of motion. Most forms of physical activity—whether cardiovascular training, resistance training, or stretching exercises—improve range of motion *as long as joints are moved through their normal ranges.* Maintaining this full range of motion results in improved functional capacity and decreased risk for injury. Additionally, activity stimulates synovial fluid production, promotes ligament and tendon pliability, and maintains muscle elasticity—all of which increase joint mobility.

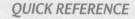

QUICK REFERENCE

According to the Centers for Disease Control and Prevention, nearly 15,000 people aged 65 and older died from falls in 2004, while close to 1.9 million were treated for fall-related injuries in emergency rooms.

Numerous studies suggest that physical activity decreases the risk of falling through its influence on balance. Consequently, many exercise programs targeted toward seniors now focus specifically on balance training. In many cases, they emphasize disciplines such as yoga, Pilates, and Tai Chi.[19] These modes of exercise improve coordination, breathing, core strength, and concentration—areas in which seniors are often deficient. They also lower blood pressure and enhance quality of sleep. Thus, combining strength exercises with balance exercises provides optimal benefits. In fact, studies show that the cumulative effects of strength and balance training are even greater than the effect of either alone.

Not only does the combination decrease the likelihood of falling, but it also increases self-confidence and improves self-esteem.

QUICK REFERENCE

A 1996 study at the Emory University School of Medicine in Atlanta found that seniors aged 70 and older who participated in a 15-week Tai Chi program reduced their risk of falling by more than 47%.

IMPROVED MENTAL HEALTH (PSYCHOLOGICAL BENEFITS)

Although researchers do not fully understand the mechanism, studies show a correlation between increased activity and better mood, improved self-confidence, elevated self-esteem, and enhanced cognitive functioning. First of all, physical activity stimulates the release of endorphins—the body's own mood-enhancing substances. Second, it decreases blood levels of cortisol, a hormone released during stressful times and thought to increase feelings of anxiety.[20] Several studies indicate that cardiovascular exercise in particular produces the greatest psychological effect, especially in those who have been exercising intensely and frequently for at least 10 weeks.[21]

In a study conducted at Duke University, researchers found that a significant number of elderly patients formerly diagnosed with major depressive disorder were no longer depressed after 16 weeks of exercise and that the effect of exercise therapy alone equaled the effect of exercise combined with drug therapy. One possible explanation for this is that 'exercise therapy' gives patients a sense of control over their outcome. It provides an active solution to the problem; whereas, taking a pill is passive. This is not meant to imply that all cases of depression can be treated without medication. It simply suggests that in *some* cases, increasing activity level improves mood and enhances psychological profile; however, this is not a guaranteed outcome for every depressed individual.[22]

TABLE 5-9   SUMMARY OF THE BENEFITS OF EXERCISE IN SENIOR ADULTS

- Lower risk of coronary heart disease and stroke
- Lower risk of hypertension
- Lower risk of diabetes
- Lower risk of overweight and obesity
- Lower risk of falls and subsequent injury
- Lower risk of some cancers (possibly colon and breast cancer)
- Improved self-esteem, elevated mood, and reduced incidence of depression
- Improved quality of life with a possible increase in lifespan
- Improved sleep, both quality and quantity

Data from the Centers of Disease Control and Prevention suggest that 28% to 34% of adults aged 65 to 74 are completely inactive. Forty-four percent of adults over the age of 75 engage in absolutely no leisure time activity, with women being less active than men. Since they can derive significant benefits from exercise, it is important to appeal to members of this population (Table 5.9).

RECOMMENDATIONS FOR EXERCISE TESTING AND EXERCISE PRESCRIPTION

People who participate in regular exercise programs throughout their lives typically continue activity into their later years. They usually modify frequency, duration, intensity, and type of activity, but essentially, their conditioned bodies are able to tolerate the challenge imposed by physical activity. What about previously sedentary seniors who want to initiate an exercise program? How do they begin?

> ### QUICK REFERENCE
>
> According to American College of Sports Medicine (ACSM), the term "older adult" refers to people who are ≥65 years old or those who are 50 to 64 years old and have clinically significant conditions or physical limitations that affect their ability to participate in activity.[23]

Exercise is potentially dangerous for the elderly population because many seniors suffer from preexisting conditions that place the body under stress. In addition, organ systems deteriorate over time, so adding exercise to the mix might put a senior at greater risk for both acute and chronic injuries. Controlled studies, however, indicate that exercise *benefits* rather than harms the senior adult. This section addresses general recommendation for senior exercisers.

The American College of Sports Medicine (ACSM) and the American Heart Association (AHA) have established screening criteria for the aging population.[23–26] Since risk for chronic disease increases with age, fitness professionals must screen potential clients for symptoms associated with cardiovascular, pulmonary, and metabolic diseases (Table 5.10). This helps determine who needs medical clearance from a physician prior to initiating an exercise program and who may begin exercising without clearance. Chapter 2 of *ACSM's Guidelines for Exercise Testing and Prescription*, 8th Ed. provides further information regarding risk stratification guidelines.

Overall, both ACSM and AHA concur that previously sedentary senior exercisers should obtain medical clearance from a physician before participating in *maximal* exercise testing or *vigorous* exercise. This includes men over the age of 45 and women over the age of 55 or anyone under the age of 45 who has risk factors for cardiovascular disease; however, "apparently healthy seniors," or those with no other risk factors, may participate in *submaximal* exercise testing and *low-to-moderate* exercise without clearance from a physician.[23–26]

TABLE 5-10 RISK FACTORS ASSOCIATED WITH CARDIOVASCULAR, PULMONARY, OR METABOLIC DISEASE
■ Chest, neck, jaw, or arm pain
■ Shortness of breath at rest or with mild exertion
■ Irregular, rapid, or fluttery heart beat
■ Dizziness
■ Inability to breathe easily unless sitting up or standing straight
■ Swollen ankles
■ Intermittent claudication
■ Unusual fatigue with usual activities
■ Known heart murmur

Source: ACSM's Guidelines for Exercise Testing and Prescription.

EXERCISE TESTING

According to ACSM, various test protocols exist for the senior population. For the generally healthy senior, standard testing procedures with slight modifications are suitable. Specialized tests have also been developed for frail elderly individuals who have physical disabilities. In general, *ACSM's Guidelines for Exercise Testing and Prescription*, 8th Ed. provides the following guidelines for exercise testing:

■ The initial workload should be 2 to 3 **metabolic equivalents (METs)** with incremental increases not exceeding 0.5 to 1.0 METs for anyone with a low work capacity.

■ If balance, coordination, or muscle weakness are problems, use a cycle ergometer rather than a treadmill. If the treadmill is used, ensure handrail support; however, adding this type of support reduces the accuracy of estimated peak MET capacity. Adjust treadmill speed based on walking ability.

■ Be prepared to extend the initial stage of testing, to restart testing, or to repeat the test if an elderly client has difficulty using the exercise equipment.

■ Be aware that exercise-induced **dysrhythmias** are more common in seniors than in any other population. In addition, elderly individuals typically take one or more medications, many of which influence heart rate and blood pressure response to exercise.

■ The exercise electrocardiogram (ECG) has higher sensitivity and lower specificity in seniors than in younger age groups. This is perhaps because of the presence of conduction disturbances or left ventricular hypertrophy among seniors.

The indications for terminating exercise testing in older adults are similar to those in other populations. Absolute indications include a drop in systolic blood pressure greater than 10 mm Hg from baseline despite an increase in workload; moderately severe angina; increasing dizziness, incoordination, or loss of consciousness; signs of poor oxygen availability (cyanosis or pallor); technical difficulties monitoring the ECG or systolic blood pressure; subject's request to stop; and sustained ventricular tachycardia.[23]

ACSM also offers advice on exercise testing for those over the age of 75 and individuals with severe mobility limitations. Instead of requiring exercise testing, request a complete medical history and physical examination to determine cardiac limitations to exercise. Stratify those with symptoms of cardiovascular disease according to standards presented in Chapter 2 of *ACSM's Guidelines for Exercise Testing and Prescription*, 8thEd. Overall, seniors over the age of 75 may initiate low-intensity exercise if they do not exhibit any symptoms of cardiovascular disease. Low-intensity exercise includes activities performed at ≤3 METs.[23]

EXERCISE PRESCRIPTION

As with other populations, an exercise program for the elderly must emphasize cardiovascular endurance, resistance training, and flexibility work. In compliance with existing literature and guidelines from ACSM, the following recommendations are considered safe for a generally healthy senior adult.

QUICK REFERENCE

Seniors should accumulate 30 to 60 minutes of moderate-intensity physical activity on at least 5 days per week.[23]

- Precede all forms of exercise with at least 5 minutes of a low-impact, low-intensity warm-up such as walking, stationary cycling, or general limbering movements. As for all exercisers, the warm-up prepares the joints and muscles for movement by increasing blood flow and heart rate. Additionally, follow each workout with at least a five-minute cooldown to return the heart rate and blood flow to normal. The cooldown is also a time for light stretching and mental relaxation.

QUICK REFERENCE

Use the 0 to 10 Rate of Perceived Exertion (RPE) Scale to measure intensity for this group. Moderate intensity is defined as a rating of 5 or 6. Vigorous intensity is defined as a rating of 7 or 8.

Intermittent claudication—an aching, cramping, and sometimes burning leg pain that comes and goes. It typically occurs with walking and goes away with rest; caused by poor blood circulation in the arteries of the legs.
Metabolic equivalent (MET)—The unit used to estimate the amount of oxygen used by the body. 1 MET equals the oxygen used by the body at rest.
Dysrhythmia—an abnormal heart rhythm.

- Seniors should participate in 30 to 60 minutes of moderate aerobic activity (RPE = 5 or 6) on at least 5 days per week. They may accumulate this in 10-minute segments throughout the day for a total of 150 to 300 minutes of activity per week. If high-intensity activity is performed (RPE = 7 to 8), frequency should be 3 days per week for 20 to 30 minutes per day, or a total of 75 to 100 minutes per week. Be advised that senior exercisers wishing to increase workload should increase duration of activity prior to increasing intensity.
- Avoid activities that have a high risk of falling since the bones of older adults are more fragile than those of younger adults. This includes activities that require rapid changes in direction.
- Low-impact exercises such as walking, stationary cycling, water aerobics, and swimming are preferred to high-impact activities like running, jumping, and bouncing. Group fitness classes are great for exercise and socializing.
- Resistance training helps preserve muscle mass, strength, functional ability, and mobility. Perform one set of 10 to 15 repetitions for 8 to 10 different exercises, each targeting a major muscle group. Intensity should be between moderate (RPE = 5 to 6) and vigorous (RPE = 7 to 8) according to the Borg Scale. As improvements are made, increase the number of repetitions prior to increasing resistance. If a client is highly deconditioned, be conservative in the initial stages of training and keep intensity and duration low.
- Perform all resistance exercises with a neutral spine and in a controlled manner. Breathe out on the exertion phase and in on the return phase. Move muscles and joints through a full range of pain-free motion for maximum effect. Include multijoint exercises to improve balance.
- The type of resistance training depends upon the capabilities of individual clients. Machines or resistance bands are preferable to free weights if balance is an issue. Machines stabilize the back and allow for more control over range of motion.
- Avoid strenuous exercise during hot, humid weather since senior exercisers have difficulty in regulating body temperature. Have clients drink plenty of fluids before, during, and after exercise to help maintain body temperature.
- Do not exercise during flare-ups of arthritis or other chronic conditions.
- Perform flexibility exercises for the hip, back, shoulder, knee, upper trunk, and neck areas. Static stretches should be performed to the point of tightness but not pain (RPE of 5 to 6). Each should be held for 15 to 30 seconds with 2 to 4 repetitions per stretch. Flexibility training is helpful for all populations, but it is especially important in the elderly since it enhances mobility, balance, and agility.

QUICK REFERENCE

If limited by physical disabilities, seniors should remain as physically active as their conditions allow.[23]

SAMPLE EXERCISES FOR SENIORS

WARM-UP

Warm-up the muscles with 5 to 10 minutes of limbering movements such as walking or stationary cycling. Light stretching is safe near the end of the warm-up.

UPPER BODY STRENGTH TRAINING

Most seniors are able to perform traditional upper body exercises. Be sure to include exercises that target the chest, back, shoulders, biceps, and triceps. A stability ball can effectively improve core strength and balance, two components often limited in the elderly individual. Most upper body exercises may be done while seated on a stability ball. Many previously sedentary seniors prefer using resistance bands rather than free weights. If using free weights, watch for possible balance issues. Tai chi, yoga, and pilates are also beneficial for developing strength, balance, and muscular endurance.

Following are examples of resistance training exercises for the senior population. These exercises incorporate several different training tools including dumbbells, elastic tubing, and weight machines. The mode chosen for a particular client will depend upon equipment availability and client fitness level.

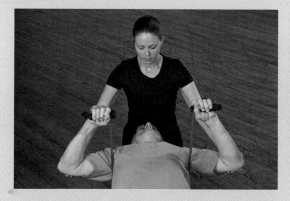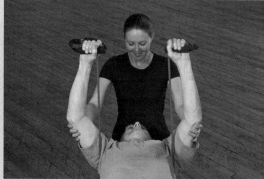

■ Chest Press with Elastic Tubing (Fig. 5.4)

Lie on a bench with tubing behind back just below the armpits and shoulder blades. Feet should be flat on floor, back in neutral alignment. Hold one handle in each hand, palms forward. Grasp the band toward the center to create resistance. Push hands up toward ceiling. Pause. Return to starting position. Repeat 10 to 15 times. This exercise can also be done in the seated position.

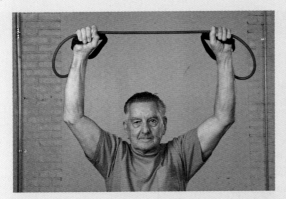
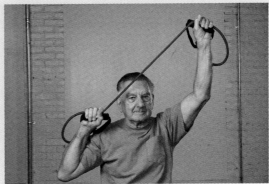
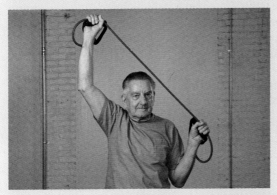

■ **Lateral Pull Downs with Elastic Tubing (Fig. 5.5)**

Hold one handle in each hand. Grasp tubing toward the center to create resistance. Bring arms up overhead while pulling shoulder blades down. Push left arm toward ceiling while pulling right elbow down until right hand is at ear or shoulder level. Pause and return to start. Repeat 10 to 15 times with right arm. Change to left arm. Alternatively, hook the tubing around a stationary fixture about 5 ft off the floor. Let the ends hang free. Sit in a chair or on a bench with toes lined up with elastic tubing. Keep feet flat on floor, back neutral, abdominals contracted. Grasp the handles, one end in each hand, palms facing each other. Pull on tubing until hands are just above shoulder level. Pause. Slowly return to starting position. Repeat 10 to 15 times.

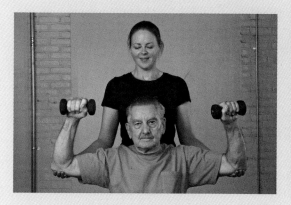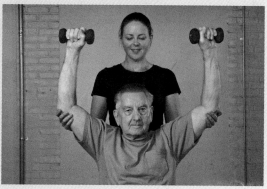

■ Shoulder Press (Fig. 5.6)

Sit on a bench with spine in neutral alignment and abdominals contracted. Hold one dumbbell in each hand, palms facing forward, arms parallel to the ground, elbows bent. Push weights up toward ceiling. Pause. Return to starting position. Repeat 10 to 15 times.

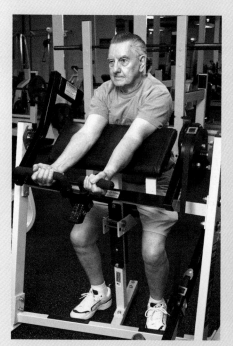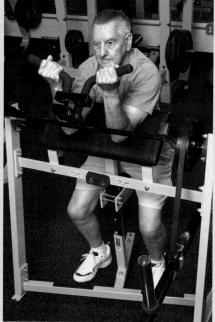

■ Biceps Curl (Fig. 5.7)

Sit in a biceps machine with back in neutral alignment and abdominals contracted. Grasp handles and slowly flex the elbows. Pause. Return to starting position. Repeat 10 to 15 times.

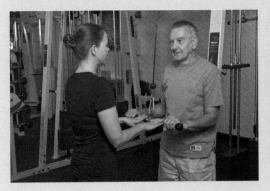 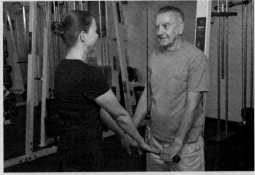

■ **Triceps Extension (Fig. 5.8)**

Stand with feet shoulder width apart, spine in neutral alignment, and abdominals contracted. Place hands on bar about shoulder width apart. Stabilize elbows without squeezing them to the sides, and push bar down until elbows are fully extended. Pause. Bring bar back up until forearms are parallel to ground. Repeat 10 to 15 times.

LOWER BODY EXERCISES

Most seniors can perform traditional lower body exercises using weight machines, resistance bands, or light dumbbells. They may also incorporate into their workouts regular daily activities that stress the lower body. The following section describes exercises that train muscles of the quadriceps femoris, hamstrings, and leg.

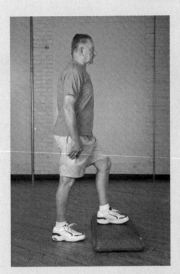 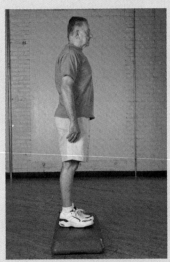 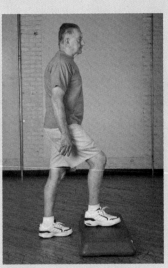

■ **Step-Ups (Fig. 5.9)**

Strengthen quadriceps, hip flexors, and hamstrings. Have client stand in front of a step (height of step should be determined as with the general population). Client should step up onto platform while making sure the entire foot lands on the step and the back is neutral. Repeat for 10 to 15 steps using the same leg. Switch legs and perform another 10 to 15 step-ups. To increase intensity, have the client hold light dumbbells during the exercise.

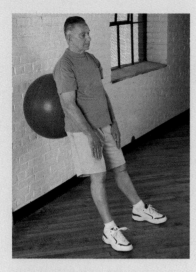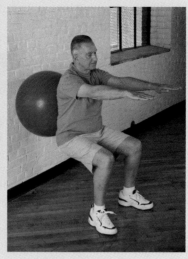

■ **Squat (Fig. 5.10)**

Strengthens quadriceps, hamstrings, and buttocks. Stand with feet shoulder width apart. Slowly bend the knees until the thighs are parallel to the floor (as in sitting down on a chair). Ensure 90 degree angles at hip and knee joints. Slowly lift the body back to the starting position while pushing through the heels. Maintain a neutral spine and contract abdominals throughout the movement. Alternatively, do squats with a stability ball (pictured). Stand with back toward a wall. Position a stability ball in between the lower back and the wall. Slowly bend the knees until thighs are parallel to the floor; then return to starting position.

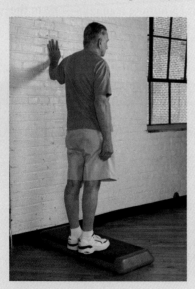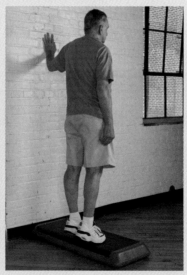

■ **Calf Raises (Fig. 5.11)**

Strengthen the lower legs. Stand on top of a platform, toes on platform, heels off. Hold onto wall with one hand if balance is an issue. Raise the heels while contracting the calf muscles. Pause. Lower heels. To increase difficulty, hold dumbbells while performing the exercise. Another alternative is to perform the exercise with one leg at a time.

EXERCISE AND THE FRAIL ELDERLY CLIENT

"Frail elderly" individuals are usually those over the age of 75 who have physical or mental impairments that interfere with their ability to perform ADLs. ADLs include self-feeding, bathing, dressing, grooming, maintaining a home, and participating in general leisure activities. Because they are unable to independently take care of themselves, the frail elderly often live in retirement communities, assisted living facilities, or nursing homes; therefore, the average fitness professional does not usually encounter them. Still, exercise professionals should understand how routine activity improves functional capacity in this group by developing muscle strength, joint flexibility, and balance.[27,28]

The goal of exercise for frail elderly individuals is to restore the ability to perform normal ADLs—or at the very least to prevent further loss of functional ability. Limit intensity and duration to avoid injury and promote compliance. Because frail elderly individuals often experience severe muscle weakness, joint pain, and balance problems, they usually have to exercise while seated, or possibly while lying in bed. Make adjustments according to individual limitations.

In general, an exercise program for frail seniors has the same basic components as a program for the general population. It should consist of a warm-up, aerobic training, resistance exercises, flexibility work, and balance training.[27] The warm-up alone is often challenging enough for the frailest of the frail, so pay attention to individual response. Some experts recommend splitting the daily workout into two 15-minute segments—one in the morning and the other in the evening.[28] Others suggest working out for 30 to 60 consecutive minutes.[27] Actual duration depends on the client's fitness level.

SAMPLE EXERCISES FOR THE FRAIL ELDERLY PATIENT

These exercises should be done in two 15-minute segments each day.

WARM-UP (3 TO 5 MINUTES)

The warm-up prepares the body by increasing blood flow to muscles. It may include gentle stretching of targeted muscles. Begin with seated marching, arms relaxed. Switch to toe taps to the front, arms relaxed. Switch to heeltaps to the front, arms relaxed. Return to marching and add normal "marching arms." Switch to toe taps with alternating front shoulder raises. Switch to heeltaps with double biceps curls. Return to marching and add shoulder abduction/adduction. Add toe taps with shoulder shrugs. End with heeltaps and triceps kickbacks.

STRENGTH TRAINING

Choose to work either the upper body or the lower body on any given day. If working the upper body for 15 minutes in the morning, work it again for 15 minutes in the evening.

Then work the lower body on the following day.[28] In some cases, the exerciser's body weight is sufficient for resistance. In other cases, fitness professionals might need to apply resistance with their own hands. Elastic tubing is also useful if greater resistance is needed.

Frail seniors often achieve significant benefits by "practicing" everyday activities rather than performing typical exercises. For example, simply moving from a sitting position to a standing position for several repetitions can be challenging enough to develop muscular strength, muscular endurance, and balance. Slowly stepping on and off a low step is also demanding. Even performing the motions of free weight exercises *without the weights* is beneficial. Most importantly consider the specific capabilities and limitations of individual clients when designing a safe and effective exercise program.

Lower Body Strengthening Exercises

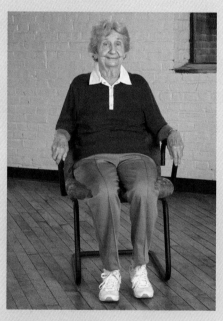 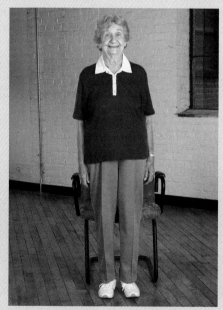

■ Sit-to-stand (Fig. 5.12)

Begin by sitting in a chair that has arms. Place hands on arm rails. Using arms and legs, stand up. Return to original position. Repeat 10 to 15 times.

Source: Petersen T. Functionally fit: The Daily Program for Frail or Dependent Seniors. 2004. American Academy of Health and Fitness.

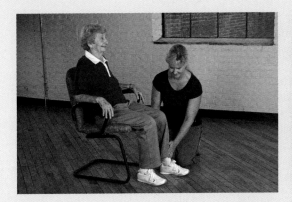 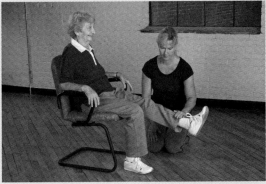

■ **Single-Knee Extension on Chair (Fig. 5.13)**

While seated, slowly extend the left knee by raising the left leg. Lower and repeat 10 to 15 times. Perform on right side. To increase intensity, fitness professional can apply resistance to lower leg during the concentric phase of contraction.

Source: Petersen T. Functionally fit: The Daily Program for Frail or Dependent Seniors. 2004. American Academy of Health and Fitness

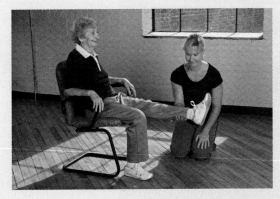 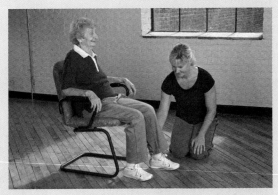

■ **Seated Single-Leg Curl (Fig. 5.14)**

Sit in a chair and extend left knee. Fitness professional should apply resistance at the back of the lower leg while client flexes left knee. Return to starting position. Repeat 10 to 15 times on the left. Perform on the right side.

Source: Petersen T. Functionally fit: The Daily Program for Frail or Dependent Seniors. 2004. American Academy of Health and Fitness

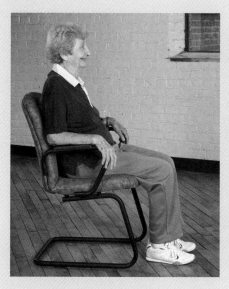 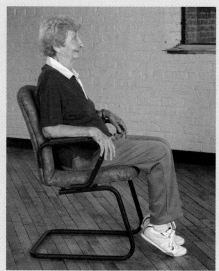

■ **Seated Heel Raises (Fig. 5.15)**

Sit in a chair. Plantarflex the ankles to raise both heels off ground. Repeat 10 to 15 times.

Source: Petersen T. Functionally fit: The Daily Program for Frail or Dependent Seniors. 2004. American Academy of Health and Fitness

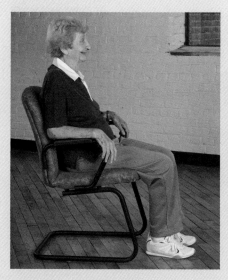 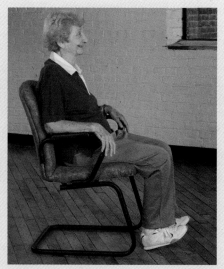

■ **Seated Toe Raises (Fig. 5.16)**

Sit in a chair. Dorsiflex the ankles to raise both sets of toes off ground. Repeat 10 to 15 times.

Source: Petersen T. Functionally fit: The Daily Program for Frail or Dependent Seniors. 2004. American Academy of Health and Fitness

Upper Body Strengthening Exercises

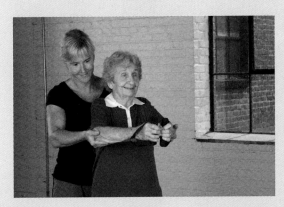 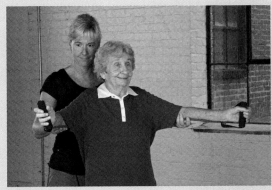

■ Chest Flies Using Elastic Tubing (Fig. 5.17)

This exercise may be done while seated or standing. Place elastic tubing around the back just below the armpits and shoulder blades. Hold one handle in each hand. Grasp tubing toward center to create resistance. Bring arms to the sides, parallel to the ground with elbows slightly bent. Palms should face one another. Keeping arms relatively straight (with only a slight bend in elbows), bring hands together in front of the chest. Pause. Return to starting position. Repeat 10 times.

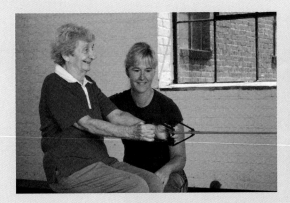 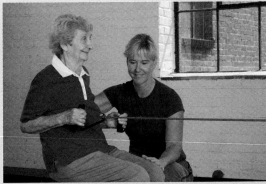

■ Seated Row Using Elastic Tubing (Fig. 5.18)

Wrap tubing around a secure bar or chair. Sit in a chair that is about a foot away from the bar. Be sure to face it. Grasp one end of the tubing in each hand. With palms down, pull tubing toward the chest. Pause. Return to starting position. Repeat 10 times.

Source: Petersen T. Functionally fit: The Daily Program for Frail or Dependent Seniors. 2004. American Academy of Health and Fitness

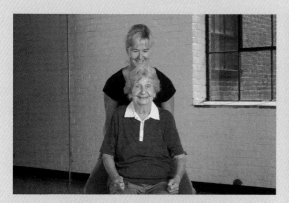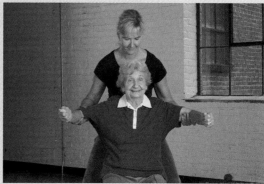

■ Lateral Shoulder Raises (Fig. 5.19)

Sit in a chair with arms to the side. Flex elbows. Fitness professional should apply resistance to middle of both arms. Have the client abduct the arms to 70 degrees. Return to starting position. Repeat 10 times.

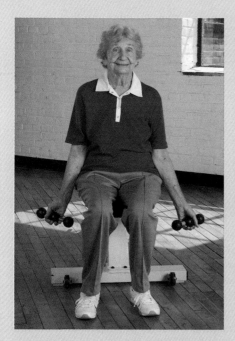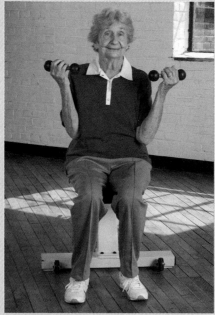

■ Bicep Curls with 1-pound Dumbbells (Fig. 5.20)

Sit in a chair with a 1-pound dumbbell in each hand, palms facing forward. Slowly curl the weights up while flexing elbows. Pause. Return to starting position. Repeat 10 times.

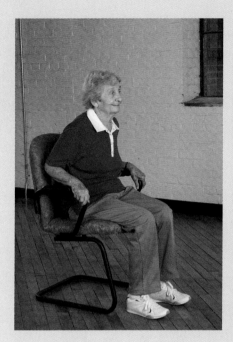 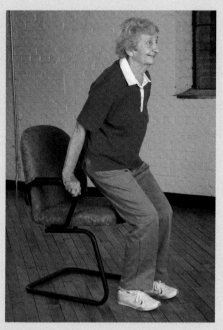

■ Triceps Dips in a Chair (Fig. 5.21)

Sit in a chair with arm supports. Grasp arm supports with hands, keep feet flat on floor. Using only the triceps, push up until the buttocks are raised off the seat. Lower and repeat 10 times.

Source: Petersen T. Functionally fit: The Daily Program for Frail or Dependent Seniors. 2004. American Academy of Health and Fitness

NUTRITIONAL CONSIDERATIONS WITH AGE

Researchers are actively investigating the relationship between diet and aging to try to discover nutrition's precise role in the aging process. Studies indicate that lifelong healthy eating and exercise reduce the risk for chronic disease, but the extent to which these lifestyle behaviors affect the rate of natural aging is not yet clear. Overall, differentiating between the effects of good nutrition versus the effects of other positive lifelong behaviors is difficult and complex. More than likely, numerous factors exert a cumulative effect that surpasses the effects of any one independent factor. Thus, delineating the roles of individual nutrients might be impossible. See additional positive lifestyle behaviors listed in Table 5.11.

Genetic predisposition, existing chronic conditions, use of medications, and lifelong avoidance of certain foods are examples of variables that affect nutritional status and needs. Seniors who have avoided dairy products throughout life likely have problems associated with a chronic calcium deficiency. Those who have neglected to consume fibrous foods might suffer the consequences of a chronic fiber deficiency. Others who

TABLE 5-11   LIFESTYLE BEHAVIORS THAT IMPROVE OVERALL HEALTH

- Eating well-balanced meals
- Participating in regular physical activity
- Not smoking
- Moderate or no use of alcohol
- Sleeping regularly
- Maintaining a healthy weight

TABLE 5-12   SPECIAL CONCERNS FOR THE ELDERLY POPULATION

- Diminished taste and smell make eating unappealing
- Poor dental health makes eating difficult
- Deterioration of the digestive, urinary, and respiratory systems impacts overall health
- Changes in cardiovascular and bone health limit physical abilities
- Use of medications can impact appetite, digestion, absorption, and nutrient action

have been consuming a varied, healthy diet might take medications that interfere with absorption, use, or excretion of different nutrients and must therefore contend with numerous vitamin and mineral deficiencies. See Table 5.12 for additional factors that influence a senior's nutritional status.

Determining the exact nutritional needs of the aging adult is not easy. However, this section discusses nutrients that appear to be of particular concern for the older adult.

WATER

Water contributes approximately 60% to an adult's body weight. Skeletal muscle in particular stores large volumes of water; therefore, people who have a greater ratio of muscle mass to fat contain more water than those who have a greater ratio of fat to muscle.

Water performs several vital functions. It participates either directly or indirectly in all metabolic reactions; it transports nutrients, wastes, and other substances throughout the body; it lubricates food passing through the digestive tract; it cushions joints and other structures; and it helps maintain normal body temperature. The body continuously loses water through sweat, respiration, kidney excretion, and feces elimination, so water must be replaced regularly (Table 5.13).

Since total body water content decreases with age, seniors can experience extreme increases in core temperature. To complicate matters, many older adults lose their sense of thirst. Some consciously reduce fluid intake because of urinary bladder problems or malfunctioning urethral sphincters. Moreover, some seniors take diuretics to control hypertension, but since diuretics increase water excretion by the kidneys, they also affect

TABLE 5-13 WATER LOSS	
Method of Loss	Amount (mL/day)
Sweat	450–900
Exits the lungs via exhaled air	200–350
Excreted by kidneys as urine	1,500
Lost in feces	100–150

TABLE 5-14   SIGNS OF DEHYDRATION

- Fatigue
- Confusion
- Dry lips
- Sunken eyes
- Increased body temperature
- Decreased blood pressure
- Constipation
- Decreased urine output
- Nausea

hydration level. No matter what the cause, if water intake does not match daily water loss, life-threatening dehydration can result (Table 5.14). Experts, therefore, suggest that elderly adults ingest a minimum of six glasses of water per day. If they are active, they should also replenish any water lost through perspiration.

QUICK REFERENCE

Seniors need to consume a minimum of six glasses of water per day to avoid dehydration. At its worst, dehydration can cause life-threatening increases in core body temperature. It can also increase the risk for urinary tract infections, pneumonia, pressure ulcers, and disorientation.

CARBOHYDRATES, PROTEIN, AND FAT: THE ENERGY-YIELDING NUTRIENTS

Average energy requirements begin to decline by about 5% per decade in early adulthood. A loss of muscle mass and a decrease in thyroid hormones cause 1% to 2% of this; the rest is attributed to reduced physical activity. No matter what the cause, older adults need to select **nutrient-dense foods** to ensure adequate nutrition since energy allowance declines over time. There is little leeway for added sugars, fats, or alcohol.

Proteins in the body provide structure, facilitate reactions, form antibodies and hormones, regulate fluid and acid balance, transport substances through fluids and cell membranes, and provide energy. Clearly, they participate in nearly every action in the body and must be consumed regularly in the diet to maintain health. When the demand for protein exceeds its dietary supply, the body strips protein from skeletal muscles—a factor that results in muscle wasting in the long term. Therefore, adequate intake can slow the loss of muscle mass at any age.

Most authorities recommend that seniors, like the general population, consume 0.8 g of protein per kilogram of body weight (or 0.36 g per pound of body weight). At least one study suggests a slightly higher intake—0.45 g per pound of body weight—but there is currently insufficient evidence to support this.

Unfortunately, many seniors consume less protein than they need. This is largely because of the age-related changes that occur in the digestive system and the false belief that meat is the only good source of protein. Consider changes in the digestive system mentioned earlier in this chapter. Many people lose teeth and must wear dentures. Dentures can interfere with the ability to chew meat, so older adults often avoid it. In addition, stomach and pancreatic cells produce fewer protein-digesting enzymes, which makes it more difficult to **catabolize** proteins in the stomach and small intestine. To avoid the accompanying GI discomfort, seniors might simply choose to avoid these high-protein foods.

The primary role of dietary carbohydrates is to provide energy. Excess carbohydrates initially fill glycogen stores; once glycogen stores are filled, carbohydrates are stored as fat.

Nutrient-dense foods—foods that have a high nutrient to kilocalorie ratio; they provide the biggest nutrient "bang" for the smallest energy "buck." As an example, skim milk is more nutrient dense than whole milk. One cup of skim or whole milk contains about 300 mg of calcium; however, the skim milk contains only 90 kcal per cup, while the whole milk contains 149 kcal per cup.

Catabolize—to break down larger molecules into smaller ones; releases energy as bonds are broken.

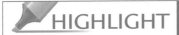

HIGHLIGHT   Fiber

Dietary fiber provides numerous benefits to the body. Fiber prevents unwanted weight gain because high fiber foods are naturally low in kilocalories but provide a sense of fullness. Fiber maintains motility of the GI tract, which decreases the risk for colon cancer. It prevents constipation by providing bulk to stools. It traps dietary cholesterol and eliminates it from the GI tract before it is absorbed (which reduces risk of heart disease). And it slows glucose absorption into the blood, which helps diabetics process glucose better. Even though fiber performs such important functions in the body, the average senior only consumes 12 g of fiber per day—a far cry from the recommended 25 to 30 g per day needed to maintain bowel functioning. Good sources of fiber include legumes, vegetables, fruits, and whole grain products.

Adequate carbohydrate intake is essential, however, to prevent the body from catabolizing muscle tissue for energy. For the average adult, a *minimum* of 50 to 100 g of carbohydrates per day provides this "protein-sparing effect" that ultimately preserves muscle mass. A minimum of 130 g per day, however, is required by the average person for proper nervous system functioning.

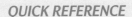

QUICK REFERENCE

The average person should consume a *minimum* of 50 to 100 g of carbohydrates per day to prevent muscle wasting. A *minimum* of 130 g per day meets the needs of the nervous system, but not the needs of active individuals.

Carbohydrate requirements depend upon overall energy demands; thus, active seniors need more carbohydrates than sedentary seniors. Since energy expenditure tends to decline with age, however, seniors should decrease simple carbohydrate intake, while they increase complex carbohydrate intake. Simple carbohydrates provide little more than **empty kilocalories** and are associated with elevated triglyceride levels, a risk factor for heart disease. Complex carbohydrates, on the other hand, are packed with fiber, essential vitamins and minerals, **phytochemicals**, and other beneficial substances.

Triglyercides, or fats, serve various purposes. In food, fat enhances flavor and provides the essential linoleic and linolenic fatty acids. In the body, fat stores energy, provides insulation, and protects organs. Consequently, there is definitely a place for fat in the diet. As with people of all ages, however, seniors need to moderate their fat intake to reduce their risk for diabetes, cancer, atherosclerosis, and other chronic diseases (Table 5.15).

Twenty to thirty-five percent of a senior's total daily kilocalorie intake can be in the form of fats. Older adults should limit saturated and trans fatty acid intake and focus on

---

TABLE 5-15   GENERAL RECOMMENDATIONS REGARDING FAT INTAKE

- Reduce total fat intake
- Replace saturated and trans fats with monounsaturated fats
- Reduce cholesterol intake to <300 mg/day
- Balance omega-6 and omega-3 fatty acids
- Increase intake of fruits, vegetables, and grains, which are naturally low in fat

---

consuming more of the essential omega-3 fatty acids. Omega-3 fatty acids are the most important members of the linolenic fatty acid family. Experts believe that they decrease the risk of heart disease by lowering blood pressure, decreasing inflammation, reducing blood triglycerides, preventing blood clots, and protecting against irregular heartbeats. The best sources of omega-3 fatty acids are fatty fish, but canola oil, flaxseed oil, soybean oil, and walnuts are also good. Omega-6 fatty acids, which are often mentioned in conjunction with omega-3s, are also essential. They are found in corn oil, sunflower oil, nuts, seeds, poultry, meats, and eggs, so they tend to be plentiful in the American diet. For those 51 years and older, the adequate intake (AI) for linolenic acid (omega-3) is 1.6 g per day for men and 1.1 g per day for women. The AI for linoleic acid (omega-6) is 14 g per day for men and 11 g per day for women. The optimal overall ratio of linoleic to linolenic acid is 6:1.

VITAMINS AND MINERALS

Because of GI tract problems, inadequate intake, or interference by medications, older adults are prone to vitamin and mineral deficiencies. The focus here is on vitamin B_{12}, vitamin D, calcium, vitamin C, and the antioxidants since these are commonly deficient in this population.

Vitamin B_{12}

Vitamin B_{12} facilitates new cell synthesis, maintains neurons, and assists in fatty acid and amino acid catabolism. A deficiency, therefore, leads to devastating results such as poor cognitive abilities, severe anemia, and major neurological dysfunctioning. Vitamin B_{12} is only found in animal products and requires intrinsic factor produced by the stomach for absorption. A deficiency of vitamin B_{12} in the elderly is not necessarily caused by

---

Empty kilocalories—foods that are high in energy but low in nutritional value; also known as junk foods. Examples include potato chips, candy, and regular soda.

Phytochemicals—nonnutritive plant chemicals that have protective properties in the human body. Recent research demonstrates that phytochemicals protect humans against diseases by acting as antioxidants, affecting enzyme action, and interfering with DNA replication in cancer cells. Lycopene in tomatoes, isoflavones in soy, and flavanoids in fruits are phytochemicals.

inadequate intake; instead, it results from atrophic gastritis, a condition that interferes with intrinsic factor production in approximately 10% to 30% of adults over age 50. If intrinsic factor is lacking, vitamin B_{12} is not absorbed. The Recommended Dietary Allowance (RDA) for seniors is the same as it is for younger adults: 2.4 μg per day with no upper limit.

QUICK REFERENCE
The RDA for vitamin B_{12} is 2.4 μg per day.

Vitamin D

The need for vitamin D tends to increase with age. Essentially, vitamin D stimulates small intestinal cells to produce calcium-binding proteins that lock onto calcium and permit absorption into blood vessels. In other words, vitamin D is necessary for calcium absorption in the GI tract. This vitamin also decreases calcium excretion by the kidneys and thus indirectly promotes bone health.

The major food source for vitamin D is fortified milk, so the fact that many seniors are lactose intolerant is a problem (see Chapter 8 for further information on lactose intolerance). Vitamin D is also made in the body when UV radiation converts a vitamin D precursor (7-dehydrocholesterol) into active vitamin D. Seniors, however, tend to avoid exposure to sunlight, a behavior that certainly reduces the risk for skin cancer but also decreases circulating blood levels of vitamin D. To prevent bone loss and to maintain vitamin D status, people over age 50 need 10 to 15 μg daily. The tolerable upper intake level is 50 μg per day since excesses result in abnormally high blood calcium, which is associated with calcification of soft tissues like the blood vessels, heart, lungs, and joints.

QUICK REFERENCE
People over the age of 50 need 10 to 15 μg of vitamin D daily. The tolerable upper intake is 50 μg per day.

Calcium

The body monitors and regulates blood calcium levels closely because of calcium's role in muscle contraction and nerve impulse conduction. If blood levels drop, neither the muscular nor the nervous system functions properly. Consequently, if a person does not ingest enough dietary calcium, the body retrieves calcium from bone. In fact, the body readily sacrifices bone tissue to maintain blood calcium levels since nervous and muscular system functioning are more important than maintaining bone integrity. Bone loss results in osteoporosis, and osteoporosis increases the risk of fracture during a fall.

The best sources of calcium are milk and milk products, but seniors often avoid these because of lactose intolerance. Other good sources include tofu, almonds, sesame seeds, turnip greens, parsley, broccoli, tortillas, wheat bread, and mineral water. Vitamin D and stomach acid enhance calcium absorption while phytates (found in seeds, nuts, and grains) and oxalates (found in rhubarb, spinach, and sweet potatoes) inhibit absorption. Those over the age of 50 need 1,200 mg per day. The tolerable upper intake is 2,500 mg per day since excess calcium causes constipation and increases the risk of urinary stones and kidney dysfunction. It can also interfere with the absorption of other minerals.

QUICK REFERENCE

People over the age of 50 need 1,200 mg of calcium per day. The tolerable upper intake level is 2,500 mg per day.

Vitamin C

Vitamin C is also necessary for bone health because it is used to synthesize the protein collagen. Collagen is an essential component of the bone matrix; in fact, lack of collagen results in fragile and unusually slender bones. Recommended amounts are discussed in the next section.

ANTIOXIDANTS

Antioxidants reduce the damage incurred by free radicals. Free radicals are unstable, highly reactive molecules that attack body cells and damage tissues; they are often referred to as oxidants. Free radicals naturally occur in the body and arise from normal metabolism. Anything that increases metabolism, therefore, increases the number of circulating free radicals. Their levels also increase with exposure to air pollution, cigarette smoke, and UV radiation.

The body capably handles normal amounts of free radicals by using its antioxidant defense system. Antioxidants inactivate existing free radicals, prevent the formation of new free radicals, and interrupt the chain of reactions that promote free radical damage. Certain vitamins and minerals have antioxidant properties. These include vitamin C, vitamin E, beta carotene,* lycopene, and selenium. The most commonly known antioxidants are vitamins C and E, so they are the focus of this section.

The RDA for vitamin C is 90 mg per day for senior males and 75 mg per day for senior females. Some experts recommend that seniors take enough supplemental vitamin C to make their total daily intake approach 250 to 500 mg per day because higher levels are thought to prevent chronic age-related diseases. The tolerable upper intake level for vitamin C is 2,000 mg; an intake above this amount causes severe diarrhea and overall GI distress.

---

*Supplements of beta carotene are not recommended because they are associated with an increased risk of death from all causes, especially heart disease and stroke. This is particularly true for smokers.

The RDA for vitamin E is 15 mg per day for senior males and females. Experts suggest taking enough supplemental vitamin E to reach a total daily intake of 100 to 800 mg. The tolerable upper intake level for this vitamin is 1,000 mg or 1,500 IU; intakes in excess of this amount cause hemorrhage.

QUICK REFERENCE
Men over the age of 50 need 90 mg of vitamin C per day. Women over the age of 50 need 75 mg per day. Senior males and females require 15 mg of vitamin E per day.

Although supplements are necessary for some people, most should try to consume adequate nutrients through a varied diet. An active lifestyle elevates metabolism, which in turn permits a greater energy intake. Those who can consume a greater quantity of food are also more likely to obtain adequate nutrients. Those who require supplements, however, should remember what the word supplement means. It means "in addition to," not "in place of." An unhealthy diet cannot be made healthy simply by taking a pill. A healthy diet begins with various nutrient-dense foods; it may then be augmented with supplements if necessary.

SUMMARY

Exercise programs for all populations must be individualized and take into consideration preexisting medical conditions, overall health status, and special needs. Nevertheless, conditioning programs should generally include exercises that focus on cardiovascular endurance, muscular strength, muscular endurance, and flexibility. Activities designed to address each of these components preserve muscle mass, maintain bone tissue, reduce excess body fat, sustain metabolic rate, and improve overall quality of life. For seniors, these components are critical for maintaining functional ability. Appropriate exercise design, including a warm-up, resistance training, cardiovascular training, flexibility, and cooldown, ensures safe activity, neutral body alignment, and gradual improvements for the aging population.

CASE STUDY

Sam, a 68-year-old man with no signs of cardiovascular or pulmonary disease, would like to start an exercise program because he does not have the energy to mow the lawn or take care of the house. He would also like to get into better shape so that he will be able to play with his 1-year-old grandson. Although he has not been very active during the past 15 years, Sam used to play college football and ran 3 miles at least 3 days per week until he developed arthritis in his knees at age 50. He has not done any resistance training since his football years, but he is willing to do whatever it takes to become more fit.

■ Describe the type of exercise program you would suggest for Sam.

THINKING CRITICALLY

1. Identify several age-related changes that occur in the integumentary system and explain how they affect a senior's ability to exercise.
2. Identify several age-related changes that occur in the nervous system and explain how they affect a senior's ability to exercise.
3. Explain how weight-bearing exercise prevents or slows the devastating effects of osteoporosis.
4. Constipation is often a problem in the senior population. What advice would you give an older client experiencing this?
5. List and explain some of the causes of nutrient deficiencies in the senior population. Identify at least three nutrients that are of particular concern in this group. What problems are associated with deficiencies of these nutrients?
6. Why is it especially important to maintain adequate calcium intake? What happens if the diet is deficient in calcium?
7. Name two forms of arthritis. Explain the differences between them. Which is an autoimmune disorder?
8. Explain the development of atherosclerosis.
9. Explain lactose intolerance. What is the cause of this problem? What are its symptoms? Why is it so dangerous? What advice would you give an elderly client who has this condition? You might need to see Chapter 8 for further information on this condition.

REFERENCES

1. Survivor's Guide to Surgical Menopause. www.sur-meno.blogspot.com/2006/03/estrogen-functions.html
2. Buckwalter J. Decreased mobility in the elderly: the exercise antidote. Physician Sportsmed 1997; 25(9):127–133.
3. Maiers M, Hartvigsen J, Schulz C, et al. Chiropractic and exercise for seniors with low back pain or neck pain. BMC Musculoskelet Disord 2007;94(8).
4. Petersen T. SrFIT: the personal trainer's resource for senior fitness. Lawrence, KS: American Academy of Health and Fitness, 2004.
5. Bell JT. The Book on Group Fitness. Tarpon Springs, FL: International Fitness Professionals Association 2000:319–380.
6. Grossman M, Stewart A. 'You aren't going to get better by just sitting around': Physical activity perceptions, motivations, and barriers in adults 75 years of age or older. Am J Geriatr Cardiol 2003; 12(1):33–37.
7. McGinnis JM, Foege WH. Actual causes of death in the United States. JAMA 1993;270(18):207–12.
8. Topolski T. The rapid assessment of physical activity among older adults. Prev Chronic Dis 2006; 3(4):A118.
9. Jancin B. Exercise classes improve function in seniors with chronic conditions. Int Med News.2004;37(23):18.
10. Garg PK, Tian M, Criqui M, et al. Physical activity during daily life and mortality in patients with peripheral arterial disease. J Vasc Surg 2007; 45(2):437.
11. Brach J, FitzGerald S, Newman A, et al. Physical activity and functional status in community-dwelling older women—a 14 year prospective study. Arc Int Med 2003;163:2565–2571.
12. Demark-Wahnefried W, Clipp E, Morey M, et al. Lifestyle intervention development study to improve physical function in older adults with

cancer: Outcomes from project LEAD. J Clin Oncol 2006; 24(20):3465–3473.

13. Luukinen H, Lehtola S, Jokelainen J, et al. Prevention of disability by exercise among the elderly: a population based, randomized, controlled trial. Scand J Prim Health Care 2006;24(4):199–205.

14. Sevick M, Bradham D. Cost effectiveness of aerobic and resistance exercise in seniors with kene osteoarthritis. Med Sci Sports Exerc 2000; 32(9): 1534–1540.

15. Ettinger WH, Burns R, Messier SP, et al. A randomized trial comparing aerobic exercise and resistance exercise with a health education program in older adults with knee osteoarthritis. The Fitness Arthritis and Seniors Trial (FAST). JAMA 1997; 277(1):25–32.

16. Fiatrarone MA, O'Neill EF, Doyle-Ryan N, et al. Exercise training and nutritional supplementation for physical frailty in very elderly people. N Engl J Med 1994;330(25):1769–1775.

17. Rowe JW, Kahn RL. Successful Aging: The MacArthur Foundation Study. New York: Dell Publishing, 1998.

18. Talbot L, Morrell C, Metter EJ, et al. Comparison of cardiorespiratory fitness versus leisure time physical activity as predictors of coronary events in men aged ≤65 years and > 65 years. Am J Cardiol 2002;89:1187–1192.

19. Province M, Hadley E, Hornbrook MC, et al. The effects of exercise on falls in elderly patients. A preplanned meta-analysis of the FICSIT trials. Frailty and injuries: cooperative studies of intervention techniques. JAMA 1995;273(17):1341–1347.

20. Dishman R. Physical activity and public health: mental health. Quest 1995;47:362–385.

21. Landers DM. The influence of exercise on mental health. President's council on physical fitness and sports research digest. 1997;2(12), http://purl.access.gpo.gov/GOV/LPS21091

22. Blumenthal J, Babyak M, Moore KA, et al. Effects of exercise training on older patients with major depression. Arch Int Med 1999;159(19):2349–2356.

23. American College of Sports Medicine. ACSM's Guidelines for Exercise Testing and Prescription. 8th Ed. Philadelphia: Lippincott Williams & Wilkins, 2010:190–194.

24. Neid R, Franklin B. Promoting and prescribing exercise for the elderly. Am Fam Physician 2002; http://www.aafp.org/afp/20020201/419.html

25. Pruitt B. Exercise progressions for seniors: take a sensible and gradual approach to improving older adults' quality of life. IDEA Health Fitness 2003;21(3):53–55.

26. Stiggelbout D, Popkema M, Hopman-Rock M, et al. Once a week is not enough: effects of a widely implemented group based exercise programme for older adults—a randomized control trial. J Epidemiol Community Health 2004;58(2):83–86.

27. Guidelines for exercise programming for the frail elderly. The results of the European Commission Framework V better aging project. 2005. Available at: www.laterlifetraining.co.uk

28. Petersen T. Functionally Fit: The Daily Program for Frail or Dependent Seniors. Lawrence, KS: American Academy of Health and Fitness. 2004.

SUGGESTED READINGS

American College of Sports Medicine. ACSM's Guidelines for Exercise Testing and Prescription. 7th Ed. Philadelphia: Lippincott Williams & Wilkins, 2006: 229–231.

Howley E, Franks BD. Fitness Professionals Handbook. 5th Ed. 2007. Human Kinetics.

EXERCISE FOR OVERWEIGHT AND OBESE INDIVIDUALS

6

For the past couple of decades, the incidences of **overweight** and **obesity** have been increasing throughout the United States. This is true for both men and women and across all age groups, races, education, and income levels. According to the Centers for Disease Control, the prevalence of obesity in the United States more than doubled between the years of 1980 and 2004.[1] An estimated 65% of adults in the United States are currently classified as overweight according to **BMI** (body mass index) standards (BMI ≥25),[2,3] 32% are considered obese (BMI ≥30), and 5% are classified as extremely obese (BMI ≥40).[2] For the BMI classification scheme, see Table 6.1. Sadly, the number of overweight children and adolescents increased as well. Nearly 14% of children between the ages of 2 and 5 and nearly 20% of those between the ages of 11 and 20 are now considered to be overweight.[1] Since excess weight during childhood strongly correlates with excess weight during adulthood, the outlook for future generations is grim.

Overweight results when individuals consume more kilocalories than their bodies expend. Yet, why some people pack on the pounds with even slight increases in energy intake while others seem to tolerate increases without gaining an ounce is difficult to understand. Is it the environment? Or are some people genetically predisposed to store extra weight? That is the million-dollar question.

There are likely many causes or contributors to excess weight gain. Certainly, genes play an important role, so researchers are investigating the effects of various hormones and other body chemicals on the propensity to gain weight. The fact that the offspring of overweight and obese parents are more likely to be overweight and obese than the offspring of normal weight parents also implicates heredity. Current evidence suggests, however, that environmental factors are the major contributors. After all, surroundings contribute to eating patterns, food preferences, and activity level, factors that ultimately influence weight.

Overweight—typically defined as an excess of weight relative to height or a BMI of 25 to 29.9.

Obesity—excess body fat or a BMI of 30 or higher.

BMI—body mass index; a measure of a person's weight relative to height. BMI is determined by dividing weight in kilograms by height in meters squared ([weight in kg] ÷ [height in meters]^2). Or it can be determined by multiplying weight in pounds by 703 and then dividing by height in inches squared ([weight in pounds × 703] ÷ [height in inches]^2). Although BMI does not give the percentage of body fat, studies show that BMI values correlate well with risk for chronic disease (i.e., risk increases as BMI increases).

TABLE 6-1 BMI CLASSIFICATIONS	
Classification	BMI
Underweight	<18.5
Healthy weight	18.5–24.9
Overweight	25–29.9
Obese	30–39.9
Extreme obesity	≥40

No matter what the cause, overweight and obesity are serious because excess weight increases the risk for coronary heart disease, diabetes, stroke, hypertension, **dyslipidemia**, gallbladder disease, osteoarthritis, and **sleep apnea**. In addition, excess weight is associated with a shorter life span and impaired quality of life. Some obese individuals report feelings of self-loathing, rejection, and isolation—factors that can foster depression and shame. Consequently, many overweight individuals are willing to try just about anything to lose a few pounds. In fact, nearly 45% of women and 30% of men are trying to lose weight at any given time. They spend an estimated $40 billion annually on weight-loss supplements, gym memberships, exercise equipment, weight-loss programs, and products that claim to "melt away fat." Not only are *obese individuals* trying to find solutions for their excess weight, but *researchers* are also investigating "treatments" that will ultimately reduce the risks for obesity-associated health complications.

Although many people hope for a magic weight-loss pill, experts agree that a combination of improved diet and routine exercise is the key to healthy weight loss and maintenance. The following chapter discusses how changes in lifestyle behaviors offer promise to overweight and obese individuals.

ANATOMICAL AND PHYSIOLOGICAL CHANGES

Excess weight is usually gained at a relatively slow rate over a long time period, so many are unaware of their expanding waistlines until their weights become dangerously high. This excess weight, typically in the form of fat, is a burden that taxes most body systems, particularly the cardiovascular, musculoskeletal, pulmonary, digestive, and endocrine systems.

CARDIOVASCULAR SYSTEM

Excess body fat increases the work load of the heart and often promotes hypertension (Fig. 6.1). Why? Adipocytes, the cells found in fat tissue, require oxygen and nutrients just like every other body cell. Consequently, when fat cell number increases, the body must make additional blood to meet the new demands. As blood volume increases, the pressure exerted against arterial walls also increases as the heart itself contracts more rapidly to meet demands. This explains the elevated heart rate often evident in those with excess

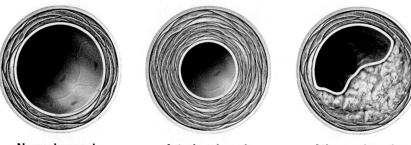

Normal vessel   **Arteriosclerosis**   **Atherosclerosis**

FIGURE 6.1 ■ Artery blockage resulting in hypertension. Sustained hypertension damages blood vessels. If blood vessels are subjected to high blood pressure for an extended period of time, they can thicken and harden, making them less flexible. This condition is called arteriosclerosis. Also, if excessive amounts of fat are found in the blood, the arteries can accumulate fatty deposits called plaques. This buildup, called atherosclerosis, causes the vessels to narrow or become obstructed. (Asset provided by Anatomical Chart Co.)

weight. Additionally, as blood volume increases, blood sodium levels also increase (primarily in response to hormone release). A greater blood sodium content promotes water retention, a factor that increases blood pressure even more. Overall, this cycle puts undue stress on the heart and taxes it even at rest. Imagine the burden caused by physical exertion—even if the activity is of low intensity. Unfortunately, an unhealthy heart has difficulty withstanding such demands.

As mentioned, excess weight often results in dyslipidemia, a condition that usually includes abnormally high blood levels of LDL and triglycerides. This promotes the formation of fatty deposits on arterial walls. These fatty deposits often develop into plaques that ultimately narrow blood vessels and increase blood pressure. Elevated blood pressure in turn promotes **aneurisms** and further damage to arterial walls. Damaged arterial walls attract additional fatty deposits, which can ultimately cause a heart attack or a stroke if the small arteries supplying the heart or the brain, respectively, are occluded.

Obese individuals often have poor circulation, so they commonly experience edema in their lower extremities. This occurs for several reasons. First of all, obese people tend to be sedentary—a lifestyle factor that interferes with efficient return of venous blood to the

Dyslipidemia—disproportionate lipid levels in the blood. It typically involves an excess of triglycerides and LDL and a deficiency of HDL. These increase the risk of developing atherosclerosis.

Sleep apnea—a condition in which soft tissues in the back of the throat block the air passageway during sleep. As a result, the sufferer stops breathing periodically throughout the night. The causes are varied.

Aneurism—a weakened wall in a blood vessel that balloons out and forms a blood-filled pouch. If an aneurism bursts, it can cause substantial blood loss, a dangerous drop in blood pressure, and possibly death.

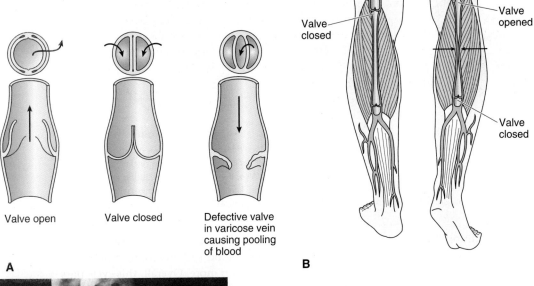

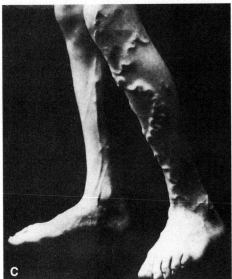

FIGURE 6.2 ■ Development of varicose veins. **A.** Function of valves in venous system. **B.** Contraction of skeletal muscle causes valves to open and close, preventing backflow of blood returning to heart. **C.** Varicose veins. (From Willis MC, CMA-AC. Medical Terminology: A Programmed Learning Approach to the Language of Health Care. Baltimore: Lippincott Williams & Wilkins, 2002.)

heart. In addition, blood traveling from the legs back to the heart has to fight gravity even in a normal weight person. Imagine the tremendous pressure that results from excess weight. Rather than moving efficiently back to the heart, fluid accumulates in lower body blood vessels. As it accumulates, it exerts pressure against venular walls. Eventually, this pressure forces more fluid into the interstitial space than the body can handle (see chapter 2 for more information on how the lymphatic system handles normal amounts of interstitial fluid). As the interstitial space fills with fluid, it restricts movement through veins. Thus, fluid accumulates in the thin-walled veins. As fluid accumulates, pressure within the veins builds and promotes the development of **varicose veins** as valves in the superficial vessels of the legs malfunction (Fig. 6.2).

QUICK REFERENCE

According to the U.S. Surgeon General, a 5% to 15% drop in weight significantly reduces the risk for heart disease because it lowers blood pressure and improves blood glucose and cholesterol levels.

MUSCULOSKELETAL SYSTEM

Since skeletal muscles act across joints to move bones of the skeleton, the skeletal and muscular systems are commonly referred to collectively as the musculoskeletal system. The five components of the musculoskeletal system are bones, muscles, **ligaments**, **tendons**, and cartilage. Tendons attach muscles to bones, while ligaments attach bones to bones. Cartilage has various functions. Hyaline cartilage, the most abundant type in the body, covers the ends of many bones to allow bone surfaces to glide over one another without friction. Elastic cartilage, which is somewhat springy, forms the structure of the ear and **epiglottis**. Fibrocartilage, the strongest type of cartilage, resists compression and prevents bone-on-bone contact. It connects the two pelvic bones anteriorly and forms the intervertebral discs of the spine and the menisci in the knees.

Excess weight stresses the musculoskeletal system and causes wear and tear of cartilage, particularly cartilage of the hips, knees, and lower back.[4] This results in pain, stiffness, and

---

Varicose veins—enlarged veins that occur due to damaged venous valves. They typically develop in the veins of the legs because of prolonged standing or excessive weight gain. The veins of the leg are already under tremendous pressure and must overcome the force of gravity to return blood to the heart. Extra body weight exacerbates the situation. Varicose veins are sometimes painful, itchy, and uncomfortable.

Ligaments—connective tissue that attaches bones to bones.

Tendons—connective tissue that connects muscle to bones.

Epiglottis—a flap of elastic cartilage that attaches at the base of the tongue. During swallowing, it prevents food from entering the trachea.

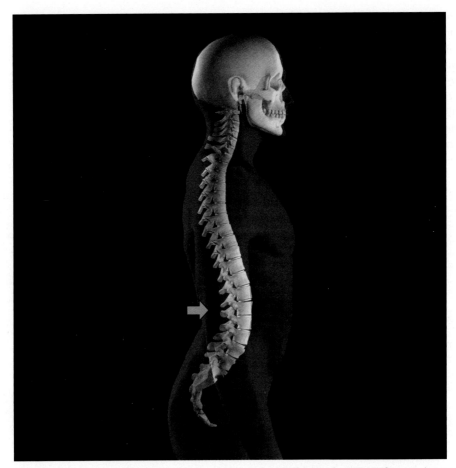

FIGURE 6.3 ■ Lordosis is the abnormal or excessive curvature of the lumbar spine, often seen in pregnancy or obesity. (LifeART image copyright ©2009 Lippincott Williams & Wilkins. All rights reserved.)

inflammation around joints that often limit mobility and develop into arthritis. In fact, statistics show that overweight and obese people experience arthritis more often than those at normal weights. Postural problems, such as **lordosis** (Fig. 6.3), might also result since excess weight shifts the center of balance and can promote spinal malformations.

Inactive joints produce insufficient synovial fluid. Recall from Chapter 2 that synovial fluid is produced by the joint capsule. It reduces friction between two articulating bones, provides shock absorption during movement, and nourishes nearby cartilage cells. As long as joints remain active, the joint capsule continues to produce synovial fluid, which in turn facilitates joint movement. As activity levels decrease, however, less synovial fluid is produced and the existing synovial fluid thickens—a factor that limits range-of-motion. Since many overweight and obese individuals are sedentary, they often produce insufficient synovial fluid and thus suffer the associated joint problems.

Whether or not obesity is an independent risk factor for arthritis is still unknown.[5,6] Certainly, the joints of obese individuals are under much more stress than the joints of healthy-weight people. Additionally, statistics suggest that those carrying excess weight often report acute pain, inflammation, and limited mobility, particularly in the knee joints. According to the U.S. Department of Health and Human Services, the risk for developing arthritis increases by 9% to 13% for every 2-lb increase in weight, with symptoms improving after even a minor weight loss. In fact, research shows that losing just 14 lb of weight likely reduces pressure on the knees by 30 lb. A study in Wisconsin also found a correlation between arthritis and BMI. In this study, 28% of arthritis sufferers had a BMI exceeding 30, which suggests that excess weight contributes to arthritis development in some individuals.[6]

Lastly, depending upon where excess weight is stored, overweight and obese individuals sometimes experience balance and locomotion problems. Extremely large thighs make walking difficult; excess arm, leg, and/or abdominal fat interferes with the ability to assume certain positions; and fat concentrated in the abdomen changes the center of balance.

RESPIRATORY SYSTEM

Obesity interferes with the functioning of the respiratory system by limiting respiratory capacity, diminishing lung volume, interfering with breathing mechanics, and impairing gas exchange. It also increases the risk for pulmonary embolism, pneumonia, and respiratory failure, all of which increase the risk of death.[7] In addition and as mentioned earlier, obese individuals experience sleep apnea more frequently than healthy-weight people. Not only is this dangerous, but it also interferes with the length and quality of sleep. Chronic sleep deprivation is associated with complications such as chronic fatigue, avoidance of physical activity, and lack of motivation, factors that set into motion the cycle of unhealthy eating, sedentary lifestyle, and continued weight gain.

For years, researchers have suspected a link between obesity and asthma since the incidence of asthma has nearly tripled simultaneously with the dramatic increase in overweight and obesity.[8,9] Although this correlation exists, experts do not yet know if it is the obesity that increases asthma risk or if having asthma increases the likelihood of developing obesity. Nevertheless, the lungs of obese individuals cannot expand normally because of excess fat, which crowds internal organs and limits their movements. This results in shorter, shallower breaths and difficulty breathing. In addition, the bodies of obese people

---

Lordosis—an excessive curvature in the lumbar spine area; also called swayback. One contributing factor is excess weight in the abdominal area as occurs during pregnancy. As the added weight succumbs to gravity, an excessive curvature in the lumbar spine develops.

tend to exist in a state of chronic low-grade inflammation that results from extra adipose. As this inflammation moves into the smooth muscle lining of the air passageways, it constricts the passageways and promotes asthma attacks. Overall, existing research is conflicting; however, it appears that weight loss dramatically decreases medication requirements and improves lung functioning, symptoms, and the overall health status of asthma sufferers.[9–12]

DIGESTIVE SYSTEM

Various digestive problems result from overweight and obesity. Acid reflux occurs more frequently because excess fat displaces the stomach and other digestive organs. The cardiac sphincter, designed to prevent stomach contents from reentering the esophagus, weakens and begins to permit acidic stomach components to move back into the esophagus—especially if the sufferer lies down soon after eating. This results in heartburn. Unfortunately, continual exposure of the esophageal lining to stomach acid increases the risk for esophageal cancer.

Gallbladder complications, including gallstones and gallbladder disease, sometimes develop in response to excess cholesterol absorbed in the small intestine or produced by the liver. These complications cause abdominal pain, vomiting, and overall discomfort that often requires gallbladder removal. Once the gallbladder is removed, tolerance for dietary fats diminishes. As a result, fat intake must be closely regulated to avoid discomfort. Another problem that occurs in response to excess weight gain is the accumulation of fatty deposits around the liver. These deposits interfere with liver functioning, and since the liver is a major metabolic organ, the results can be devastating.

Lastly, obese individuals often suffer frequent bouts of constipation as fat buildup interferes with GI tract motility. Further contributing to this problem is the fact that the diets of overweight people often lack sufficient fiber, so stools are less bulky and more difficult to pass. Constipation, in turn, promotes hemorrhoid development since sufferers typically have to strain to eliminate.

HORMONE LEVELS

Hormones are regulatory substances produced by endocrine tissue. Normally, the body precisely controls the release of these substances to maintain optimal conditions within each organ system. When hormone levels deviate from normal, problems result.

Interestingly—and contrary to popular belief—few cases of obesity result from faulty glands. On the contrary, the state of obesity seems to interfere with the proper release and performance of several hormones such as **leptin**, **adiponectin**, **insulin**, and **estrogen**.

Leptin and adiponectin are hormones produced and released by adipocytes. Leptin, released in response to food consumption, signals the body to stop eating. It also increases energy expenditure to burn the extra kilocalories. In addition, it acts as an inflammatory agent. Obese individuals typically have unusually high leptin levels, a condition that promotes low-grade inflammation and airway constriction (as discussed earlier). Obesity is also associated with low levels of adiponectin, a hormone that has an anti-inflammatory effect on blood vessels and is associated with a reduced risk of heart attack.

Researchers still do not fully understand the relationship between obesity and insulin. Insulin is a hormone released in response to the increasing blood glucose levels that develop whenever a person consumes food. Insulin binds to receptors on body cells and essentially acts as a key that opens a door to permit glucose entry. This is vital to survival since glucose is the primary substance used by body cells to fuel cellular processes. Without access to circulating glucose, cell functioning ceases and cells starve. The problem with obesity is that cell receptors become unresponsive to insulin in the presence of excess adipose; thus, insulin is unable to function and glucose accumulates in the blood. In an effort to lower blood glucose levels, the pancreas continues to produce and release progressively greater quantities of insulin, but the insulin cannot function. Ultimately, this promotes hyperglycemia and noninsulin dependent diabetes mellitus.

Insulin's role is not limited to glucose transport; it also stimulates fatty acid movement into adipocytes, which increases overall fat storage. Consequently, high levels of blood insulin predispose the body to weight gain. Weight loss, on the other hand, normalizes insulin levels and insulin response.[13,14]

Estrogen levels are anywhere from 60% to 219% higher in obese women than in healthy-weight women. Why? Because obese women have an abnormally large number of adipocytes, cells that produce and release estrogen. Studies suggest that this higher estrogen contributes to the increased risk for breast cancer experienced by women with high BMI values. In fact, one study estimates that breast cancer risk increases by 18% for every 5-point increment on the BMI scale.[15]

Ghrelin, a relatively recently discovered hormone produced by the stomach, stimulates appetite, decreases energy expenditure, and increases energy storage. Levels typically increase prior to a meal and decrease after a meal. Interestingly, obese people tend to produce lower amounts of ghrelin—possibly because their bodies are constantly

---

Leptin—a hormone produced by fat cells that inhibits the desire to eat and increases energy expenditure in an attempt to maintain body weight. Obese individuals have high leptin levels indicating that their bodies are struggling to suppress appetite and burn kilocalories to avoid further weight gain. Leptin levels decrease with weight loss as the body attempts to preserve body mass. Leptin also acts as an inflammatory agent.

Adiponectin—a hormone produced by fat cells that acts as an anti-inflammatory. It also decreases the risk for heart attack. Levels tend to diminish as weight increases.

Insulin—a hormone released by the pancreas in response to increasing blood glucose levels.

Estrogen—a hormone produced by the ovaries and by adipocytes. High levels are associated with an increased risk for breast cancer.

Ghrelin—a hormone produced by stomach cells that stimulates appetite and increases energy storage.

in an energy-surplus situation. Leaner people, on the other hand, produce greater amounts of ghrelin, likely because their energy stores are low. Thus, they could benefit from an increased energy intake. The precise relationship between ghrelin and obesity is not yet clear; however, researchers are enthusiastically investigating it.

PRECAUTIONS DURING EXERCISE

Because excess weight already tremendously strains the body, the added stress of exercise can be detrimental if response is not monitored and intensity adjusted to ensure safety. This is especially true given that obese individuals have a decreased work tolerance and extreme variability in their initial health status. Hypothetically, exercise could cause a cardiac event, a stroke, debilitating joint injuries, or a dangerously high body temperature. This section explores the issues of particular concern for overweight or obese exercisers.

Since obese individuals often have co-existing risk factors that preclude certain types of exercise, they should seek medical clearance prior to beginning an exercise program. Certain groups are particularly vulnerable to adverse side effects during exercise. These include overweight or obese men who are over the age of 40; overweight or obese women who are over the age of 50; those with heart disease, lung disease, asthma, arthritis, or osteoporosis; those experiencing chest pressure or pain with exertion; those who easily develop shortness of breath; those with hypertension, diabetes, or high blood cholesterol; those who smoke cigarettes; or those with a family history of heart attacks or coronary heart disease.

INCREASED RISK FOR A CARDIAC EVENT OR STROKE

As mentioned earlier, the heart of an overweight or obese person has to work harder than the heart of a healthy-weight person during normal daily activities, even when those activities are of low intensity. Thus, heart rate and blood volume are elevated even at rest. Since an obese person's arteries are often full of fatty streaks and plaque, blood pressure can reach dangerously high levels. Moreover, vessels are often weak and prone to aneurisms. Adding the demands of exercise can potentially result in life-threatening events. Therefore, a qualified fitness trainer properly plans exercise and monitors tolerance as described later in this chapter.

DEBILITATING JOINT INJURIES

Excess body weight unduly stresses joints, so obese individuals frequently experience weak or even damaged knee, hip, or lower back joints before they even think of beginning an exercise program. Since exercise itself stresses joints and sometimes causes joint injuries in healthy-weight people, overweight and obese individuals need to be especially cautious to avoid exacerbating preexisting joint conditions. They might need to avoid certain activities altogether, but it all depends upon the specific joint(s) involved. Furthermore, obese clients should cautiously approach cardiovascular training; they need to focus on protecting the hips, knees, and ankles. Since high-intensity training can overstress these joints—particularly in the initial stages of exercise—overweight participants need to include nonweight-bearing activities such as stationary cycling or water aerobics. These nonimpact activities allow joints to slowly adapt to increased impact and work loads.

HYPERTHERMIA: A DANGEROUS INCREASE IN CORE BODY TEMPERATURE

All metabolic processes release heat as a by-product. In fact, skeletal muscle contraction produces most of the heat that maintains core body temperature at 98.6°F. During exercise, core body temperature rises as skeletal muscles contract more frequently. Under normal circumstances, the body effectively cools itself to prevent a dangerous rise in temperature. It accomplishes this primarily through evaporative and radiative cooling. More specifically, the brain stimulates sweat glands to release sweat onto the body's surface. As sweat evaporates from the body it carries a tremendous amount of heat along with it. If body temperature continues to climb, the brain also stimulates dilation of blood vessels in the dermis. This diverts warm blood from internal organs to the dermis, which permits heat to radiate into the environment.

Overweight and obese people tend to produce excessive amounts of heat, so their cooling mechanisms are sometimes overwhelmed during physical exertion. Additionally, overweight and obese people have large subcutaneous fat stores that help insulate the body and retard heat loss. These factors promote hyperthermia during exercise and increase the risk for heat illness.

BARRIERS TO EXERCISE

Barriers to exercise exist in every population; therefore, fitness professionals are accustomed to discovering and addressing them. Not only is it important to be aware of barriers, but it is also essential to treat clients with respect while helping them overcome these barriers.

Standard exercise equipment, such as stationary cycles and resistance-training machines, are not designed for large body frames. Be sensitive to an obese client's needs and avoid embarrassing situations. If wider seats or larger pieces of equipment are available, use them. When uncertain as to whether or not a client will fit on a particular machine, avoid it completely and choose an alternative in advance. Keep in mind that many obese people have had previous unpleasant experiences with exercise, so they might give up if they have another.

A second barrier to exercise is the overall low physical capacity associated with most obese individuals. Those carrying excess weight often claim to lack the energy to get through the day, so how could they possibly begin exercising? Emphasize that regular exercise actually increases energy, improves sleep, and decreases overall discomfort, so it ultimately minimizes lethargy.

Lack of time, a barrier common to all populations, also affects this special needs group. Setting aside 30 to 60 minutes per day for exercise might seem impossible, so initially keep duration short and encourage clients to become more active during their typical daily activities. They can park their cars farther away from the grocery store, use the stairs rather than the elevator, and walk to a coworker's office rather than calling or e-mailing. Simply adding these activities into the daily routine can increase energy expenditure, improve cardiorespiratory functioning, and increase muscular strength and endurance.

BODY FAT DISTRIBUTION AND ITS EFFECTS ON HEALTH

Body composition and fat distribution are more reliable predictors of chronic disease risk than body weight. According to Dr. C. Everett Koop, former Surgeon General of the United States and Senior Scholar at the C. Everett Koop Institute at Dartmouth, men under the age of 39 should have a body fat percentage from 8% to 19%; women under the age of 39 should have a body fat percentage from 21% to 32%; men over the age of 39 should aim for 11% to 24% body fat; and women over the age of 39 should strive for 23% to 35% body fat. Hydrostatic weighing, dual-energy x-ray absorptiometry, and magnetic resonance imaging are laboratory techniques that precisely measure body fat percentage relative to lean mass. In the field, skinfolds, bioelectrical impedance, and anthropometry are common.

The distribution of body fat is actually an easier and just as reliable predictor for chronic disease risk. **Intra-abdominal fat**, which surrounds organs within the abdominal cavity, increases the risk for heart disease, stroke, high blood pressure, diabetes, and several other chronic diseases when compared to **lower body fat**. Lower body fat, or fat stored primarily around the hips and thighs, does not appear to increase the risk for chronic diseases. Consequently, men, who commonly store extra intra-abdominal fat, have a higher risk for cardiovascular events than women since women tend to store fat in the hips and thighs.

BENEFITS OF EXERCISE

Although exercise imposes some risks, it improves the health of this special population in various ways. The following section discusses some of the specific benefits experienced by overweight and obese exercisers.

IMPROVED CARDIOVASCULAR AND RESPIRATORY FUNCTIONING

Studies confirm a negative correlation between activity level and risk for cardiovascular disease. According to the National Health and Nutrition Examination Survey I (NHANES I), sedentary obese individuals have a risk for cardiovascular death that is three times that of active healthy-weight people.[1,16] Additionally, cardiovascular death rates among women were positively correlated with BMI in the Nurses' Health Study.[16,17] In other words, women in this study experienced more cardiac events as BMI increased.

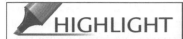 **HIGHLIGHT** Determining Risk for Chronic Disease Using Waist Circumference

An easy and inexpensive method of assessing a client's risk for chronic disease is to measure the waist circumference. Since the risk for developing heart disease, stroke, and diabetes increases in those with central obesity, the waist circumference is a valid indicator. In general, the risk for chronic diseases increases for the following:

Men who have a waist circumference greater than 35 in.

Women who have a waist circumference greater than 40 in.

Exercise improves cardiovascular risk by lowering blood pressure, increasing HDL levels, decreasing LDL and triglyceride levels, and improving heart and lung functioning—even in the absence of weight loss.[9,16,18] Since excess weight is an independent risk factor for cardiovascular disease, however, any weight loss accompanying increased activity dramatically decreases risk as well. In fact, a mere 5% to 10% loss in body weight significantly improves blood pressure, blood lipids, and glucose tolerance.[2]

Lung functioning tends to improve as abdominal fat diminishes. The lungs, whose actions are inhibited by excess body fat, are able to fully inflate with weight loss, so breathing rate and depth return to normal. In addition, maximal oxygen uptake improves.

DECREASED RISK FOR TYPE 2 DIABETES

Overweight and obese individuals have an increased risk for developing insulin resistance even though insulin levels are usually in the normal-to-high range. Insulin resistance results in elevated blood glucose levels, the first indicator of diabetes. As mentioned earlier, the pancreas of an obese person typically produces insulin, but body cells become

Intra-abdominal fat—fat stored around the abdominal organs; also known as central obesity. Often referred to as an "apple shape." Fat stored in this area increases the risk for chronic diseases such as cardiovascular disease, diabetes, stroke, hypertension, and certain types of cancers. Men and postmenopausal women commonly have high levels of intra-abdominal fat.

Lower body fat—fat stored in the hips and thighs. Often referred to as a "pear shape." This pattern of fat distribution is common in women and does not appear to increase the risk for chronic disease.

less responsive. This is possibly because excess adipose alters the shape of insulin recep-tors thereby preventing them from binding with insulin. As blood glucose levels climb (since glucose cannot enter cells), the pancreas produces more and more insulin until insulin levels are uncharacteristically high—a state called hyperinsulinemia. Eventually, all of this work overstresses the pancreas, but blood glucose and insulin levels continue to rise. Consequently, the blood becomes more viscous, which can damage blood vessels, increase blood pressure, interfere with blood clotting, and promote the development of type 2 diabetes.

Because type 2 diabetes, or noninsulin dependent diabetes, positively correlates with obesity, it makes sense that fat loss decreases risk. In fact, even moderate weight loss sig-nificantly improves insulin response, which prevents blood glucose from reaching dangerously high levels. Moreover, weight loss accompanied by regular exercise nearly eliminates glucose intolerance and insulin resistance in most people.[16]

QUICK REFERENCE
Obese people are three times more likely to develop type 2 diabetes than healthy-weight people.

REDUCED OVERALL DISCOMFORT

Carrying excess fat mass is difficult and uncomfortable, particularly for those with low percentages of muscle mass. Activities that are simple for healthy-weight individuals become difficult, if not impossible, for the obese. They often struggle to breathe while sitting. Trying to go from a seated position to a standing position is difficult. Move-ment into and out of automobiles becomes strenuous. And tasks such as cleaning, cooking, and doing laundry are exhausting. Accompanying weight loss is a renewed vigor and stamina that enables the formerly obese person to once again engage in normal activities. Additionally, changes in body composition—or, more specifically, an increase in muscle mass and a decrease in fat mass—decrease stress during all activ-ities. Work loads seem lighter, recovery times are shorter, and perception of effort completely changes—all of which encourage continued exercise.

IMPROVED MOOD AND DECREASED ANXIETY

Whether accompanied by weight loss or not, physical activity elevates mood, improves self-esteem, and decreases the incidence of anxiety.[19] This is true whether the physical pursuits are in the form of regimented exercise programs or whether they simply involve more movement in normal daily activities. Improvements in mood and anxiety level then encourage obese people to get more involved with their lives and to seek out social settings—factors that further encourage activity.

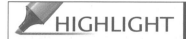

HIGHLIGHT   Metabolic Syndrome

According to the American Heart Association, metabolic syndrome is on the rise in the United States and now affects over 50 million Americans. It is indicated by a cluster of symptoms that increases the risk for cardiovascular disease and diabetes. These symptoms include the following:

Intra-abdominal fat

- Men with a waist circumference ≥40 in. (>102 cm)
- Women with a waist circumference ≥35 in. (>88 cm)

High triglycerides

- Blood triglyceride level ≥150 mg per dL

Low HDL level

- Men with an HDL level <40 mg per dL
- Women with an HDL level <50 mg per dL

Hypertension

- Blood pressure ≥130/85 mm Hg on more than three consecutive readings

Insulin resistance or glucose intolerance

- Indicated by elevated fasting glucose ≥110 mg/dL

Intra-abdominal obesity and physical inactivity seem to be the strongest predictors formetabolic syndrome. According to the American College of Sports Medicine (ACSM) and the National Cholesterol Education Program, interventions should focus on weight control, physical activity, and treatment for coexisting cardiovascular disease risk factors.[2,20] The best methods for managing metabolic syndrome include losing enough weight to decrease BMI to <25; increasing physical activity to achieve a minimum of 30 minutes or more of moderate intensity activity per day; and reducing the intake of saturated fat, cholesterol, and trans fat.

When working with clients diagnosed with metabolic syndrome, base risk stratification upon the presence of dyslipidemia, hypertension, and hyperglycemia. If indicated, obtain a medical screening by a physician before initiating exercise testing. Since many people with metabolic syndrome are also overweight or obese, follow general guidelines offered in this chapter for the overweight population. Additionally, strictly monitor blood pressure before and during exercise since most sufferers have high blood pressure.[2]

In general, exercise prescription guidelines for this population are similar to those for the general population. Consider all cardiovascular risk factors and adjust recommendations accordingly (see chapter 7 for more information on exercise guidelines for those with cardiovascular disease). Initial exercise intensity should be moderate (40% to 60% VO_{2R}) with a gradual progression to more vigorous intensity (50% to 75% VO_{2R}). Because many people suffering from metabolic syndrome carry excess weight, they should strive to lose weight by slowly increasing the duration of exercise to 300 minutes per week—or 50 to 60 minutes of activity on 5 days per week. Exercise can be continuous—or it can be separated into several 10-minute segments of daily exercise if necessary. Some research suggests that individuals actually have to exercise for 60 to 90 minutes per day to lose and then maintain weight loss.[2]

TREATMENT PLANS FOR OBESITY

Drugs

The search for a pharmacological treatment of obesity intensified once obesity was classified as a chronic disease. The overall goal is to find an effective medication with minimal side effects that results in long-term weight loss that does not require continued medication use. Although several existing drugs satisfy one or two of these criteria, no drug meets all of them. Sibutramine, marketed as Meridia, works by suppressing the appetite. Side effects include headache, constipation, rapid heart rate, and increased blood pressure. Orlistat, marketed as Xenical, promotes weight loss by inhibiting the small intestine's ability to digest dietary fats. Undigested dietary fats cannot be absorbed. Orlistat reduces fat absorption by 30% and is the only medication approved for use by adolescents. Side effects include frequent bowel movements and reduced absorption of fat-soluble vitamins.

Weight-loss drugs work; they often result in a 10% reduction in weight in people who also exercise and reduce their energy intake. The problem with most weight-loss drugs is that they are only approved for short-term use. Once a person stops using them, weight is typically regained. Furthermore, most have uncomfortable side effects that are sometimes hazardous, so drugs are not the answer for everyone.

Surgery

An increasing number of clinically obese people (BMI > 40) are seeking surgical procedures to help in their fight against obesity. In most cases, these procedures are designed to decrease the size of the stomach. A smaller stomach capacity forces patients to consume fewer total kilocalories, which promotes a negative energy balance and weight loss. In addition, this type of surgery also limits the amount of ghrelin released into the blood stream. Lower ghrelin levels diminish the appetite and inhibit fat storage. Examples of surgeries commonly performed include gastric bypass surgery, gastric lap band surgery, and stomach stapling. All forms of surgery have risks of complication to include infection, dehydration, nausea, constipation, and vomiting. In addition, patients risk nutrient deficiencies since they must drastically reduce food intake following surgery.

Diet and Exercise

Obese individuals need to closely monitor their diets to lose weight and maintain weight loss. They need to limit their intake of **empty kilocalories**, while they increase their intake of **nutrient-dense foods** to create an overall energy deficit that does not result in nutrient deficiencies. Although a lower kilocalorie diet is necessary for weight loss, diet alone (in the absence of exercise) tends to promote the loss of metabolically active muscle tissue and a concurrent drop in metabolic rate. This lowered metabolic rate then makes it difficult to maintain weight loss. In essence, dieting alone does not result in significant or sustained weight-loss.

Moderate exercise alone often does not result in significant weight loss in obese individuals. In fact, most studies find that the greatest amount of weight loss occurs in response to *vigorous* exercise done for long durations. Unfortunately, most obese people cannot sustain high intensities because of weak musculoskeletal systems or their elevated risk for cardiovascular events, so a safer approach that encourages more moderate activity is usually taken. Overall, a combination of moderate exercise and diet seems to be the key for successful and healthy weight loss in the obese population.

RECOMMENDATIONS FOR EXERCISE

EXERCISE TESTING

The ACSM suggests that overweight and obese individuals with no other complications may safely undergo standard exercise testing protocols without serious risk, provided that they have been cleared for exercise by a medical professional. As mentioned earlier, however, tolerance for work load diminishes with increasing body weight, so initial work load should be limited to 2 to 3 metabolic equivalents (METs) with small incremental increases of 0.5 to 1.0 METs per testing stage.[2] Any additional conditions such as joint injuries, limited range-of-motion, hypertension, or preexisting heart conditions warrant further adjustments and might interfere with the accuracy of test results. A cycle ergometer with an oversized seat is probably easier for testing than the treadmill, but exercise testing should be individualized based on the client's current health status.

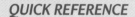

QUICK REFERENCE

Standard termination criteria might not apply to this special population because overweight and obese people have difficulty reaching the typical physiological criteria of maximal exercise testing.[2]

EXERCISE PRESCRIPTION

After determining an obese client's goals, design an exercise program that helps meet those goals and takes into consideration the precautions discussed earlier. Weight loss is always a primary goal for this particular population. (Table 6.2 shows general tips for weight loss.) In most cases, however, severely obese clients who participate in exercise do not lose tremendous amounts of fat, so fitness professionals should emphasize the health improvements that occur even in the absence of weight loss. These include a

---

Empty kilocalories—an empty kilocalorie food is one that provides energy but little or no vitamins and minerals. Candy bars, potato chips, and sugary sodas are examples.

Nutrient-dense foods—these are foods that have a high nutrient value relative to their kilocalorie content. As an example, skim milk (300 mg of calcium, 0 g of fat, and 80 kcal per serving) is more nutrient-dense than whole fat milk (300 mg of calcium, 8 g of fat, and 146 kcal per serving).

TABLE 6-2   GENERAL TIPS FOR WEIGHT LOSS

- Strive for a 5%–10% weight loss over 3–6 months
- Change diet and exercise behaviors for long-term weight loss
- Create an energy deficit of 500 kcal/day for a weekly loss of 1 lb. Create a deficit of 1,000 kcal/day for a weekly loss of 2 lb. This deficit is created by reducing energy intake and increasing energy expenditure.
- Progressively increase weekly activity to a minimum of 150 minutes. Strive for up to 300 minutes of activity per week or a total of 2,000 kcal/week.

Source: American College of Sports Medicine. ACSM's Guidelines for Exercise Testing and Prescription. 8th Ed. Philadelphia: Lippincott Williams & Wilkins, 2010:253–256.

reduced risk for cardiovascular disease, improved joint functioning, increased energy for daily activities, and better sleep. In addition, since weight loss is often slow, stress the importance of *gradual* improvements that last. After all, it takes longer than two weeks to put on 40 lb of fat, so it is impossible to take it off in two weeks. In addition, since studies suggest that exercise alone leads to disappointing results in the obese population, strongly encourage clients to combine increased activity with improved eating.[21]

According to current research and recommendations, exercise prescription for the overweight or obese population should adhere to the following guidelines:

- Since most obese individuals have additional risk factors for chronic diseases, they should receive medical clearance prior to initiating an exercise program.
- As with the general population, obese exercisers should precede all activity with a 5 to 10 minute warm-up to prepare the body for activity and follow up with a 5 to 10 minute cool-down to return the body to a resting state.
- General guidelines pertaining to type, frequency, duration, and intensity of aerobic exercise are similar to recommendations for the general population.
    □ According to ACSM, aerobic exercise should be the primary focus for this population. The type of exercise chosen needs to effectively work large muscle groups to ensure adequate kilocalorie expenditure. Low-impact activities that minimize trauma to the joints are ideal. Walking, which requires no special skills and is easy on the joints, is usually the best choice in the initial stages of an exercise program. Water aerobics is another viable option that is easy on the joints and helpful for thermoregulation.
    □ A frequency of 5 to 7 days per week of moderate intensity activity for 30 to 60 minutes optimizes energy expenditure and helps achieve the minimum of 150 minutes of activity per week suggested by experts. Members of this population should gradually progress to 300 minutes of activity per week. Initial intensity should be moderate (40% to 60% VO_{2R}) since obese people are unconditioned and at an increased risk for musculoskeletal injuries. As improvements in cardiovascular and respiratory functioning occur, these clients may increase intensity (up to 50% to 75% VO_{2R}) as long as the increase does not cause musculoskeletal

problems. In many cases, it is actually better to increas *intensity* to reduce some of the risk. Exercise can be (increments in cases where continuous exercise cannot '

☐ The Department of Health and Human Services, the D and ACSM indicate that some individuals need to st 90 minutes of moderate-to-vigorous activity to effec tain weight loss. Clients exercising for this longer du... cautious to avoid overuse injury.

■ According to ACSM, resistance training in this population does not effect vent the loss of fat-free mass that occurs as large amounts of weight are lost. Obe... people who include resistance training in their exercise regimen, however, increase muscular strength and endurance, improve functional capacity, and enhance neuromuscular functioning. In addition, strength-training increases bone mass, a benefit that decreases long-term risk for osteoporosis. Overall, these changes reduce physiological stress during everyday activities. To be effective, the frequency of resistance training should be two to three times per week. A minimum of 8 to 10 exercises should target all major muscle groups, just as ACSM suggests for healthy-weight exercisers. Exercisers should use a resistance that fatigues the muscle in 8 to 12 repetitions, and they should perform a minimum of one set per exercise.

■ Because obese exercisers have a high risk for elevated body temperature during activity, proper hydration before, during, and after activity is essential.

■ Change the goal of exercise from weight loss to mood enhancement or fatigue reduction. Ask clients how they feel after a workout. Inquire about their quality of sleep a couple of weeks after initiating exercise. Find out if normal activities of daily living—such as unloading the groceries from the car or giving a toddler a bath—are easier since exercise initiation. In other words, *give clients a method of measuring their success that does not depend upon the scale, the tape measure, or even the amount of resistance.*

QUICK REFERENCE

Individuals in this special population can have quite different functional capacities. Obese clients with normal mobility can usually engage in most traditional resistance exercises and cardiovascular training. Those with restricted abilities because of limited range-of-motion or pain in different joints might need to concentrate on simpler movements. An exercise program for the more functional obese client would resemble that of a healthier weight client—with some modifications in duration and frequency. The less mobile obese client, however, might need simple aerobic activities. These clients should avoid traditional strength exercises until overall functional capacity improves.

One final point: never underestimate the benefit of increased daily activities at home or at work. Encourage clients to walk and use the stairs more to increase energy expenditure. Since exercise adherence is often low in this particular population, creating additional means by which these clients can burn energy is priceless.[22]

MPLE EXERCISES FOR THE OVERWEIGHT OR OBESE CLIENT

To lose weight, overweight and obese clients should focus on reducing kilocalorie intake and engaging in cardiovascular exercise that optimizes energy expenditure. This combination is the most effective means of weight loss. Walking and water aerobics are easy on the joints, but stationary bicycles or recumbent cross trainers are also viable modes. Resistance training, which builds muscular strength and endurance, can also be a beneficial adjunct to the program.

The types of resistance exercises appropriate for any individual obese client vary depending upon level of functioning and comorbidities. Regardless of the level of functioning, however, the exercise program should develop the core, upper back, iliopsoas, and adductors. Why? Because obese individuals, who often carry extra weight in the midsection, develop an excessive anterior pelvic tilt—a position that puts undue stress on the spine and leads to back pain.[23]

Use a combination of free weights, elastic bands or tubing, and weight machines to train the overweight client. In cases where clients are extremely large, avoid weight machines to preclude embarrassing and discouraging experiences.

TRAINING CORE MUSCLES USING THE STABILITY BALL

The stability ball is effective at improving core strength and balance in nearly all populations as long as proper size is chosen. Models available in retail stores typically support up to 250 lb. For obese clients, use better quality, stronger brands designed to withstand a large amount of weight. In addition, invest in balls that are burst-resistant. This means that if punctured, they lose air slowly and do not pop.

QUICK REFERENCE

When working with a stability ball, size matters. To determine appropriate size, have the client sit on the ball with feet flat on the floor and weight evenly distributed. There should be a 90-degree angle at the hips and knees so that the thighs are parallel to the floor. The following chart provides suggestions for various heights:

Height	Stability Ball Size (cm)
4'6" to 5'0"	45
5'1" to 5'7"	55
5'8" to 6'1"	65
6'1" to 6'7"	75

Stability balls from different manufacturers are made of different materials and, therefore, have different firmnesses. In general, the firmer the ball, the more challenging the exercise.

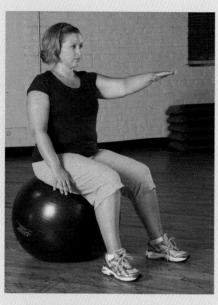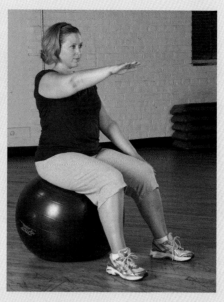

■ **Seated Ball Bounce with Alternating Front Shoulder Raises (Fig. 6.4)**

Sit on the ball with feet firmly planted on the floor shoulder width apart. Contract abdominals and maintain neutral spine. Rhythmically bounce up and down while maintaining balance. Alternately, lift arms to the front slowly. Continue for approximately 2 minutes. This exercise warms up the muscles, improves balance, and helps alleviate lower back pain.

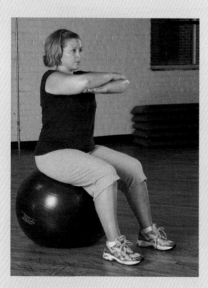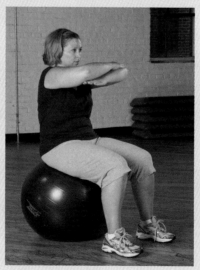

■ **Seated Pelvic Tilt (Fig. 6.5)**

Sit on the ball with feet firmly planted on the floor shoulder width apart, abdominals contracted, and spine in neutral alignment. Rotate the pelvis forward and back with minimal ball movement. Repeat for 10 to 20 repetitions. This exercise improves balance and trains the abdominals and gluteals.

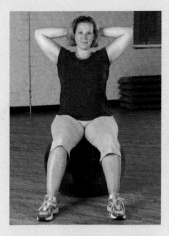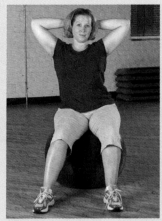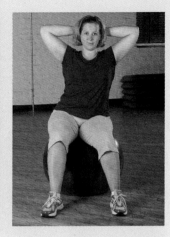

■ Seated Lateral Glides (Fig. 6.6)

Sit on ball with feet firmly planted on the floor shoulder width apart, abdominals contracted, and spine in neutral alignment. Shift hips to the right and then to the left with minimal ball movement. The upper body should remain upright. This exercise improves balance and strengthens the abdominals, gluteals, and lower back. Alternatively, perform seated circles from same position. Hands may be on the ball for more stability, on the thighs for more of a challenge, or on the head (as in an abdominal crunch) for the greatest challenge. Slowly roll the hips in a circle to the right making small circles initially. Make larger circles as balance improves. Do 10 to 20 repetitions to the right. Then repeat to the left.

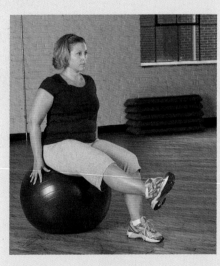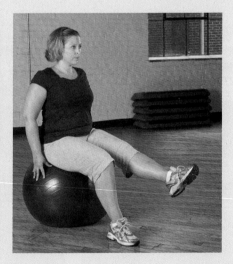

■ Seated Leg Extension (Fig. 6.7)

Sit on the ball with feet firmly planted on the floor and closer together than shoulder width, abdominals contracted, and spine in neutral alignment. Slowly kick one leg out while the other remains firmly planted. Return foot to floor and repeat with the other leg. This exercise is easier when the leg is lifted higher. It is more challenging when the leg is barely lifted. This exercise improves balance and trains the abdominals, gluteals, quadriceps, hamstrings, hip flexors, and lower back.

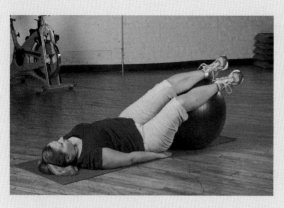 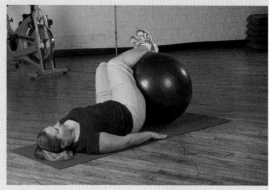

■ Lumbar Rotation in Supine Position (Fig. 6.8)

Lie with back on the floor and both legs supported by the ball. Slowly roll both legs back and forth to allow rotation of the lumbar spine. Only rotate through a comfortable range of motion. This exercise targets the oblique muscles.

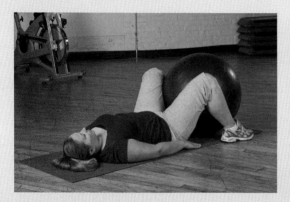 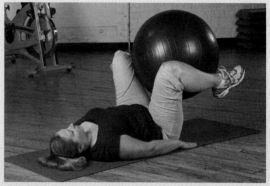

■ Thigh Adduction with Stability Ball Lift (Fig. 6.9)

Lie on the floor with feet flat on the floor and arms extended at side with palms down. The ball should be between the legs. Grip the ball with the knees and squeeze. Contract abdominals and lift feet off floor while bringing ball toward torso. Hold for 5 to 10 seconds. Release and repeat for 10 to 20 repetitions.

Many obese individuals have weak upper backs that promote poor posture because they have to support so much weight in the upper anterior torso. Furthermore, they tend to have tight chest and anterior shoulder muscles because gravity pulls the excess weight down toward the front. Training the rhomboids and stretching the chest help alleviate the resulting discomfort. To train the rhomboids, have the client perform the seated row. Either use a seated cable row machine or resistance bands or tubing.

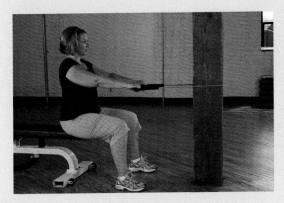 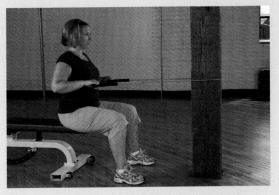

■ Seated Row with Elastic Tubing (Fig. 6.10)

Wrap tubing around a secure bar or chair. Sit in a chair that is about a foot away from the bar. Be sure to face it. Grasp one end of the tubing in each hand. With palms down, pull tubing toward the chest. Pause. Return to starting position. Repeat 8 to 15 times. Ensure a neutral spine and proper breathing (exhale on exertion, inhale on return phase).

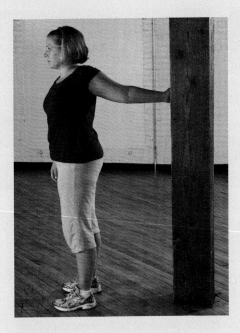

■ Chest Stretch Using a Wall (Fig. 6.11)

Have the client stand next to a wall with the arm closest to the wall extended. The hand of the extended arm should touch the wall. Using the wall as resistance, have the client turn in the opposite direction until a stretch is felt in the chest.

The iliopsoas muscles, which help form the hip flexors, often become shortened and subsequently tight in obese people because of the anterior pelvic tilt that results with excess abdominal weight. This forces the lower back muscles to contract and often results in varying degrees of lower back pain. Stretching the hip flexors alleviates much of this pain.

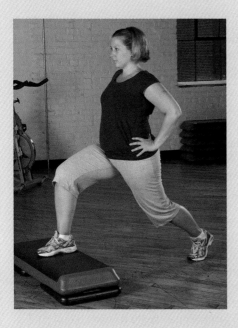

■ Hip Flexor Stretch (Fig. 6.12)

Stand behind a step or elevated platform that is a comfortable distance away. Place one foot completely on the step and slowly lunge forward by bending the forward leg. Push hips slightly forward and hold. Repeat on the other side. Be sure to keep the torso upright during the stretch.

Because of excess adipose tissue in the thighs, obese people often stand with their legs wider than shoulder width apart, so the adductors become weak and misaligned. This often results in knee and hip pain, so train the adductors to address this problem. Figure 4.11 gives instructions on how to train the adductors using a stability ball. If available, an adductor/abductor machine can be more challenging as the client progresses.

Add different resistance exercises as clients become stronger. Use elastic bands or tubing to perform the lat pull down, chest press, shoulder press, lateral shoulders, biceps, and triceps if desired. See chapter 5 for guidelines on how to properly perform these. Once clients fit into traditional resistance machines, use machines for variety.

NUTRITIONAL CONSIDERATIONS

To maintain weight, energy consumed must equal energy expended. Therefore, to effectively lose weight, obese individuals must create an overall energy deficit by combining exercise with a restricted kilocalorie intake. Careful diet planning is necessary because diets that severely limit energy intake tend to decrease metabolism, an effect that interferes with long-term weight loss. In addition, as people lose weight, they lose a combination of fat *and* muscle. Since muscle is metabolically active, which means it burns kilocalories and promotes a higher metabolism, a loss of muscle mass ultimately slows metabolism. Consequently, an obese person trying to lose weight, eat a healthier diet, and improve body composition must strive for balance.

Contrary to the claims of many current weight-loss programs, no special food combination or magic nutrient supplement ensures weight loss. Rather than relying on popular **fad diets**, obese people should begin making small improvements in their current diets. These changes should be feasible in the long term since maintenance of weight loss is a life-long endeavor.

ENERGY-YIELDING NUTRIENTS

When it comes to weight loss, total energy intake is more important than the proportion of carbohydrates, protein, and fat in the diet. In fact, healthy weight, overweight, and obese individuals require the same percentages of the energy-yielding nutrients.

Carbohydrates

Carbohydrates should constitute 45% to 65% of total daily kilocalorie intake. The obese individual should limit simple carbohydrate intake and increase the intake of whole grains, fruits, and vegetables. These foods are not only low in fat and kilocalories, but they are also packed with vitamins and minerals and contain nonnutrient substances such as **phytochemicals** that appear to improve health. In addition, foods high in fiber provide a feeling of fullness since fiber slows absorption and keeps food in the stomach longer than usual. The American Dietetic Association suggests an intake of 20 to 35 g of fiber per day to regulate blood cholesterol levels, promote regular bowel movements, and avoid constipation.

Proteins

Protein should comprise 10% to 35% of the total daily kilocalorie intake for those on a weight-loss diet. Some sources suggest limiting intake to 15% since many high protein foods are also high in saturated fat. Obese people should include various plant-based proteins in the diet and choose lean cuts of meat to limit saturated fat and cholesterol. Baked skinless chicken, broiled fish, and ground turkey are healthy choices.

Fat

Fat is both necessary and acceptable in a weight-loss diet. Fat adds flavor to foods and provides a source of concentrated energy. It also delays the movement of food through the small intestine, a factor that perhaps postpones hunger and delays glucose absorption.

Fat becomes problematic when consumed in excess. Some experts have observed that overweight and obese individuals tend to eat at restaurants more frequently than healthy-weight people. Not only do chefs use fat to enhance the flavors of favorite dishes, but they also serve enormous portions that provide excess kilocalories from all three energy-yielding nutrients. It seems that people no longer respond to internal hunger and satiety clues. Instead, they ignore signals to stop eating and attempt to completely consume these huge portions. To be successful at weight loss, obese people need to decrease their weekly trips to their favorite restaurants, and they need to decrease the quantity of food consumed at each meal. Ordering small serving sizes is one easy method to reduce total energy and fat intake. Making healthier, low fat, and low kilocalorie choices at restaurants is another. Having the waiter box-up half of an order before bringing it to the table will also encourage portion control.

Fat provides 9 kcal per gram, more than twice the number of kilocalories provided per gram of carbohydrate or protein. Those on a high fat diet, therefore, can ultimately end up with a huge surplus of energy. Unfortunately, the body easily stores any extra energy as adipose. Incidentally, it requires very little energy to convert the fat found in foods into the fat stored in adipose; in fact, the body becomes more efficient at storing fat when continuously supplied with fat. Furthermore, dietary fat is not satiating like dietary protein. Moreover, fat intake actually stimulates the appetite, so those on a high fat diet tend to consume larger quantities than those who limit fat intake.

Everyone, including overweight and obese individuals, should limit total fat intake to 20% to 35% of total kilocalorie intake. Saturated fats should contribute no more than 8% to 10% to the diet, while polyunsaturated and monounsaturated fats should make up the bulk of fat intake. Cholesterol intake should not exceed 300 mg per day, which is the same recommendation for healthy-weight people.

Energy Intake

Obese individuals need to be realistic about their energy intake. They must consume fewer kilocalories than they expend to lose weight; however, a severe kilocalorie restriction is rarely recommended. Drastically reducing energy intake can promote excessive lean tissue loss, a lowered basal metabolic rate (BMR), and eating disorders. To lose 1 lb per week, an adult needs to increase physical activity and reduce energy intake enough to create a 500-kcal deficit each day. To lose 2 lb per week, an adult needs to increase physical activity and reduce energy intake enough to create a 1,000-kcal deficit each day. An energy deficit of more than 1,000 kcal per day is nearly impossible; therefore, a weight loss of more than 2 lb per week is unlikely.*

---

*A safe rate of weight loss is ½ to 2 lb per week. Some obese individuals experience a greater loss of weight in the initial stages of their exercise and weight-loss program. This loss, however, typically tapers off to no more than 2 lb per week after the first couple of weeks. The initial drop in weight includes some water and lean muscle loss that will hopefully slow down in time.

Fad diet—a "temporary" diet that promises rapid weight loss. Americans spend nearly $40 million each year on weight-loss and exercise programs, many of which include fad diets. Fad diets often promise extreme weight loss in a short period of time, suggest that certain foods must be eliminated from the diet because they are "bad," and suggest supplements to replace nutrients missing from the diet (which dieters may conveniently purchase from those advocating the diet).

Phytochemicals—substances found in plants that seem to have protective effects in the body. Examples include lycopene found in tomatoes, isoflavones found in soy, and flavanoids found in various fruits. There are over 100 different phytochemicals, each of which has a different mode of action. Some act as antioxidants and fight free radicals; others have effects similar to hormones; some stimulate enzymes; others inhibit enzymes; some act as antibacterials; and others interfere with cancer cell replication.

Obese clients should be weary of foods that claim to be "fat-free" or "low-fat" because most of these still contain a large number of kilocalories, often in the form of simple carbohydrates. Unfortunately, knowing that a food is "low in fat" often compels consumers to eat more than a serving size. Since a box of no-fat cookies contains lots of kilocalories, consuming an entire box can sabotage a weight-loss diet.

QUICK REFERENCE

Alcohol also provides energy. Alcohol, however, is not considered a nutrient since it actually destroys cell membranes and ultimately kills cells. Reducing the intake of alcoholic beverages, however, is an easy way to decrease energy intake since 1 gram of alcohol contributes 7 kcal. Furthermore, in addition to the energy contributed by the alcohol itself, many alcoholic beverages contain other empty kilocalories that drastically increase the total amount of energy in the beverage. Cutting out or limiting alcoholic drinks, therefore, often results in a relatively large energy deficit.

VITAMINS AND MINERALS

It is difficult to obtain an appropriate vitamin and mineral intake on fewer than 1,200 kcal per day. Therefore, unless supervised by a doctor, no one should ever begin a weight-loss program that suggests fewer than this minimal daily amount. Many diets for severely obese people, however, recommend 1,000 to 1,200 kcal per day for women and 1,200 to 1,600 kcal per day for men, so food choice is critical. Individuals on such restrictive diets need to consume nutrient-dense foods that have a high nutrient content and low energy content. In many cases, people on weight-loss diets benefit from a multivitamin/mineral supplement supplying no more than 100% of the Recommended Daily Allowance (RDA).

QUICK REFERENCE

Individuals on weight-loss diets need to consume various nutrient-dense foods; regulate portion sizes to control energy intake; consume high fiber foods to control hunger; and include enough protein, fat, and carbohydrates for repair and maintenance of tissues (while simultaneously decreasing overall intake to achieve an energy deficit).

WATER

Adequate hydration is important for all exercisers, whether they are trying to lose weight or not. Water, however, indirectly helps with weight loss by providing a feeling of fullness to the stomach during meals; by satisfying thirst without adding any kilocalories; and by easing the passage of high-fiber foods through the digestive tract. Water intake is particularly important to the obese exerciser since increased activity often results in hyperthermia.

Like everyone else, obese clients should drink a minimum of 64 oz of water daily. In addition to this minimum amount, they should consume enough water to replace any water lost from sweating during exercise. A simple plan suggests that exercisers drink two to three 8-oz glasses of water 2 hours prior to exercise, another one to two cups 10 to 15 minutes before exercise, and then one to one-and-a-half cups every 15 minutes during exercise to avoid dehydration. After exercise, two to three cups per pound of body weight lost helps restore normal fluid levels.

SUMMARY

Although countless numbers of people have managed to shed unwanted pounds, only 5% maintain their weight loss for over one year. Those who are successful beyond a year permanently change lifestyle behaviors. They realize that a long-lasting commitment to healthier habits, rather than a reliance on short-term programs and fad diets, is the key to a healthier body. Thus, obese individuals must combine life-long exercise with a long-term healthy, reduced kilocalorie diet to be successful.

Establishing realistic goals and deadlines are a part of being successful on the weight-loss journey. A rapid rate of weight loss rarely produces long-term results and often results in feelings of fatigue, hunger, and depression. Most people who try to "starve" themselves so that they lose weight quickly decidedly give up and put on more weight than they had before they attempted to lose weight. In general, most people can safely lose ½ to 2 lb per week, or up to 10% of their total body weight over a 6-month period of time. This ensures a sufficient nutrient intake that maintains normal functions within the body.

Participation in exercise provides many rewards, including weight loss and improved physical appearance. More importantly, however, routine exercise enhances cardiovascular fitness and increases longevity independently of weight loss. In fact, an active overweight person often has a healthier cardiorespiratory system than a sedentary, normal weight person. Why? Because exercise affects variables such as blood pressure, blood lipids, glucose tolerance, and various other conditions in such a way that improves cardiovascular health. This is reason enough to get moving!

CASE STUDY

A 29-year-old sedentary man arrives for his initial appointment with you. He is 5'8" tall and weighs 285 lb. He has decided to begin exercise at the advice of his doctor who has told him that he has high cholesterol, high blood triglycerides, high blood pressure, and is prediabetic.

- Calculate his BMI and discuss his BMI classification.

- What type of exercise testing would you perform?

- Describe what you would have this client do during his first training appointment.

THINKING CRITICALLY

1. Define BMI and explain how it is calculated. What are the advantages and disadvantages of using BMI?
2. Describe the impact of overweight and obesity on the cardiovascular system. How do these factors affect the ability to exercise?
3. Define hyperthermia and explain why an obese person has a greater risk of hyperthermia during exercise.
4. What are some of the barriers to exercise seen by this population? How would you address these concerns?
5. What are the recommendations for carbohydrates, protein, and fat?
6. Why do obese individuals often suffer from lower back problems?
7. What is the range of safe weight loss? Describe the energy deficit that would result in a safe rate of weight loss.
8. Discuss the importance of water in weight loss.

REFERENCES

1. Centers for Disease Control. www.cdc.gov
2. American College of Sports Medicine. ACSM's Guidelines for Exercise Testing and Prescription. 8th Ed. Philadelphia: Lippincott Williams & Wilkins, 2010:253–256.
3. Dansinger M, Tatsioni A, Wong J, et al. Meta-analysis: the effect of dietary counseling for weight loss. Ann Intern Med 2007;147:41–50.
4. Anandacoomarasamy A, Caterson I, Sambrook P, Fransen M, March L. The impact of obesity on the musculoskeletal system. Int J Obesity 2007;32(2): 211–212.
5. Leveille S, Wee C, Iezzoni L. Trends in obesity and arthritis among baby boomers and their predecessors, 1971–2002. Am J Public Health 2005; 95(9):1607–1613.
6. Mehrotra C, Chundy N, Thomas V. Obesity and physical inactivity among Wisconsin adults with arthritis. Wisconsin Med J 2003;102(7):24–28.
7. Koenig S. Pulmonary complications of obesity. Am J Med Sci 2001;321(4):249–279.
8. Elamin M. Asthma and obesity: a real connection or a casual association? Chest 2004;125:1972–1974.
9. Schachter LM, Salome CM, Peat JK, Woolcock AJ. Obesity is a risk factor for asthma and wheeze but not airy hyper responsiveness. Thorax 2001;56:4–8.
10. Chin S, Downs SH, Anto JM, et al. Incidence of asthma and net change in symptoms in relation to changes in obesity. Eur Respir J 2006;28: 763–771.
11. Shaw K, Gennat H, O'Rourke P, et al. Exercise for overweight or obesity. Cochrane Database Syst Rev 2006;(4): CD003817.
12. Stenius-Aarniala B, Poussa T, Kvarnstrom J, et al. Immediate and long term effects of weight reduction in obese people with asthma: randomized controlled study. Br Med J 2000;320: 827–832.
13. Kahn B, Flier J. Obesity and insulin resistance. J Clin Invest 2000;106(4):473–481.
14. Lazarus R, Sparrow D, Weiss S. Temporal relations between obesity and insulin: longitudinal data from the normative aging study. Am J Epidemiol 1998;147(2):173–179.
15. Key T. Body mass index, serum sex hormones, and breast cancer risk in postmenopausal women. J Natl Cancer Inst 2003;95(16):1218–1226.
16. Hambrecht R, Gielen S. Hunter-gatherer to sedentary lifestyle. Lancet 2005;366:560–561.
17. National Heart, Lung, and Blood Institute. www. nhlbi.nih.gov
18. Lee CD, Blair SN, Jackson AS. Cardiorespiratory fitness, body composition, and all-cause and cardiovascular disease mortality in men. Am J Clin Nutr 1999;69:373–380.
19. Sarsan A, Ardic F, Ozgen M, et al. The effects of aerobic and resistance exercises in obese women. Clin Rehabil 2006;20:773–782.
20. National Cholesterol Education Program. Third Report of the National Cholesterol Education

Program (NCEP) Expert Panel on the Detection, Evaluation, and Treatment of High Blood Cholesterol in Adults (Adult Treatment Panel III). 2002. Bethesda, MD. NIH Publications No. 02-5215.

21. Jakicic JM, Otto A. Treatment and prevention of obesity: what is the role of exercise. Nutr Rev 2006;64(2):S57–S61.

22. Perri M, McAllister D, Gange J, et al. Effects of four maintenance programs on the long-term management of obesity. J Consul Clin Psychol 1988;56: 529–534.

23. Rice R. Program design for life. IDEA Fitness J 2007; 4(1):1–5.

SUGGESTED READINGS

Ashmore A. Torque and training overweight clients. IDEA Fitness J 2005;2(1):51–57.

Dahlberg CP. Living large. Yoga J 2003;178:88–95.

Kraus SJ, Madden SK. Unlocking barriers for heavy clients. IDEA Fitness J 2005;2(1):46–55.

7

EXERCISE FOR INDIVIDUALS WITH CARDIOVASCULAR DISEASE

According to the American Heart Association (AHA), nearly 871,000 Americans died of cardiovascular disease (CVD) in 2004—a number that represents 36% of all deaths during that year. It affects both genders and does not discriminate based upon race or ethnicity. This makes CVD the number one killer in America today. In addition to claiming so many lives, CVD is also a leading cause of disability in the United States according to data from the Centers for Disease Control and Prevention. Overall, $300 billion is spent annually on CVD-related healthcare expenses, medications, and lost work time. Obviously, prevention would not only curb this financial burden, but it would also decrease both the morbidity and the mortality associated with this disease.

CVD refers to various conditions that result from deterioration of the heart and blood vessels. Examples include coronary artery disease, **arteriosclerosis, atherosclerosis**, heart valve disease, arrhythmia, hypertension, peripheral artery disease (PAD), and congenital heart disease. Coronary artery disease, also known as coronary heart disease, is responsible for the greatest number of deaths. This chapter explores many forms of CVD and offers suggestions on risk reduction (see Table 7.1).

ANATOMICAL AND PHYSIOLOGICAL CHANGES ASSOCIATED WITH CVD

MAJOR COMPONENTS OF THE CARDIOVASCULAR SYSTEM

To understand the anatomical and physiological changes that occur as CVD develops, it is helpful to review how this system functions at its best. The cardiovascular system consists of blood, the heart, and blood vessels.

Blood

Blood consists of a liquid portion called plasma that contains dissolved substances such as glucose, amino acids, glycerol, vitamins, minerals, carbonic acid, bicarbonate, and water. It also contains formed elements, which include red blood cells, white blood cells, and platelets.

Red blood cells are biconcave-shaped discs filled with hemoglobin. Hemoglobin is a large protein molecule that consists of four **polypeptide chains** (which constitute the "–globin" portion) and four iron-containing portions (which constitute the "heme–" portion). The heme– portion of hemoglobin attaches to and transports 98% of the body's

TABLE 7-1 GENERAL STRATEGIES TO REDUCE THE RISK FOR CVD

- Quit, or never start, smoking
- Maintain a healthy weight
- Participate in regular physical activity
- Control high blood pressure
- Control blood cholesterol levels
- Eat a healthy diet low in saturated fat and high in fiber

oxygen to body cells. Oxygen is essential for cell functioning because oxygen is necessary to completely break down carbohydrates, triglycerides, and proteins. By completely breaking down these molecules, cells produce large amounts of ATP, or adenosine triphosphate. ATP, in turn, is used to fuel metabolic processes such as muscle contraction, tissue repair, and protein synthesis. Cellular respiration is the major means for producing large quantities of ATP; it requires a continuous oxygen supply.

Various white blood cells travel through the blood and lymph and primarily protect the body from potentially harmful substances called pathogens. Macrophages and neutrophils are important **phagocytes**, white blood cells that engulf, digest, and destroy pathogens. Other white blood cells, called B-cells and T-cells, are involved with specific defense and immunity. They seek out and destroy the specific pathogens for which they have receptors.

Platelets are actually fragments of much larger cells called megakaryocytes. Although they are not actually cells, they play an important role in blood clotting and platelet plug formation.

Heart

The heart is a muscular pump responsible for creating the force that drives blood through blood vessels. In addition, it pumps blood low in oxygen to the lungs where the blood

---

Arteriosclerosis—any condition in which the arteries become less flexible and more rigid. Healthy arteries are pliable and permit free flow of blood; rigid blood vessels do not. Normal aging, diabetes, smoking, obesity, and hypertension are contributing factors to arteriosclerosis development. Three types exist: atherosclerosis (defined next), Monckeberg's arteriosclerosis (hardening of the arteries characterized by calcium deposits in the blood vessel wall; usually occurs in peripheral arteries), and arteriolosclerosis (hardening of small vessels called arterioles).

Atherosclerosis—a type of arteriosclerosis that results from plaque buildup on the inner lining of arteries. Plaque narrows vessels and restricts blood flow to areas supplied by the affected vessel. Although the words "atherosclerosis" and "arteriosclerosis" are often used interchangeably, they technically have different meanings.

Polypeptide chain—a long chain of amino acids.

Phagocyte—a type of white blood cell that engulfs and destroys cells, foreign matter, and debris.

picks up oxygen and rids itself of carbon dioxide, a by-product of metabolism. Cardiac muscle tissue is the primary type of tissue found in the heart.

The heart contains four chambers. They include two upper atria and two lower ventricles. The heart also contains four valves that facilitate blood flow and prevent backflow. The tricuspid valve is located between the right atrium and the right ventricle; the pulmonary semilunar valve is located between the left ventricle and the pulmonary trunk (the vessel that branches and transports blood low in oxygen from the right ventricle to the lungs); the bicuspid valve is located between the left atrium and the left ventricle; and the aortic semilunar valve is located between the left ventricle and the aorta (Figs. 7.1 and 7.2). As long as

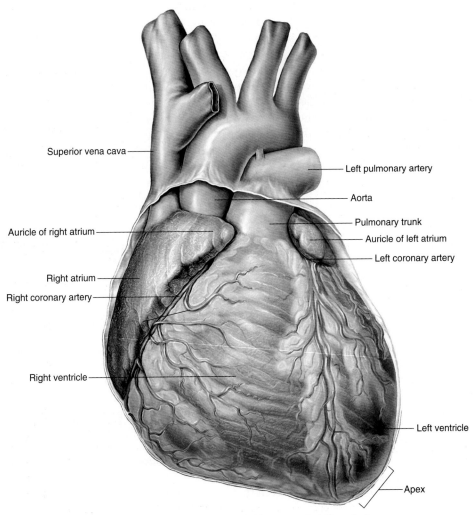

FIGURE 7.1 ■ Anterior view of the heart. (Asset provided by Anatomical Chart Co.)

the heart and its valves function properly, blood is efficiently pumped throughout the body. The right side of the heart acts as the pump for pulmonary circulation since it transports oxygen-poor blood to the lungs to be reoxygenated. The left side of the heart, on the other hand, acts as the pump for systemic circulation since it transports oxygen-rich blood to all body tissues. Because it has to pump blood farther than the right ventricle, the left ventricle has a much thicker and stronger wall.

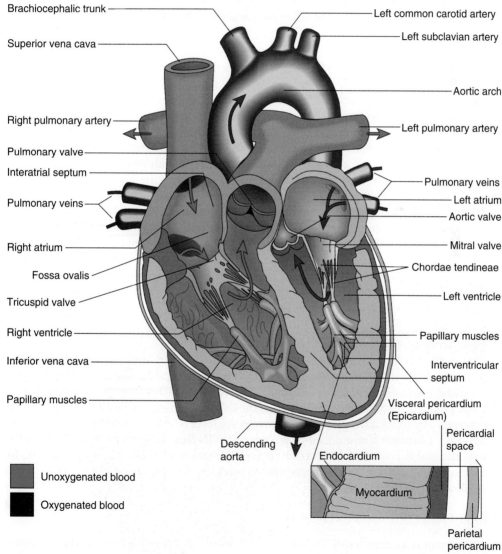

FIGURE 7.2 ■ Internal structures of the heart. (From Smeltzer SCO, Bare BG. Brunner and Suddarth's Textbook of Medical-Surgical Nursing. 9th Ed. Philadelphia: Lippincott Williams & Wilkins, 2002.)

As mentioned, the heart is a muscle, so it needs an uninterrupted supply of blood to function. The heart cannot obtain nutrients or oxygen from the blood within its chambers. Instead, it receives oxygen-rich blood from the right and left coronary arteries, vessels that branch from the initial segment of the aorta. These two coronary arteries continue to branch repeatedly as they surround the cardiac muscle. This ensures that the heart receives an adequate supply of freshly oxygenated blood in between each heartbeat. Basically, the right coronary artery and its branches supply blood to the right atrium, right ventricle, and lower portion of the left ventricle, while the left coronary artery and its branches supply blood to the left atrium and the remainder of the left ventricle.

Blood Vessels

Blood vessels are the conduits for blood. They are found in most body tissues and include arteries, arterioles, capillaries, venules, and veins. Arteries are relatively thick-walled vessels that transport blood away from the heart, and in most instances, the blood they transport is rich in oxygen. The pulmonary arteries are an exception; they transport oxygen-poor blood away from the heart toward the lungs. The aorta is the body's major artery. It connects to the left ventricle and branches into numerous smaller arteries that supply major body regions. These arteries continue to branch into smaller vessels called arterioles, which ultimately connect to capillaries. Capillaries are exceedingly thin-walled vessels that act as the sites of gas exchange; they are plentiful in most tissues. They allow oxygen to be exchanged for carbon dioxide. Venules are small veins that form from capillaries and unite to form larger veins. Veins are relatively thin-walled vessels that deliver blood toward the heart, and in most cases, the blood they contain is low in oxygen. Again, an exception occurs in pulmonary circulation where the pulmonary veins transport oxygen-rich blood toward the left atrium of the heart. Two major veins, the superior vena cava and the inferior vena cava, connect directly to the right atrium of the heart and deliver oxygen-poor blood to the heart.

Functions of the Cardiovascular System

Overall, blood contains the nutrients and oxygen required by body cells, but it also picks up waste products released by them. Two major jobs of the cardiovascular system then are to ensure adequate distribution of oxygenated blood throughout the body and to deliver waste products to excretory organs such as the kidneys, lungs, and skin where they can be removed. The heart is the pump that provides the force to drive blood through blood vessels. Each heartbeat is stimulated by electrical signals that travel through a specific pathway and cause coordinated contraction and relaxation of the atria and ventricles. In essence, this enables all three components to work together to accomplish the tasks of the cardiovascular system (Fig. 7.3).

RISK FACTORS AND CVD

A risk factor is a characteristic or behavior that increases a person's likelihood of developing a disease. As with other chronic conditions, the probability of developing CVD correlates with the number of risk factors present and to the length of time that they have

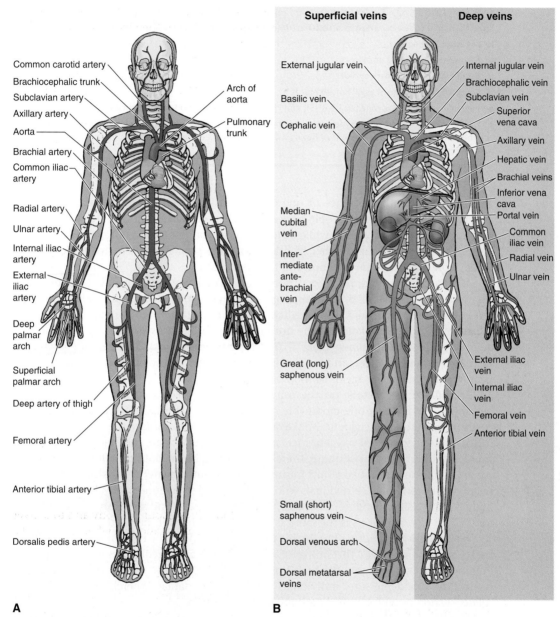

Superficial veins

Deep veins

Common carotid artery

Brachiocephalic trunk

Subclavian artery

Axillary artery

Aorta

Brachial artery

Common iliac artery

Radial artery

Ulnar artery

Internal iliac artery

External iliac artery

Deep palmar arch

Superficial palmar arch

Deep artery of thigh

Femoral artery

Anterior tibial artery

Dorsalis pedis artery

Arch of aorta

Pulmonary trunk

External jugular vein

Basilic vein

Cephalic vein

Median cubital vein

Inter-mediate ante-brachial vein

Great (long) saphenous vein

Small (short) saphenous vein

Dorsal venous arch

Dorsal metatarsal veins

Internal jugular vein

Brachiocephalic vein

Subclavian vein

Superior vena cava

Axillary vein

Hepatic vein

Brachial veins

Inferior vena cava

Portal vein

Common iliac vein

Radial vein

Ulnar vein

External iliac vein

Internal iliac vein

Femoral vein

Anterior tibial vein

A

B

FIGURE 7.3 ■ Cardiovascular system. **A:** Principal arteries. **B:** Principal veins. (From Moore KL, Dalley AF II. Clinical Oriented Anatomy. 4th Ed. Baltimore: Lippincott Williams & Wilkins, 1999.)

TABLE 7-2   RISK FACTORS FOR CVD

- Cigarette smoking
- Men who are 45 years or older
- Women who are 55 years or older
- Low HDL levels (defined as HDL < 40 mg/dL)
- High blood pressure (defined as ≥140/90 mm Hg) or taking high blood pressure medication
- Family history of heart disease (defined as having a first degree male relative who was under the age of 55 when diagnosed with heart disease or having a first degree female relative who was under the age of 65 when diagnosed with heart disease)

---

existed; however, the presence of one or more risk factors does not guarantee disease development. In fact, some people have absolutely no risk factors for CVD but still experience cardiovascular problems, while others have several risk factors but never suffer. Nevertheless, the greater the number of risk factors, the stronger the chance of developing CVD. Table 7.2 lists some common risk factors for CVD.

In general, risk factors that contribute to CVD development include smoking, obesity, inactivity, high blood pressure, high LDL levels, low HDL levels, high cholesterol levels, diabetes, age, gender, and heredity. Some of these factors are nonmodifiable, which means they cannot be changed. The nonmodifiable risk factors are age (men over age 45 are at a greater risk; women older than 55 are at greater risk), gender (men have an increased risk at any age), and family history (having a family member diagnosed with heart disease before the age of 60 increases risk).

Modifiable risk factors, on the other hand, can be controlled by altering lifestyle behaviors. The number one modifiable risk factor for CVD is cigarette smoking. Components in cigarettes and cigarette smoke raise blood pressure, damage the inner arterial lining, deprive the heart of oxygen, increase the heart's workload, increase heart rate, and interfere with platelet functioning, thereby promoting blood clot formation. Incidentally, passive inhalation of smoke results in similar effects. Since cigarette smoking strongly correlates with heart attack, individuals who smoke should stop immediately. Fortunately, the body is quite resilient and responds almost instantly to smoking cessation. In fact, the risk for CVD in *former* smokers is the same as it would have been if they had never smoked.

Hypertension is another modifiable risk factor for CVD. The mechanical force of high blood pressure damages the lining of blood vessels and predisposes them to plaque buildup. In fact, the higher the blood pressure, the greater the risk for heart disease. By controlling blood pressure, individuals can minimize damage thereby decreasing risk. A later section provides more details about hypertension.

High blood cholesterol is another risk factor for CVD. Blood cholesterol consists of cholesterol derived from the diet as well as cholesterol produced by the liver. Interestingly, the liver makes far more cholesterol than the average person consumes. It produces 800 to 1,500 mg per day, an amount much greater than the average dietary intake of 250 to 350 mg per day. Unfortunately, some people are sensitive to dietary cholesterol, so they experience dramatic changes in blood cholesterol levels in response to diet. Since cholesterol collects on the lining of *damaged* vessels, the more cholesterol present, the greater

TABLE 7-3 VALUES FOR THE BLOOD LIPID PROFILE			
Measure	Optimal	Borderline	High Risk
LDL level	<100 mg/dL	130–159 mg/dL	160+ mg/dL
HDL level	>60 mg/dL	35–45 mg/dL	<35 mg/dL
Total cholesterol	<200 mg/dL	200–239 mg/dL	>240 mg/dL
LDL to HDL ratio	4	5	6
Triglycerides	<150 mg/dL	150–199 mg/dL	>200 mg/dL

the risk. Surprisingly, a high dietary intake of saturated fat elevates blood cholesterol levels *more* than a high dietary intake of cholesterol; consequently, those with high blood cholesterol levels should be even more concerned about their saturated fat intake than their cholesterol intake.

Obesity and overweight are additional risk factors for CVD. As mentioned in Chapter 6, excess weight strains the heart because the heart must work harder to provide nutrients and oxygen to the extra fat cells. Because their hearts are already challenged during regular daily activities, obese people typically have more difficulty withstanding the added stress of exercise than normal weight people. Therefore, they often avoid exercise and become less active or perhaps completely sedentary. A sedentary lifestyle is actually an additional risk factor for CVD. Sedentary individuals tend to have a cluster of risk factors for CVD including overweight or obesity, an unhealthy blood lipid profile, reduced cardiovascular and respiratory health, and unhealthy blood vessels (which often causes hypertension). Furthermore, obese and sedentary people are at an increased risk for developing type 2 diabetes—a condition that increases the risk for atherosclerosis. As mentioned in Chapter 9, diabetics also have elevated blood glucose levels, a factor that damages blood vessels and exacerbates atherosclerosis.

High blood LDL levels also increase the risk for CVD. As mentioned, free radicals oxidize LDL. Macrophages then engulf oxidized LDL and form foam cells, which thicken arterial plaque and further obstruct arteries. A blood lipid profile ascertains LDL level and ultimately determines the risk for CVD. It typically includes a measure of total blood cholesterol, HDL, LDL, and triglyceride levels. Table 7.3 lists suggested values for the blood lipid profile.

HOMOCYSTEINE, C-REACTIVE PROTEIN, AND FIBRINOGEN

In addition to the risk factors mentioned earlier, high blood levels of homocysteine, C-reactive protein (CRP), and fibrinogen are also associated with an increased risk of CVD. Homocysteine is an **amino acid** formed whenever the body removes a methyl group

> **Amino acids**—the basic building blocks of proteins. Proteins are long chains of amino acids arranged in a precise order. Twenty amino acids combine in various ways to form all of the proteins in the body (just as 26 letters of the alphabet make up all of the words in the English language).

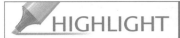

HIGHLIGHT Cholesterol, HDL, and LDL

Exactly what is cholesterol? Are HDL and LDL really two different types of cholesterol? If so, why does the amount of HDL plus LDL not equal the total amount of cholesterol in a person's blood? And what do all of these letters and numbers really mean?

Most individuals have a vague and oftentimes incorrect understanding of the words "total cholesterol," "HDL," and "LDL." This is not surprising given that TV advertisements, magazine articles, and even physicians incorrectly suggest that there are two different types of cholesterol. They refer to these as "HDL cholesterol" and "LDL cholesterol." In fact, doctors teach patients that HDL is "good cholesterol," while LDL is "bad cholesterol."

In reality, only one type of cholesterol exists—and it has vital functions in the body. For instance, cholesterol is an important component of every cell membrane in the body. Without it, the membranes would be unstable and prone to collapse. Additionally, the body uses cholesterol as a foundation for making estrogen, testosterone, vitamin D, and several other hormones. To meet these needs, the liver produces approximately 800 to 1,500 mg of cholesterol per day—an amount far more than what the average person consumes in the diet.

Cholesterol itself consists of four interlocking rings of carbon and hydrogen that are arranged identically in each cholesterol molecule. Since cholesterol has only one shape,

there is only one type of cholesterol which looks like this:

HDL and LDL are not forms of cholesterol at all! Instead, they are cholesterol transporters called lipoproteins. A lipoprotein consists of both a lipid portion, which is insoluble in water but soluble in other lipids, and a protein portion, which is insoluble in lipids but soluble in water. The lipoprotein positions itself so that its water-soluble portion faces the external fluid, while its lipid portion faces the interior. This arrangement enables it to transport other lipids such as triglycerides and cholesterol throughout water-based blood. Consequently, lipoproteins have totally different molecular structures than cholesterol, and are thus not types of cholesterol.

Based on density, there are four general types of lipoproteins. Density is determined by the relative proportion of lipids versus proteins present in the molecule. Since proteins are much denser than lipids, lipoproteins that have a higher protein to fat ratio are called dense lipoproteins.

(continued)

from methionine, an **essential amino acid**. Under normal circumstances, homocysteine rarely accumulates because the body usually converts it into another product. In some circumstances, homocysteine reaccepts a methyl group to reform methionine, while at

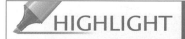

HIGHLIGHT   Cholesterol, HDL, and LDL (*continued*)

Chylomicrons are the largest lipoproteins. They primarily transport dietary triglycerides throughout the body. In fact, they consist of over 80% triglycerides, a small amount of cholesterol, and a negligible amount of protein. Essentially, chylomicrons ensure that body cells receive an adequate supply of triglycerides for the aerobic production of ATP. As chylomicrons circulate throughout the body, they become smaller and smaller as their contents dwindle. Eventually, the liver removes depleted chylomicrons from circulation and recycles their components.

The liver also makes a second type of lipoprotein—the very-low-density lipoprotein, or VLDL. VLDL continues to transport triglycerides to body cells, but they only contain about 50% triglycerides. They carry a larger amount of cholesterol than the chylomicrons and a slightly greater amount of protein. Thus, they are somewhat denser than chylomicrons. As the VLDL molecules move through body fluids, cells remove triglycerides thereby making VLDL smaller as the proportion of cholesterol and proteins increases relative to the proportion of triglycerides. Eventually, the VLDL becomes low-density-lipoprotein, or LDL.

LDL continues to circulate throughout the blood making its cholesterol available to body cells. As mentioned, cells need cholesterol to reform cell membranes and to produce hormones, so LDL addresses this need. The problem with LDL, however, is that it easily "spills"

cholesterol into blood vessels. If the blood vessels are damaged, cholesterol can stick to affected areas and promote plaque formation. Plaque buildup then restricts blood flow and causes high blood pressure. High blood pressure then stresses the heart and triggers a cascade of events that results in further blood vessel damage. (Think of LDL as an open hay cart. Instead of hay, LDL transports cholesterol. As the hay cart moves through blood vessels, its cholesterol easily spills and might collect on arterial walls.)

The liver makes a fourth type of lipoprotein that consists of over 50% protein. This high-density-lipoprotein, or HDL, travels through blood vessels and mops up excess cholesterol spilled by LDL. HDL then transports the excess cholesterol back to the liver where the liver recycles or disposes of it. (Think of HDL as a vacuum cleaner. It vacuums up and transports excess blood cholesterol to the liver. Essentially, it cleans up after LDL; therefore, a high level of HDL offers important protection against plaque buildup on arterial walls. In fact, an HDL level of >60 mg/dL is considered a "negative risk factor." In other words, it reduces the risk of CVD.)

Overall, only one type of cholesterol exists and that cholesterol is necessary for a healthy body. It only becomes destructive when it accumulates on the inner linings of arteries where it interferes with blood flow and oxygen delivery (Fig. 7.4).

Essential amino acid—an amino acid that the body cannot make and must, therefore, be obtained in the diet.

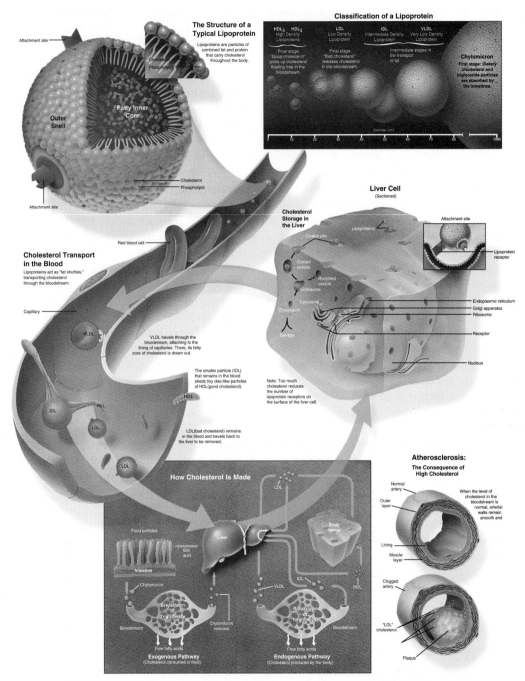

FIGURE 7.4 ■ Understanding cholesterol. (Asset provided by Anatomical Chart Co.)

other times the liver metabolizes it into cysteine, a **nonessential amino acid**. Both pathways require specific **enzymes** to facilitate the reaction. Unfortunately, a small percentage of people lack the enzyme necessary to convert homocysteine into other forms, so homocysteine accumulates in the blood. This condition, recognized over 25 years ago, is called homocystinuria. Studies show that those suffering from homocystinuria typically have an elevated risk for heart attack and stroke that appears to result from homocysteine's effect on arterial linings. More specifically, excess homocysteine damages the arterial lining, promotes cholesterol buildup, and interferes with clotting factors. Research shows that lowering blood homocysteine levels in those with homocystinuria effectively lowers CVD risk as well.

Since high homocysteine levels predispose those with homocystinuria to premature heart attack and stroke, researchers hypothesize that elevated homocysteine levels in anyone, even those without the enzyme deficiency, might also increase risk for heart attack and stroke. Indeed, several clinical trials have confirmed this positive correlation, but it is still unknown whether reducing blood homocysteine levels in those without homocystinuria actually diminishes CVD risk or not.[1-3]

Homocysteine levels rise for various reasons. Some people are genetically predisposed to elevated homocysteine levels even though they do not suffer from homocystinuria, while others simply have lifestyle behaviors that increase blood levels. For instance, those who consume diets low in folic acid, vitamin B_{12}, and vitamin B_6 tend to have elevated homocysteine levels. This is because these vitamins are necessary to convert homocysteine into methionine or cysteine. Deficiencies, therefore, allow homocysteine to accumulate in the blood. It seems reasonable then to assume that folate, vitamin B_{12}, and vitamin B_6 supplements might actually reduce homocysteine levels and subsequently lower the risk for CVD. Indeed, a 2002 study found that a control group that took a B-vitamin supplement had a one-third lower risk for heart attack and death than those taking a placebo.[1-3]

C-reactive protein (CRP) is a plasma protein that indicates inflammation. Levels of CRP increase in response to systemic inflammation that can result from various conditions including coronary artery disease, cancer, infection, or trauma. Studies show that CRP levels independently predict risk for heart attack and should, therefore, be tested along with blood lipids when determining risk.[4]

An elevated level of fibrinogen, a plasma protein involved with blood clotting, is also an independent risk factor for CVD. Fibrinogen makes blood more viscous, a factor that interferes with blood flow, increases the heart's workload, and promotes excessive platelet

---

Nonessential amino acid—an amino acid that is not required through the diet since the body can make an adequate amount to meet its needs (as long as a nitrogen source is available).

Enzyme—a protein that acts as a catalyst to speed up chemical reactions.

C-reactive protein—a protein released during inflammation that promotes an immune response. High levels suggest a heart attack.

TABLE 7-4   HOW TO REDUCE FIBRINOGEN LEVELS

- Quit smoking
- Exercise
- Eat a healthy diet low in saturated fat and high in fruits and vegetables
- Reduce stress
- Increase intake of omega-3 fatty acids
- Take a low dose of aspirin each day

clumping. If platelets clump uncontrollably, they can form blood clots, which might cause heart attack or stroke. In addition, viscous blood can damage blood vessel walls, a condition that increases the risk of atherosclerosis (discussed later in this section). One study even showed that those with high fibrinogen levels were twice as likely to die from a heart attack as those with lower levels.[5,6] Table 7.4 lists behavior factors that can reduce fibrinogen levels.

The risk for heart disease actually increases with each additional risk factor and the length of time each risk factor is present; thus, individuals should make as many positive lifestyle changes as possible to reduce the likelihood of developing cardiovascular problems.

DISEASES OF THE CARDIOVASCULAR SYSTEM

Atherosclerosis

Atherosclerosis, which causes the most common forms of CVD, is a condition that develops as fatty deposits consisting of cholesterol, calcium, and other substances accumulate on the inner lining of arterial walls. This accumulation ultimately narrows blood vessels and interferes with oxygen and nutrient delivery to areas supplied by affected vessels. As mentioned earlier, oxygen delivery to metabolically active cells is crucial since most cells produce energy through cellular respiration, a process that requires a continuous oxygen supply. When deprived of oxygen, cells stop functioning and die. Unfortunately, atherosclerosis does not always elicit symptoms during its early stages.

Surprisingly, atherosclerosis begins during childhood. Babies are born with clear, smooth arteries, but fatty streaks begin to appear on the inner lining as early as age 10. As they develop, these fatty streaks enlarge, attract deposits, and begin forming raised lesions called plaques. Lesions repeatedly regress and regrow until they eventually stiffen as calcium and other materials accumulate. Additionally, a network of fibrous connective tissue forms around and encapsulates the plaque. Some of these capsules are sturdy, while others are fragile. Once plaque stiffens, it narrows the affected artery and permanently restricts blood flow. Unfortunately, the arteries of most people contain well-developed plaques by the age of 30. The risk associated with plaque, however, depends upon plaque location and pervasiveness throughout the body.

What exactly promotes the initial formation of fatty streaks in blood vessel linings? To answer this, understand that the lining of all but the smallest blood vessels consists of three layers (Fig. 7.5). Consider an artery. The outermost layer is the tunica externa, which anchors

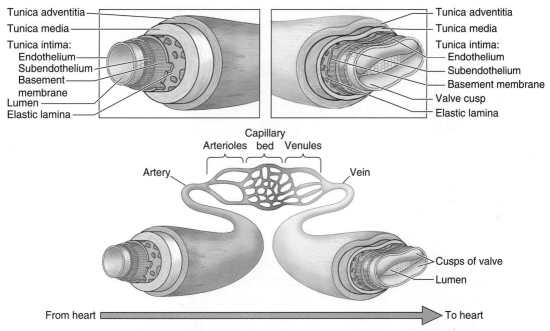

FIGURE 7.5 ■ Structure of blood vessel wall. (From Moore KL, Dalley AF II. Clinical Oriented Anatomy, 4th Ed. Baltimore: Lippincott Williams & Wilkins, 1999.)

the vessel to surrounding structures. The middle layer is the tunica media. It is composed of varying amounts of smooth muscle and elastic connective tissue, a combination that enables it to stretch, recoil, constrict, and dilate. The innermost layer, called the tunica interna or tunica intima, is the only layer that contacts blood; it plays a significant role in atherosclerosis development. The tunica interna is an exceedingly thin layer of very flat cells. It is easily damaged by high blood pressure, cigarette smoking, high LDL and triglyceride levels, elevated homocysteine, infection, and diabetes. Damage to this layer increases the blood vessel's permeability and elicits inflammation. In fact, experts believe that widespread inflammation is at the core of atherosclerosis. During inflammation, blood flow to the damaged area increases to bring macrophages to clear the area of debris and to provide supplies necessary for repair. As this occurs, cells in the area release chemicals, some of which make the area sticky and others that stimulate smooth muscles cells in the tunica media to grow. As smooth muscle cells grow, the vessel hardens and thickens. Simultaneously, the sticky lining traps circulating substances, particularly LDL, which are then oxidized by free radicals. To clear the area of debris, macrophages slip under the tunica interna and engulf oxidized LDL. As they continue to engulf more and more LDL, macrophages enlarge and develop into what are called foam cells, fat-filled cells that create the fatty streaks along the arterial lining. Some evidence suggests that a chronic infection enhances plaque development since plaque also often contains various bacteria and viruses.[7] Current research is investigating this (Fig. 7.6).

Normal coronary artery

Fatty streak

Fibrous plaque

Complicated plaque

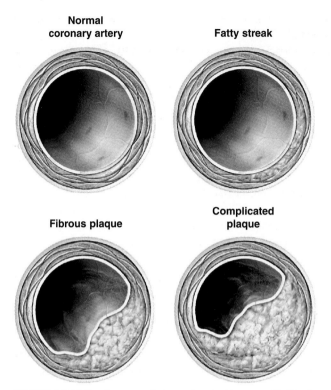

FIGURE 7.6 ■ Development of atherosclerosis. (Asset provided by Anatomical Chart Co.)

QUICK REFERENCE
Blood levels of CRP rise in response to inflammation and are reliable indicators for an impending heart attack.

As mentioned, plaque is surrounded by a fibrous capsule. Some capsules are rather thin and weak, so any sudden surge in blood pressure could conceivably crack and dislodge a portion of the plaque. If this happens, the lipid-rich core of the plaque is exposed, and the body responds as it would to any tissue damage. It sends platelets to the area to form a blood clot to prevent further bleeding. The clot, also known as a thrombus, further narrows the vessel and restricts oxygen delivery. Ultimately, this series of events sets into motion a self-perpetuating cycle that can systematically increase blockage and eventually restrict blood flow completely.[8–12]

The detached portion of the plaque—called an embolus—is left to travel freely through blood vessels. As it travels, it can cause additional damage to blood vessel linings. Moreover, if it lodges in a small blood vessel, it can totally obstruct blood flow to an organ. In fact, if it obstructs a coronary artery, a heart attack occurs. If it obstructs a vessel supplying the brain, a stroke occurs. Overall, the consequences of atherosclerosis depend upon which blood vessels are affected.

Chronic inflammation and atherosclerosis weaken arterial walls, so they can cause **aneurisms**. Aneurisms result when artery segments are dilated and enlarged and thus form bulging sacs. They are dangerous because they can rupture and result in severe bleeding. Imagine the damage that would occur if an aortic aneurism ruptures.

Coronary Artery Disease (or Coronary Heart Disease)

Coronary artery disease (CAD), which occurs when the coronary arteries develop atherosclerosis, is the most common form of heart disease. It affects nearly 13 million American men and women and is responsible for over 500,000 heart attacks each year.

As mentioned, the coronary arteries are vessels that deliver oxygen-rich blood and nutrients to the heart. If plaque buildup obstructs blood flow through either or both of these vessels, heart tissue is deprived of oxygen. If oxygen delivery is not restored quickly, cardiac tissue dies as the person experiences a heart attack. Interestingly, cardiac arrest can occur with as little as 50% blockage.[13]

Some CAD sufferers experience an early warning sign called **angina pectoris** that typically occurs during exertion. The two major forms of angina are stable angina and unstable angina. **Stable angina** is the most common type and is described as tightness in the chest that tends to spread into the arms, neck, back, or jaw. It usually lasts for only 3 to 20 minutes and subsides with rest or with oral nitroglycerin. It ultimately results from inadequate oxygen delivery to portions of the heart, a condition called **ischemia**. Stable angina is not a heart attack, but it suggests that a heart attack is likely in the future.

QUICK REFERENCE

If a heart attack occurs, obtain help within the 1st hour after the incident to improve survival rate and limit long-term damage.

Aneurism—a weak and unusual saclike bulge in a blood vessel; it fills with blood and can be dangerous because it can rupture and cause severe bleeding.

Angina pectoris—a feeling of tightness or pressure in the chest; results from inadequate oxygen delivery to the heart.

Stable angina—tightness in the chest that spreads into the arm, neck, back, and jaw. Usually alleviated with rest or oral nitroglycerin. According to the ACC and the AHA, treatment includes controlling hypertension, taking lipid-lowering medications, refraining from smoking, beginning exercise training, managing diabetes, and reducing weight in the overweight or obese.

Ischemia—an insufficient blood supply, and therefore oxygen delivery, to an organ; usually caused by the blockage of an artery.

Unstable angina occurs with or without physical exertion and is unpredictable. In addition, it is not relieved during rest and does not respond to medication. Because unstable angina is often a strong predictor of an impending heart attack, sufferers need *immediate* medical attention to circumvent a heart attack. After obtaining a complete medical history, a physician listens to the heart through a stethoscope and orders several tests to determine heart function. Common tests include an **electrocardiogram** (ECG), **blood tests**, and **coronary angiography**. Sometimes physicians prescribe a daily dose of aspirin to treat the angina. The aspirin acts as a blood thinner that decreases blood clot formation at the site of blockage. In other cases, physicians prescribe nitroglycerin to dilate the arteries and improve blood flow. Thrombolytic medicines, also known as clot busters, dissolve blood clots in the coronary arteries, but they must be taken within one hour after heart attack symptoms begin. Beta-blockers essentially reduce the heart's need for oxygen by interfering with pathways that stimulate the heart to work harder. By "blocking" these pathways, beta-blockers reduce the heart's workload, provide relief from symptoms, alleviate irregular heartbeats, and help prevent a subsequent heart attack. Calcium channel blockers relax the smooth muscle lining of the tunica media. In essence, they lower blood pressure and allow for easier blood flow, both of which reduce the heart's workload.[14]

QUICK REFERENCE

The body is remarkable! If a coronary artery is occluded, additional blood vessels can "sprout" from the damaged one to form collateral circulation. In a sense, the body ensures blood delivery to the heart by creating an alternate route. Unfortunately, collateral circulation rarely delivers adequate oxygen during times of exertion, so it cannot completely resolve issues that result from coronary artery disease.

Once they diagnose a patient with coronary artery disease, physicians focus on lowering blood LDL levels since clinical trials have shown that lowered LDL levels directly reduce the risk of a cardiac event. Before prescribing medications, physicians suggest lifestyle changes including dietary modifications, exercise[15], and smoking cessation. If these changes do not reduce LDL levels, they resort to drug therapy.

Heart Attack

Each year, nearly 1.1 million people in the United States experience a heart attack. Furthermore, every 20 seconds, a person dies of a heart attack. A heart attack, also known as a myocardial infarction, results when a portion of the heart is deprived of oxygen for so long that cells die. The major cause of ischemia is coronary artery disease. As mentioned in the previous section, the right and left coronary arteries and their branches supply the heart muscle with oxygen and nutrients. Whenever plaque buildup narrows any of these branches, the specific section of the heart that they serve is denied oxygen. If the blockage is not treated quickly, the cardiac tissue begins to die. Normally, damaged cardiac tissue is replaced with fibrous connective tissue (or scar tissue), and since this scar tissue lacks contractile properties, it cannot function like cardiac tissue. The consequences depend upon the extent of heart tissue damage and the length of time before oxygen supply is restored. Quick treatment that opens the affected artery significantly decreases long-term damage. Once cardiac tissue dies, the heart, however, loses some of its functional capacity, particularly during physical exertion.[8,16]

In addition to coronary artery blockage, a severe spasm of a coronary artery can also cause a heart attack. Although this is a much less common cause of myocardial infarction, spasm can effectively block oxygen delivery to specific sections of the heart thereby causing permanent heart damage. Spasms can occur in those with or without CAD, but the results are the same—blood flow to heart tissue is restricted, the heart is deprived of oxygen, cardiac muscle is damaged, and the damaged tissue dies and is replaced by scar tissue. The exact causes of spasms are unknown, but they are related to exposure to cigarette smoke, certain drugs like cocaine, and extreme pain or emotional upset.

Recent research has uncovered a third contributor to heart attack called coronary microvascular dysfunction. This condition is particularly prevalent in women. Years ago, investigators noted that women with a positive stress test were 4.5 times more likely to have an angiogram that showed absolutely no coronary artery blockage than men with a positive stress test. This led them to believe that the stress test was an unreliable predictor of heart disease in women; however, as more studies focused on female subjects and as new diagnostic techniques became available, researchers discovered that many of these women had abnormal vascular function tests—even in the absence of blocked arteries. Abnormal vascular function suggests poor microcirculation to the heart; in other words, the small coronary artery branches do not dilate properly. This malfunction occurs whether the larger coronary arteries are occluded or not. This discovery explained why so many cases of heart disease in women formerly went undiagnosed. It also explained why women typically do not experience the same heart attack symptoms as men. Instead of the cold sweat, nausea, and crushing chest pain that often radiates down the left arm in male sufferers, women with coronary microvascular dysfunction experience exhaustion, overall discomfort, shortness of breath (SOB), and depression prior to a cardiac event. Rather than the traditional stress test and coronary angiography used to diagnose men, women need the stress test and functional vascular imaging for proper diagnosis.[17–19]

Unstable angina—chest pain that occurs during exertion as well as during rest. Does not respond to medication and is a serious indicator of impending heart attack.

Electrocardiogram—a test that records the heart's electrical activity; it can indicate a heart attack or irregular heart rhythms.

Blood tests—various blood tests can determine the composition of blood. When heart cells die, as occurs in a heart attack, the cells burst and release their proteins. Elevated levels of certain blood proteins indicate a heart attack.

Coronary angiography—an x-ray of the heart and its surrounding blood vessels. Helps determine the area of blockage and damage. Often followed by an angioplasty.

TABLE 7-5 COMMON SIGNS AND SYMPTOMS OF A HEART ATTACK

- Angina pectoris—an uncomfortable tightness, squeezing, pressure, or fullness felt in the center of the chest. It may be intermittent and typically subsides when activity ceases
- Pain that radiates into the arms, back, neck, or jaw
- Shortness of breath
- Cold sweat
- Nausea, vomiting, or lightheadedness

What is the cause of coronary microvascular dysfunction? Inflammation is one of the major culprits. Inflammation in males tends to cause plaque formation and vessel rupture often followed by a heart attack. Inflammation in women, however, causes slow blood vessel erosion. As the body attempts to repair this erosion, further damage and inflammation occur in the tiny blood vessels serving the heart. Additionally, heredity, elevated LDL, low HDL, high triglycerides, hypertension, inactivity, obesity, and high blood glucose levels increase risk for microvascular dysfunction.

QUICK REFERENCE

Women who have anemia along with microvascular dysfunction experience poor outcomes following a heart attack. This is perhaps because anemic individuals have fewer red blood cells with which to deliver blood to cardiac muscle cells.[18,20]

Heart attack does not have to result in death. Unfortunately, many people experiencing a heart attack ignore the signs (Table 7.5) and wait too long to go to the hospital. Surveys show that over 50% of those who actually die from a heart attack die before they reach the emergency room because they chose to ignore their symptoms. Seeking treatment within one hour following symptom onset, however, dramatically improves outlook and increases the likelihood of living an active, fulfilled life.

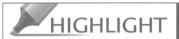 HIGHLIGHT   Metabolic Syndrome and Risk for Heart Disease

According to the National Heart, Lung, and Blood Institute, people suffering from metabolic syndrome are twice as likely to develop heart disease and five times as likely to develop type 2 diabetes as those without metabolic syndrome. Metabolic syndrome consists of a group of risk factors that significantly increase the risk for heart disease and stroke. See Chapter 6 for more information on metabolic syndrome, which is also known as syndrome X, insulin resistance syndrome, and dysmetabolic syndrome.

TABLE 7-6 GROUPS AT GREATER RISK OF DEVELOPING HYPERTENSION

- Those with a family history of hypertension
- Those who are over the age of 35
- Those who smoke
- African Americans
- Women who take birth control pills
- Those with excess weight
- Sedentary individuals
- Those who consume fatty diets

Hypertension

According to the AHA, hypertension, also known as high blood pressure, affects more than 73 million Americans over the age of 20. It killed more than 54,000 people and was responsible for more than 1 million heart attacks and half a million strokes in 2004.[8] The risk for hypertension increases with age. Risk is higher in men than in women and in blacks than in whites.[21] See Table 7.6 for a list of those who have a higher than average risk for developing hypertension, defined as a blood pressure ≥140/90 mm Hg.[8] High blood pressure itself is a risk factor for additional disorders including kidney disease, peripheral vascular disease (PVD), and congestive heart failure (CHF). In reality, the risk for these disorders actually increases at a pressure below 140/90 mm Hg; therefore, any decrease in blood pressure, even if blood pressure is within the "healthy" range, reduces the risk for hypertension-related complications.[21]

Unfortunately, hypertension is also known as a "silent disease" since nearly 30% of sufferers are completely unaware of their condition.[8] Being unaware of their elevated blood pressure increases their risk for a major cardiovascular event.

What is Blood Pressure? Blood pressure is the force that blood exerts against the inner lining of the blood vessel wall; it largely results from the pumping action of the heart and the resistance that blood encounters as it moves through vessels. Even though all vessels are under some pressure, arterial pressure is much higher than venous pressure, so a blood pressure reading measures pressure within arteries.

Why is pressure in an artery so much higher than it is in a vein? Consider the function of arteries versus veins. Arteries are the vessels that receive blood from the heart and transport blood *away* from the heart. In fact, one major artery connects directly to each ventricle and transports blood to another location. More specifically, contraction of the right ventricle forces blood into an artery that carries the blood away from the heart and toward the lungs. Contraction of the left ventricle forces blood into another artery that carries blood away from the heart and toward the rest of the body. Because these arteries directly connect to the heart, their blood is under high pressure. As blood moves farther from the heart, however, pressure diminishes. By the time blood reaches veins, blood pressure is relatively low and plays only a minimal role in the return of blood to the heart.

Because they are such low-pressure vessels, veins rely on *valves* and the actions of the *skeletal* and *respiratory pumps* to return blood back to the heart.

QUICK REFERENCE
The risk for CVD doubles for each 20 mm Hg increment increase in systolic blood pressure or for each 10 mm of Hg increment increase in diastolic blood pressure.[21]

Valves operate by preventing the backflow of blood. They are scattered throughout the venous system and are particularly plentiful in superficial veins. Once blood passes a valve, the valve closes to prevent the blood from seeping back into the section through which it just passed. As long as valves are intact, they ensure that blood moves in one direction only—toward the heart.

The *skeletal pump* functions because of the pressure exerted on deep veins by the alternating contraction and relaxation of surrounding skeletal muscles. In a sense, this kneading action squeezes blood through valve sections and moves it toward the heart. The *respiratory pump* acts in a similar manner. It involves pressure changes in the thoracic cavity during breathing. Just prior to inhalation, pressure within the thoracic cavity drops, but pressure within the abdominal cavity increases as the diaphragm contracts and flattens. This action squeezes blood from veins within the abdominal cavity into veins in the thoracic cavity. During exhalation, pressure within the abdominal cavity drops allowing the abdominal veins to fill again with blood. Together, the skeletal and respiratory pumps promote the return of blood to the heart.

As mentioned, a large artery connects to each ventricle and transports blood away from the heart. The vessel that connects to the right ventricle is the pulmonary trunk. The pulmonary trunk branches into the right and left pulmonary arteries, each of which travels to a lung. Along the way, each pulmonary artery branches repeatedly until it eventually forms pulmonary capillaries. Pulmonary capillaries surround the alveoli, microscopic air sacs that form lung tissue. Gas exchange occurs across the membranes of the pulmonary capillaries and the alveoli. More specifically, oxygen moves from the inner space of alveoli into surrounding capillaries, while carbon dioxide moves from capillaries into the alveolar space. During exhalation, the respiratory system eliminates carbon dioxide, while blood vessels deliver oxygen-rich blood to body cells. The small pulmonary capillaries of one lung merge to form pulmonary venules, which then merge to form two pulmonary veins. Ultimately, four pulmonary veins, two from each lung, transport blood to the left atrium of the heart.

The major vessel that connects to the left ventricle is the aorta. The aorta branches much more than the pulmonary arteries because the aorta is responsible for delivering blood to cells scattered throughout the body. Blood pressure is highest in the aorta, which has a large amount of elastic connective tissue in its tunica media to accommodate blood ejected from the left ventricle during each contraction. Therefore, blood pressure within the aorta and nearby arteries increases each time the left ventricle contracts—just as blood pressure within the pulmonary trunk increases each time the right ventricle contracts.

The maximum pressure reached inside each of these major arteries during ventricular contraction is the **systolic blood pressure**. The lowest pressure inside each of these vessels, which occurs when the ventricles relax, is the **diastolic blood pressure**. As the ventricles contract, the arterial walls expand to receive blood; as the ventricles relax, the arterial walls recoil to maintain blood pressure within the vessels. This alternating expansion and recoiling can be felt as a pulse in various superficial arteries such as the carotid artery, radial artery, brachial artery, and femoral artery.

Determinants of Blood Pressure. Blood pressure varies at any given time depending upon the strength of heart contraction, demands on the heart, blood volume, arterial wall elasticity and recoil, blood flow resistance, blood viscosity, and overall health status. In general, the condition of the heart, overall health status, and current demands determine the volume of blood discharged from each ventricle during each contraction (**stroke volume**), the volume discharged per minute (**cardiac output**), the number of times the heart contracts per minute (**heart rate**), and the percentage of its contents that each ventricle ejects during contraction (**ejection fraction**).

Blood volume affects blood pressure because blood pressure is directly proportional to the quantity of blood contained within vessels. Changes in blood volume, therefore, affect blood pressure in the short term. For example, water is a major component of blood, so blood pressure usually drops in the initial stages of dehydration. In cases of dehydration, ingesting liquids easily restores normal blood volume and subsequently normal blood pressure, but the body also has various mechanisms that temporarily restore blood pressure when blood volume is low and fluid intake is inadequate. These mechanisms rely on proteins such as antidiuretic hormone, renin, angiotensin, and aldosterone.

Blood viscosity refers to how easily blood moves through blood vessels. The more viscous a fluid, the more sluggish it flows. A viscous fluid, therefore, requires more pressure to move. The viscosity of blood is influenced by the relative number of red blood cells, proteins, and water in blood. It is normally consistent, but when viscosity increases, the heart must work progressively harder to move this "thicker" blood. This elevates blood pressure.

Systolic blood pressure—the top number in a blood pressure reading that represents the maximum amount of pressure exerted on the arterial walls during contraction.

Diastolic blood pressure—the bottom number in a blood pressure reading that represents the maximum amount of pressure exerted on the arterial walls during relaxation.

Stroke volume (SV)—the amount of blood ejected from the left ventricle with each contraction.

Cardiac output (CO)—the amount of blood ejected each minute; equals SV × HR.

Heart rate (HR)—the number of times the heart contracts (beats) per minute.

Ejection fraction—the percentage of blood discharged from each ventricle with each contraction.

Peripheral resistance describes the relationship between blood and blood vessel walls. Blood vessel walls provide a resistance that works against blood flow, so blood pressure must overcome this resistance. Many factors change peripheral resistance and subsequently influence blood pressure. For instance, when smooth muscle in the tunica media contracts, it narrows the blood vessel's lumen and increases resistance. As this smooth muscle relaxes, resistance decreases. In addition, the natural recoil of large, elastic arterial walls increases resistance during ventricular diastole to maintain blood pressure and blood flow from the heart. Overall, blood pressure equals the product of cardiac output and peripheral resistance (BP = CO × PR).

Healthy Versus Unhealthy Blood Pressure. A normal or healthy blood pressure is defined as less than 120/80 mm Hg. Hypertension, or high blood pressure, is a condition in which blood pressure is persistently elevated. Although it can go undetected for decades if overt symptoms are absent, it is a strong risk factor for heart attack, stroke, heart failure, kidney failure, and aneurisms. Hypertension is diagnosed when a person's blood pressure reading on at least three consecutive occasions is ≥140/90 mm Hg. A blood pressure reading ranging from 120/80 to 139/89 mm Hg indicates a condition called "prehypertension." Those with prehypertension have a high risk of developing hypertension, so they need to practice lifestyle behaviors that reduce risk. Although high blood pressure is not considered an illness on its own, it takes its toll on the inner lining of the arterial wall and thereby promotes plaque buildup. Over time, the vessel narrows, additional damage occurs, and the likelihood of an acute event increases.

Hypertension can be classified as essential or secondary. Secondary hypertension is the least common. This form of hypertension has a definite, identifiable cause such as kidney disease, adrenal gland disorders, or use of certain medications.

Essential hypertension, on the other hand, has no obvious cause and is experienced by over 90% to 95% of all hypertensive individuals. Contributing factors include cigarette smoking, excess weight, sedentary lifestyle, excess sodium in the diet for salt-sensitive individuals, drinking more than one to two alcoholic beverages per day, older age, and heredity. Since many of these are controllable behaviors, lifestyle modifications are viable treatment options for essential hypertension. In fact, results from the Framingham Heart study suggested that 65% to 75% of all hypertensive cases were directly attributable to overweight and obesity.[20] Losing excess weight, therefore, reduces the heart's workload, improves circulation, and usually decreases blood pressure. Routine exercise is another lifestyle factor that enhances the efficiency of oxygen delivery by increasing the number of blood vessels and red blood cells. It also improves coordination between the lungs and the heart, strengthens the heart muscle, and reduces blood pressure in the long term. Together, weight loss and increased physical activity are integral components of the long-term treatment and prevention of high blood pressure.[21]

For the 60% of hypertensive individuals who are salt sensitive, restricting dietary sodium decreases blood pressure.[8] Reducing daily sodium intake to no more than 2,400 mg of sodium, or 6,000 mg of sodium chloride, can reduce systolic blood pressure by 2 to 8 mm Hg.[21] Consuming a diet high in fruits and vegetables and low in saturated fat and cholesterol also improves blood pressure, as does eliminating tobacco and limiting alcohol intake.

TABLE 7-7 COMMON ANTIHYPERTENSIVE MEDICATIONS

Antihypertensive Medication	Mechanism of Action
ACE inhibitors	Also known as angiotensin-converting enzyme inhibitors; prevent vasoconstriction by interfering with the enzymes necessary for the formation of angiotensin II, a powerful blood vessel constrictor. Examples include benazepril (Lotensin), enalapril (Vasotec), and lisinopril (Prinivil, Zestril).
Angiotensin II receptor antagonists	Like ACE inhibitors, these inhibit the action of angiotensin II. Angiotensin II receptor blockers, however, prevent the action of angiotensin II by blocking receptors. Examples include losartan, valsartan, and irbesartan.
Alpha-blockers	Interfere with the action of the hormone norepinephrine. Norepinephrine constricts blood vessels. Alpha-blockers prevent this effect and thereby keep blood vessels dilated. Examples include doxazosin (Cardura), Prazosin (Minipress), and Terazosin (Hytrin).
Beta-blockers	Lower heart rate by blocking the effects of the hormone epinephrine. Some also dilate blood vessels. Examples include atenolol (Tenormin), metoprolol (Lopressor, Toprol-XL), and propranolol (Inderal, Inderal LA).
Calcium channel blockers	Dilate blood vessels by preventing calcium entry into smooth muscle cells of the tunica media. Also prevent calcium entry into cardiac muscle. Examples include amlodipine (Norvasc), diltiazem (Cardizem, Dilacor XR), nifedipine (Adalat, Procardia), and verapamil (Calan, Isoptin, Verelan, Covera).
Direct renin inhibitors	Block the action of renin. Renin is released when blood volume drops. It triggers a series of events that increases blood pressure. By interfering with this mechanism, renin inhibitors dilate blood vessels and lower blood pressure. An example is aliskiren (Tekturna).
Diuretics	Increase water excretion by the kidneys. This reduces blood volume, which in turn reduces blood pressure.

If lifestyle factors alone do not effectively decrease blood pressure, several antihypertensive drugs are available. These include angiotensin-converting enzyme (ACE) inhibitors, angiotensin II receptor antagonists, alpha-blockers, beta-blockers, calcium channel blockers, direct renin inhibitors, and diuretics. Although these drugs are important in controlling hypertension, a complete discussion of each is beyond the scope of this book. Instead, their basic mechanisms of action are presented in Table 7.7.

More than 30% of Americans have high blood pressure. Because many people are unaware of their condition, hypertension goes uncontrolled for years as it wreaks havoc on the heart and blood vessels. In some cases, chronic hypertension results in heart failure as the heart weakens in response to chronic overload. In other cases, hypertension might cause aneurisms in arteries supplying various body regions. Overall, the consequences depend upon the extent of damage and the specific vessels affected. For instances, if high blood pressure impairs the vessels supplying the kidneys, kidney damage results. If it affects vessels supplying the eyes, vision impairment occurs.

Unfortunately, blood pressure tends to increase with age. Furthermore, certain health conditions and medications drastically increase the rate at which it develops. Although it rarely, if ever, simply goes away, hypertension can be successfully managed through diet, exercise, routine care, and adherence to treatment prescribed by a physician.

Stroke

According to the American Stroke Association, a stroke occurs every 40 seconds and affects up to 780,000 Americans each year. This total includes both new and recurrent stroke incidences. Overall, nearly 150,000 people die each year from stroke, making stroke the number three killer of Americans. In addition, Americans invest over $65 billion for medical costs and disability related to incidences of stroke. Obviously, those at risk need to implement lifestyle changes to reduce their risk of stroke.

A stroke results when a part of the brain is deprived of oxygen. Ischemic stroke, the more common type, usually occurs when one of the major arteries supplying the brain develops atherosclerosis. In this case, a plaque forms, enlarges, and possibly ruptures. A ruptured plaque attracts platelets to the area, which further narrows the vessel until the vessel is completely blocked. This condition is called **cerebral thrombosis**. A **cerebral embolism** results if a clot forms at another location in the body (such as in the coronary arteries), breaks off, travels to the tiny vessels supplying the brain, and lodges in the narrow passageway. No matter the source, the results are the same: blood supply to the brain is interrupted and brain tissue receives inadequate oxygen. If deprived of oxygen for too long, permanent damage results. In fact, strokes can cause long-term weakness, numbness, tingling, slurred speech, or walking difficulty. Treatment for ischemic strokes involves clot-dissolving medications that must be taken within three hours following symptom onset. Preventive measures include anticoagulants such as warfarin, antiplatelet agents such as aspirin, surgical removal of the blocked artery, or **angioplasty** in which surgeons insert balloons or stents to open up a clogged vessel.

Hemorrhagic stroke, which only accounts for 17% of all strokes, is a different form of stroke that occurs if a vessel supplying the brain bursts. Once a vessel bursts, blood escapes and fills the spaces in the brain. Accumulating fluid puts pressure on and possibly destroys fragile brain cells. Aneurisms are common causes of hemorrhagic stroke. Treatment involves clamping or removing the damaged portion of a vessel. A less invasive method entails inserting a catheter through a major artery in the leg or arm and depositing a mechanical structure to stabilize the aneurism.[22]

A transient ischemic attack, or TIA, occurs when an area of the brain is temporarily deprived of oxygen. During TIAs, normal blood flow is restored before any permanent damage occurs. Neurological symptoms do present (such as tingling, weakness, numbness, and difficulty walking); however, they last for only minutes or maybe hours. Eventually, normal functioning returns. Sometimes referred to as a "light stroke," a TIA should not be ignored. It is often an early warning sign of an impending ischemic stroke.[22,23]

The resulting consequences of stroke depend upon the side of the brain compromised, the specific area of the brain affected, and the extent of damage. Strokes affecting the right side of the brain interfere with functioning on the left side of the body and the right side of the face. They often cause paralysis, vision problems, and memory loss. Strokes affecting the left side of the brain interfere with functioning on the right side of the body and the left side of the face. This often causes paralysis, speech and

TABLE 7-8   SIGNS OF A STROKE

If any of these signs are present, seek immediate medical attention

- Sudden numbness or weakness of the face, arm, or leg
- Sudden loss of sensation
- Sudden confusion, trouble speaking, difficulty understanding others
- Sudden difficulty seeing
- Sudden difficulty walking
- Sudden dizziness, loss of balance, loss of coordination
- Sudden severe headache

language problems, and memory loss. Table 7.8 lists common signs and symptoms of stroke.[22–24]

Peripheral Vascular Disease

Peripheral vascular disease (PVD) is any disorder that affects blood vessels found outside of the brain and heart. It usually results from atherosclerosis of the vessels in the upper extremities, lower extremities, or viscera. Although it can affect either arteries or veins, arteries are typically the target of this disease. In particular, PVD often affects the arteries supplying the arms, legs, feet, kidneys, and stomach. Overall, artery blockage interrupts oxygen and nutrient delivery, which often results in pain or numbness. If oxygen deprivation is long in duration, tissue death, also known as gangrene, occurs. Gangrene sometimes requires amputation, and sadly, PVD is the number one cause of leg amputation.[8,10,25]

Although symptoms are only present in 50% of those suffering from PVD, early warning signs include cramping or unusual fatigue of the legs and buttocks during exertion. Typically, cramping subsides when activity is stopped. This transient cramping is called intermittent claudication.[10] Additional symptoms include a weak or absent pulse in the legs, sores on the feet that heal slowly, heaviness and numbness in the muscles, and poor nail or hair growth. These, of course, are also symptoms for a myriad of other disorders.

As with other forms of arterial blockage, PVD is diagnosed with a complete health history, a physical examination, an ultrasound, x-ray angiography, and magnetic

---

Cerebral thrombosis—formation of a blood clot within a blood vessel supplying brain tissue.

Cerebral embolism—occurs when a portion of a blood clot from any vessel in the body breaks off, travels to the vessels supplying the brain, and lodges in one of these vessels. It obstructs blood flow and oxygen delivery to the part of the brain served by the affected vessel.

Angioplasty—a procedure that often follows a coronary angiography. It restores blood flow through an affected artery.

resonance angiography. Even though PVD is relatively prevalent, it is often overlooked because symptoms are frequently absent or because the symptoms are often attributed to normal aging. If diagnosed, however, initial treatment targets lifestyle factors. Sufferers should stop smoking, control diabetes and blood pressure, eat a healthy diet low in saturated fat and cholesterol, and increase physical activity. Although activity might initially be difficult and limited, one study showed that consistent exercise increased maximal walking distance by nearly 150% by the end of the testing period.[26] Additionally, medications exist that can increase walking distance, reduce platelet aggregation, and lower cholesterol levels—factors that improve overall blood vessel health. If these modifications do not reduce symptoms, angioplasty or stent insertion is an alternative.[8,10] Typically, a vascular physician participates in establishing exercise programs for those with moderate to severe PVD.

PVD affects about 10 million Americans, most of whom are over the age of 50. Risk continues to increase with age. Nearly 30% of those over the age of 75 have PVD, while close to 60% of those over the age of 85 experience it. PVD is slightly more common in men than in women and is a major contributor to the disability associated with diabetes. PVD is serious because it increases risk for heart attack, stroke, and TIA. In fact, the 10-year mortality rate for cardiovascular events is three to six times greater in those suffering from PVD than in those without it.[8,27]

Congestive Heart Failure

Congestive heart failure (CHF) results when the heart can no longer adequately pump blood. It can affect the right side of the heart, the left side of the heart, or both sides. According to the AHA, CHF results from coronary artery disease, extensive scar tissue from previous heart attacks, hypertension, valve disease, valve infection, or congenital heart defects. Although the heart continues to pump, stroke volume and ejection fraction decrease, which promotes blood pooling in blood vessels. As blood pools, pressure builds and forces excess fluid into the interstitial space. This results in **edema**, which is particularly evident in the lower extremities. It can also cause edema in the lungs. Edema is the major indicator for CHF, a condition diagnosed from a series of tests (such as an echocardiogram, chest x-ray, chest CT scan, cardiac MRI, ECG, and blood tests).

The treatment protocol for CHF involves rest, modified activities, proper diet, and medications such as ACE inhibitors, beta-blockers, diuretics, and vasodilators. ACE inhibitors and vasodilators dilate blood vessels to reduce resistance to blood flow. Diuretics eliminate excess fluid to reduce swelling, while beta-blockers improve the functional capacity of the left ventricle. Treatment effectiveness ultimately depends upon the root cause of heart failure. The two most frequent causes include hypertension and coronary artery disease. Hypertension overstresses the heart and can result in long-term damage. Coronary artery disease deprives the heart of oxygen, thereby causing tissue death. Additional contributors include valve disease, congenital heart problems, heart tumor, and lung disease. If a leaky valve is the culprit, valve replacement is the answer; however, if the heart is covered with scar tissue, heart transplant is the only possible option. Overall, CHF is a life-threatening condition that typically reduces life expectancy and worsens with both physical and mental stress. Table 7.9 lists some symptoms of CHF.

TABLE 7-9 SYMPTOMS OF CHF

- Swelling of the feet, ankles, and/or stomach
- Weight gain (as a result of water weight)
- Rapid or irregular heart rate
- Loss of appetite
- Indigestion
- Shortness of breath and reduced ability for exertion
- Nausea and vomiting
- Severe muscle weakness and fatigue
- Decreased urine output
- Persistent cough or wheezing, sometimes accompanied by pink phlegm

PRECAUTIONS DURING EXERCISE

MEDICATIONS

Cardiac patients often take medications to help control their condition. This is true for those with CHF, recent heart attack, and hypertension. Different medications affect exercise response differently. Consequently, methods used to determine exercise intensity for the healthy population might not be suitable for this special population. The rate of perceived exertion is often more reliable than heart rate since many cardiac drugs lower heart rate.

Health and fitness professional must know which medications their clients are taking to ensure a safe and effective exercise program. They should be aware that ACE inhibitors lower blood pressure. Antiplatelet drugs (or blood thinners) reduce the risk for blood clots. Beta-blockers lower heart rate, blood pressure, and oxygen requirements of the heart. Calcium channel blockers relax arterial walls, lower overall blood pressure, and decrease the workload of the heart. Diuretics decrease blood volume and lower blood pressure. And statins reduce blood levels of cholesterol.

SHORTNESS OF BREATH

Many forms of CVD result in shortness of breath (SOB), a symptom that interferes with exercise ability. It sometimes results from fluid accumulation in the lungs, which can suggest heart failure or an impending heart attack. Clients experiencing SOB should immediately stop activity and seek medical attention. Be aware that there *is* a difference between SOB and the normal breathlessness associated with exertion.

Edema—accumulation of interstitial fluid.

CHEST PAIN AND EXERCISE-INDUCED ISCHEMIA

All clients should cease exercise if they experience chest pain. Chest pain often develops in response to ischemia in heart muscle tissue. Recall that ischemia is a condition in which working cells receive inadequate oxygen. Chest pain, therefore, is often the first sign that heart cells are not receiving enough oxygen to meet the increasing demands of exercise. Since cardiac patients are at an even greater risk for cardiac arrest than the average healthy person, they should avoid exercising at vigorous intensities because higher intensities dangerously increase the heart's workload. Clients experiencing chest pain prior to beginning exercise should avoid exercise and see a physician. If clients feel fine at the onset of exercise but develop chest pain during the activity, encourage them to stop the activity immediately and seek medical attention.

HIGH BLOOD PRESSURE

Blood pressure response to cardiovascular training differs from blood pressure response to resistance training. For many years, experts claimed that cardiovascular training was the only safe means of exercise for those with high blood pressure. They believed that resistance training was dangerous because it causes acute but extreme increases in blood pressure even in healthy individuals. Current opinion, however, suggests that both forms of exercise are safe for those with hypertension and those suffering from most forms of CVD as long as certain guidelines are followed.[28,29]

During cardiovascular training, systolic blood pressure increases while diastolic blood pressure remains relatively constant. The increase in systolic pressure varies depending upon overall conditioning, resting blood pressure, exercise intensity, and environmental temperature. A typical systolic pressure reading is anywhere from 160 to 220 mm Hg during intense aerobic training. If it exceeds 240 mm Hg or does not increase with increases in intensity, the client should stop the exercise and seek medical attention. If the diastolic pressure increases by 20 mm Hg or exceeds 120 mm Hg, exercise should also be stopped.[21,29,30] Of course, not all exercisers know what their blood pressure changes are during exercise because blood pressure monitoring is not practical for most types of exercise.

Although it should not be the primary mode of exercise for hypertensive clients, resistance training can provide benefits when offered as a part of an overall training program. Blood flow to a contracting muscle actually decreases during the contraction phase of exercise as the muscle fibers shorten, bulge, and ultimately collapse the smaller vessels supplying the working muscle. This temporarily deprives the muscle of oxygen, a condition that leads to minor pain in the contracting muscle. To counteract this hypoxia, or temporary oxygen deprivation, overall blood pressure increases because the heart pumps harder as it tries to deliver more blood to the working muscle in an attempt to correct the temporary oxygen deficiency. The magnitude of increase varies depending upon contraction intensity and activity duration. The elevated blood pressure, however, can be life threatening in those with preexisting heart disease because it can overload the heart, decrease blood flow to the heart itself, and possibly rupture existing aneurysms. Therefore, clients who have preexisting hypertension must practice care to avoid a cardiac event.

Normal breathing is essential! Clients with high blood pressure must avoid holding the breath because this habit increases blood pressure, interferes with the return of blood to the heart, and overtaxes the heart muscle as it works.[28,30]

Overall, hypertensive clients should avoid isometric exercises and any other sustained or heavy resistance training. Be aware that hypertensive exercisers often experience an abrupt drop in blood pressure soon after exercise. This rebound hypotension can be dangerous and result in dizziness and fainting; therefore, a gradual cooldown is crucial. In addition, many high blood pressure medications affect heart rate, so heart rate response to exercise might not be as expected. As in those with other forms of CVD, perceived exertion is the preferred method for determining intensity.[21,30]

SPECIAL PRECAUTIONS FOR THOSE WHO HAVE HAD A RECENT HEART ATTACK OR HEART SURGERY

Exercise is necessary to strengthen the heart, so many heart attack survivors are put into cardiac rehabilitation programs soon after their cardiac event. The timing depends upon the condition of the heart. Cardiac rehabilitation programs are a wonderful means of reentering the world of activity since they are tailored to meet the needs of cardiac patients and are staffed with highly qualified medical professionals. Most likely, a physician will perform a stress test prior to designing an exercise program. Personal trainers and other health professionals need to follow physician guidelines closely to ensure exercise safety. Changes to the program should only be made with physician approval.

Those who have undergone surgery must allow their incisions to heal. Excessive pulling or undue stress on sutures can cause bleeding, infection, and delayed healing. These patients need to closely monitor heart rate response to exercise to ensure that palpitations or arrhythmias do not develop.

SPECIAL PRECAUTIONS FOR THOSE WITH CHF

The hearts and lungs of those with CHF do not respond to exercise like the hearts and lungs of healthy people. Therefore, those with CHF should only participate in mild to moderate cardiovascular exercise. Sufferers often report SOB, fatigue, rapid or irregular heartbeat, and swelling during times of *little* or *no* exertion, so physical activity can be difficult. The goal, however, is to try to challenge muscles without overloading the heart.[31,32]

Resistance exercise is important for this group because it strengthens skeletal muscles and bone. It should consist of low-intensity exercises targeted toward small, isolated muscle groups rather than high-intensity multijoint exercises. Keep repetitions low and have a longer rest-to-work-ratio than normal. Lightweights or elastic bands may be safely used by this group for strength training. Aerobic exercise trains body tissues to extract oxygen from blood more efficiently. In a sense, this lessens the burden of the heart and reduces the risk for a cardiac event. In addition, cardiovascular exercise can ease symptom severity, reduce stress, enhance mood, increase energy levels, and improve circulation and blood pressure. Walking or stationary cycling is probably the safest mode of aerobic exercise. All physical activity should be stopped if the client experiences dizziness, chest pain, or a more pronounced SOB.[8,10,28,31,32]

A physician should design the exercise prescription while considering the extent of heart failure and the results of stress tests. CHF patients should avoid exercise if exercise worsens edema, or if they feel ill and have a fever. They should stop exercise if they have any pain in the extremities or if heart palpitations occur. In addition, they should avoid exercise on days when they feel extremely fatigued and weak.

Many CHF patients participate in cardiac rehabilitation programs prior to venturing out on their own. These rehabilitation programs typically occur in hospitals or clinics, allow the patient to begin at a very mild intensity, and are supervised by highly qualified medical professionals. Therefore, they tend to be quite safe and effective.

SUMMARY OF PRECAUTIONS

The specific precautions for exercise vary depending upon the particular preexisting cardiovascular condition. Because their heart and blood vessels are already functioning less than optimally, however, those suffering from CVD have an increased risk of an acute event during exercise training. Acute events include but are not limited to heart attack and death. As long as exercise intensity is kept at low to moderate levels, however, risk is minimal. As intensity becomes more vigorous, the risk for an acute cardiovascular incident increases.[33,34] Overall, however, exercise is important for those diagnosed with CVD. They just need to be aware of four major warning signs during exercise: new or recurring angina; unusual SOB; dizziness or lightheadedness; and heart arrhythmias. If any of these exist, cease exercise and seek immediate medical attention.[21]

BENEFITS OF EXERCISE

Regular exercise reduces the risk of developing chronic diseases such as those associated with the cardiovascular system. It is generally accepted that a lifelong commitment to cardiovascular and strength training minimizes, or perhaps even prevents, the age-related decline in the cardiovascular system. Even if CVD develops in those who have been relatively active throughout life, the consequences seem to be less severe and recovery more likely. Therefore, the next logical question is the following: Does exercise provide any benefits for those who are already living with CVD? And is it ever too late to start exercising after some sort of cardiac event?[34,35]

As with all other populations, most people living with CVD experience dramatic improvements with consistent exercise training. According to the AHA, inactivity is one of the five major contributing risk factors for the initial development of CVD. It is, therefore, reasonable to assume that continuing a sedentary lifestyle after developing CVD increases the risk for a major cardiac event, worsens the outcome of existing conditions, and decreases quality of life overall. In fact, statistics show that 35% of all deaths from CVD are attributed to a sedentary lifestyle.[36] This section explores some of the health benefits and discusses the importance of exercise for those with CVD.

INCREASED MAXIMAL OXYGEN UPTAKE

Maximal oxygen uptake, or VO_{2max}, is the maximum amount of oxygen a person can take in and use. Fitness professionals often use it to assess an individual's cardiovascular health and aerobic endurance. In most cases, VO_{2max} increases with consistent cardiovascular training. A higher VO_{2max} is important not only during athletic training, however. It also lessens the burden during normal activities of daily living. Essentially, body cells become more adept at accessing blood oxygen, and this decreases the heart's workload.

VO_{2max} typically declines in those with CVD and/or hypertension, and this decline is associated with an increased risk for death. Cardiovascular exercise helps improve maximal oxygen uptake, even in those with preexisting cardiac conditions, and can decrease the risk of death while it improves quality of life.[37] The heart is a muscle, so it responds to increasing workloads like other muscles. In a study by Hambrecht et al., men with diseased coronary arteries who underwent a one-year exercise-training program increased maximal oxygen uptake by 16% and improved exercise tolerance by 20%. Eighty-eight percent did not experience a heart attack, stroke, or worsening of angina.[38] These are encouraging results! Of course, the intensity of training must be low-to-moderate to avoid complications, but the results are impressive.

IMPROVED HEART FUNCTIONING AND REDUCED ANGINA

Overall, the hearts of those suffering from CVD deteriorate. In part this is because many people are afraid to place physical demands on their bodies once they are diagnosed with CVD. They fear a heart attack, stroke, or other complications associated with CVD, so they simply avoid activity. Unfortunately, cardiac muscle responds to disuse just like any other organ in the body. It becomes less able to meet demands and begins to lose functional ability.

Just as exercise improves the condition of a healthy heart, it also improves the functional capacity of a less-than-healthy heart. As the diseased heart adapts to challenges, albeit more slowly than a healthy heart, its workload lessens as stroke volume increases, resting heart rate drops, and overall body weight drops. The heart itself becomes more efficient and learns to overcome challenges with less stress and more efficiency.[39-41]

IMPROVED HEALTH OF BLOOD VESSELS

Cardiovascular exercise improves circulation, lowers blood pressure, and minimizes plaque buildup, factors that contribute to blood vessel health. *Improved circulation* occurs as new capillaries develop in tissues in response to increased oxygen and nutrient demands. Therefore, a trained body has more blood vessels than an untrained body. In addition, the number of red blood cells, and therefore the oxygen-carrying capacity of blood, improves with long-term training. This further enhances oxygen delivery and waste removal. Simultaneously, metabolically active cells, such as skeletal muscle cells, develop more mitochondria and myoglobin, organelles that enable them to meet their rising demands for ATP. In a sense, muscle cells develop the equipment to work longer without fatigue. Lastly, as more blood vessels develop, additional lymphatic vessels form in the same areas. This improves fluid removal from the interstitial space and facilitates its return to blood. As a result, edema is less likely. The contractions of skeletal muscles also assist in fluid movement. As mentioned earlier, these contractions help move blood through veins and back to the heart. They also facilitate movement into the lymphatic vessels and through the lymphatic system.[8,41]

Another benefit of regular exercise is that it lowers blood pressure in the long term.[8,41] The effect might even be more dramatic in those with hypertension.[42] Studies show that aerobic exercise can actually decrease systolic pressure by 7.4 mm Hg and diastolic pressure by 5.8 mm Hg, results that usually occur when training at 40% to 70% VO_{2max} for 30 to 60 minutes, 3 to 5 days per week. Amazingly, this drop in blood pressure is independent of the weight loss that accompanies training.[21] As mentioned earlier, high blood pressure is often the beginning of arterial lining deterioration, a factor that promotes atherosclerotic plaque buildup and the subsequent interruption in blood flow to areas supplied by affected vessels. In addition, a portion of a plaque might rip off and travel to areas of the body served by smaller vessels. If this embolus lodges in a coronary artery, heart attack ensues. If it lodges in a vessel supplying the brain, a stroke occurs. Obviously, lowering blood pressure improves the outlook for those with hypertension.

IMPROVED BLOOD LIPID PROFILE

Numerous men and women have low HDL levels and elevated LDL and triglyceride levels, factors that predispose them to CVD. According to the National Cholesterol Education Program, two lifestyle factors that greatly improve the blood lipid profile include exercise and weight loss (in overweight and obese individuals).[43] Exercise is associated with reduced blood triglycerides, elevated HDL levels, and slightly reduced LDL levels, factors that reduce CVD risk and limit plaque buildup. These benefits accrue even in those with preexisting CVD. In fact, they can slow its progression and prevent an acute cardiac incident. When combined with a healthy diet low in saturated fat and high in whole grains, fruits, and vegetables, exercise can significantly improve the blood lipid profile.[8,36]

IMPROVED RECOVERY FROM HEART ATTACK

According to the AHA, several studies show that people who initiate an exercise program after a heart attack have much better survival rates than those who remain sedentary.[44] This is likely because of the impact of cardiovascular training on the heart and blood vessels. The heart becomes more efficient at delivering blood; therefore, it accomplishes its job with less strain. The blood vessels, most importantly the coronary arteries, remain clear and unobstructed, so the heart itself receives an adequate blood supply.

IMPROVED MOOD AND REDUCED ANXIETY

According to the American Academy of Family Physicians, nearly one out of every three heart attack survivors experiences some level of depression after the event. This depression can affect anyone and often interferes with recovery. The AHA suggests that participation in physical activity often prevents feelings of sadness and despair, so the AHA encourages exercise as a treatment option for depression. How does exercise affect depression? Consider cardiac rehabilitation programs as an example. These programs integrate people into society and prevent them from isolating themselves. Social interactions often elevate mood and improve feelings of self-worth. In addition, exercise actually alters brain chemistry, primarily through its effect on serotonin and endorphins, so it can improve overall outlook on life.

IMPROVED INSULIN SENSITIVITY

According to the American Diabetes Association, two out of every three people with diabetes die of heart disease or stroke. Therefore, reducing the incidence of diabetes could decrease the prevalence of CVD. One factor that contributes to the development of type 2 diabetes is insulin resistance. Several studies have shown that regular exercise improves insulin sensitivity and often prevents progression to type 2 diabetes. Perhaps this is because of the weight loss that often accompanies exercise.[36]

REDUCED RISK OF DEATH

Although those suffering from CVD are at a higher risk for death than those who are not, exercise seems to reduce the risk substantially. Some studies estimate a 20% to 25% reduction in both all-cause and cardiovascular mortality among patients attending cardiac rehabilitation programs after a heart attack.[41] A meta-analysis of over 8,440 patients participating in cardiac rehabilitation programs found that participation in structured programs reduced the risk for cardiac death by over 31%, and programs that included an education component and psychological support were even more effective. The overall goal of these programs is to restore as much health as possible. According to existing data, this goal is being met. Although more research is needed, the reduced mortality rate would likely remain, and possibly improve, if patients continued mild-to-moderate exercise after rehabilitation.[45,46]

RECOMMENDATIONS FOR EXERCISE

The heart is a muscle that needs to be challenged to improve its ability to function. Because those with CVD have weakened systems, strict precautions are advised; however, under most circumstances, the benefits of exercise far outweigh the risks.

EXERCISE TESTING

Before participating in exercise, anyone diagnosed with CVD should undergo exercise testing. A team of experts that includes a physician, a nurse, an exercise physiologist, a physical therapist, and medical technicians should be available since heart attacks have occurred during the testing procedure on numerous occasions.[47] In fact, surveys confirm that as many as 10 myocardial infarctions or deaths can be expected per 10,000 tests of those with CAD.[40] In general, exercise testing is important to diagnose disease, determine the extent of disease, predict prognosis for those with coronary artery disease, establish the likelihood of myocardial infarction, determine overall health, ensure effectiveness of current treatment, and ascertain exercise tolerance.[8,40,47,48]

According to a task force formed by the American College of Cardiology (ACC) and the AHA, members of this special population should undergo a cardiovascular stress test while monitored by an ECG. They can safely use either a treadmill or a bicycle, but they should have their blood pressures and heart rates monitored. The panel of experts from the ACC and AHA constructed a new stratification scheme to determine if exercise is appropriate for a given person. The classifications are noted in Table 7.10. Table 7.11 lists the absolute and relative contraindications according to the ACC/AHA standard guidelines.[40,47]

Unless working as part of a cardiac rehabilitation team, personal trainers are unlikely to actually conduct exercise testing on those with advanced CVD. Instead, they must rely on data collected by the group of qualified medical personnel. Consequently, this section

TABLE 7-10   ACC/AHA CLASSIFICATION SCHEME

Class I	Conditions for which there is evidence and/or general agreement that a given procedure or treatment is useful and effective.
Class II	Conditions for which there is conflicting evidence and/or a divergence of opinion about the usefulness of a procedure or treatment.
Class IIa	Weight of the evidence is in favor of its usefulness.
Class IIb	Usefulness is not as well established by evidence.
Class III	Conditions for which there is evidence and/or general agreement that the procedure/treatment is not useful and in some cases may be harmful.

TABLE 7-11   ABSOLUTE AND RELATIVE CONTRAINDICATIONS TO EXERCISE ACCORDING TO ACC/AHA GUIDELINES

Absolute Contraindications	Relative Contraindications
Acute myocardial infarction within the past 2 days	Left main coronary stenosis
Unstable angina	Moderate stenotic valvular heart disease
Uncontrolled cardiac arrhythmias	Electrolyte imbalances
Symptomatic aortic stenosis	Severe arterial hypertension
Uncontrolled symptomatic heart failure	Tachyarrhythmias or bradyarrhythmias
Acute pulmonary embolus or pulmonary infarction	Hypertrophic cardiomyopathy and other forms of outflow tract obstruction
Acute myocarditis or pericarditis	Mental or physical impairment that interferes with ability to exercise
Acute aortic dissection	High degree atrioventricular block

does not explore all parameters of exercise testing for each type of cardiovascular patient. For more details, please see the ACC/AHA Guidelines at www.acc.org/clinical/guidelines/exercise/dirIndex.htm.

EXERCISE PRESCRIPTION

After clients with CVD receive medical clearances from their physicians, they may begin an exercise program tailored to meet personal needs and abilities. In most instances, the first step back into activity is a cardiac rehabilitation program. Throughout cardiac rehabilitation, medical professionals trained for emergencies and experienced in working with various conditions establish and lead exercise. During these initial stages, professionals slowly challenge, closely monitor, and routinely evaluate their patients. After their patients complete inpatient programs, physicians typically encourage them to begin supervised outpatient exercise programs as they reenter the workforce and prepare for independent exercise. Physicians encourage independent exercise when cardiac symptoms are stable or absent, response to exercise meets stipulated guidelines, patients demonstrate knowledge of proper exercise techniques, patients know when to stop exercise, and motivation to continue exercising is present. It is during the independent phase that the typical personal trainer encounters members of this special population.

Designing safe and effective exercise programs for cardiac patients requires continued communication between the physician and the fitness expert. Fitness professionals must closely follow physician guidelines to reduce the risk for a cardiac event. Individualized exercise programs are crucial for this population given the various forms of CVD and the various complications possible. The following sections present exercise guidelines from the American College of Sports Medicine (ACSM).

ACSM's Guidelines for Outpatient Exercise Programs

As mentioned, patients who have experienced a cardiac event or procedure typically participate in inpatient rehabilitation programs to preserve functional capacity and prepare the body for a safe return to normal activities of daily living. In general, rehabilitative activities should be done two to four times per day for the first 3 days of a hospital stay and then two times per day thereafter. Intensity should be as high as can be tolerated without eliciting symptoms (usually rate of perceived exertion, or RPE ≤ 13 on a 6–20 scale). For those who have experienced a myocardial infarction or who have CHF, heart rate should not exceed 120 beats per minute. Following surgery, heart rate should not exceed 30 beats per minute above resting heart rate. Clinicians advise a work-to-rest ratio of 2 to 1 where duration is kept at 3 to 5 minutes and is followed by a rest period. When activity is easily sustained for 10 to 15 minute segments, gradually increase intensity.[21]

Once they complete the inpatient program and usually within one to two weeks following hospital dismissal, cardiac patients usually begin clinically supervised outpatient rehabilitation. Increased activity is generally safe as long as participants are appropriately assessed, stratified according to risk, educated, and trained. See ACSM's Guidelines for

Exercise Testing and Prescription, 8th edition, Chapter 2 or the AHA's Exercise Standards for Testing and Training: A Statement for Healthcare Professionals for the risk stratification criteria.

- Collect a medical and surgical history. Ensure that a recent physical examination has been performed evaluating the cardiorespiratory and musculoskeletal systems. Review recent cardiovascular tests and procedures, including the most recent stress test. Identify current medications and all CVD risk factors.
- Precede all activity with a 5 to 10 minute low-intensity (<40% VO_{2R}) warm-up. Follow each exercise session with a 5 to 10 minute cooldown. Warm-up and cooldown can include static stretching and range-of-motion exercises.
- Exercise intensity needs to be high enough to induce a training response but low enough to avoid provoking abnormal signs or symptoms (such as angina, dramatic changes in blood pressure, increased frequency of dysrythmias, or other signs of exercise intolerance). Exercise intensity associated with ratings of 11 to 13 (fairly light to somewhat hard) on a 6–20 scale should be the upper limit early in treatment. A rating of 14 to 16 is appropriate with continued training as long as this intensity does not elicit heart dysrhythmias or angina. Alternately, have clients work out at 40% to 60% of heart rate reserve or VO_{2R}. Or prescribe exercise at a heart rate below the ischemic threshold if this value is available.

QUICK REFERENCE
Myocardial ischemia is indicated when angina develops during exertion but subsides with rest.

- Aim for a frequency of 4 to 7 days per week.
- Strive for 20 to 60 minutes of exercise per session. If recovering from a recent cardiac event, begin with 5 to 10 minute sessions and gradually progress by increasing duration by 10% to 20% per week. Clients with very limited exercise capacities should probably participate in several 1 to 10 minute segments throughout the day. Determine duration based on initial fitness level, current symptoms, and physical limitations.
- Include various cardiovascular activities that exercise large muscle groups. Suggest walking, bicycling, stair climbing, elliptical trainers, or rowing machines. Walking is probably the best alternative early in a program since even slow walking has improved heart functioning in unfit subjects.
- Progress slowly. Gradually increasing frequency, duration, and intensity offers a safe means of improving physical conditioning.
- In addition to a regimented exercise program, these clients should increase participation in normal activities of daily living (such as walking upstairs instead of using the elevator; gardening; doing housework; etc.). All of these improve overall functional ability and heart health.

- Resistance training can effectively increase muscular strength and endurance so that cardiac patients are more capable of performing activities of daily living. Strength training is generally safe provided clients have no evidence of congenital heart failure, uncontrolled dysrhythmias, severe valvular disease, uncontrolled hypertension, or unstable symptoms. Low-to-moderate risk patients may typically begin a strength training program 5 weeks after their heart attack or surgery provided they have completed at least 4 weeks of supervised endurance training. Clients who have undergone a transcatheter procedure may begin training two to three weeks postprocedure provided they have completed at least two weeks of supervised endurance training.

  □ Most cardiac patients can safely perform resistance training using elastic bands, 1 to 5 lb hand weights, 1 to 5 lb free weights, cables, or resistance machines.
  □ Train on 2 to 3 days per week with at least 48 hours in between each workout.
  □ Train each of the 8 to 10 major muscle groups. Perform two to four sets of each exercise.
  □ Intensity should be 11 to 13 on the RPE 6–20 scale. Choose a resistance that allows 12 to 15 repetitions (about 30% to 40% 1-RM for upper body exercises and 50% to 60% 1-RM for lower body exercises). Increase loads by 5% increments when appropriate—or by 2 to 5 lb per week for the upper body and 5 to 10 lb per week for the lower body.
  □ Maintain alignment at joints. Control all movements, breathe regularly, and grip bars loosely. Tight gripping can cause dangerous blood pressure increases.
  □ Work large muscle groups first and then proceed to small muscle groups.
  □ Stop exercising if dizziness, SOB, dysrhythmias, or angina develop.

Guidelines for Those With CHF

During CHF, the heart becomes so weak that it cannot adequately eject blood. If the right side of the heart is affected, fluid accumulates in body tissues and results in systemic edema. If the left side of the heart is affected, fluid backs up into the lungs leading to pulmonary edema. Anyone experiencing acute or unstable CHF needs to avoid physical activity and stay in bed. Once their condition stabilizes, however, many may safely participate in exercise. Exercise can minimize symptoms and improve exercise tolerance—factors which improve the overall quality of life. Improvements in exercise tolerance result because of increases in mitochondria, myoglobin, and capillaries in muscle cells—not because of improvements in heart functioning.

- CHF patients must be cleared for exercise from a team of medical professionals and should have an exercise capacity of over three METs.
- CHF patients need longer warm-ups and cooldowns of at least 10 to 15 minutes each.
- Cardiovascular training including walking, stationary cycling, and other nonimpact exercises are appropriate. Resistance training is acceptable as a means of reducing fatigue and dyspnea and improving functional capabilities. CHF patients, however, should avoid isometric contractions and holding their breath since these dangerously increase blood pressure.

- CHF patients need to start slowly. Initial training duration might be 10 to 20 minutes of interval training, which consists of 2 to 6 minute exercise intervals followed by 1 to 2 minutes of rest. Each exercise bout may be increased as tolerance improves.
- CHF patients need to build up to 20 to 40 minutes of activity on 3 to 7 days per week very gradually. Intensity should be based on the results of a treadmill or cycle ergometer test at 40% to 75% VO_{2max}. This test can determine the level at which symptoms begin to appear so that intensity is kept below that level. The rate of perceived exertion is probably a better means of monitoring intensity. CHF patients can safely work out at an RPE of 11 to 14.
- Water intake is important, but these clients should talk to their physicians about the exact amount. In some circumstances, water intake might need to be limited. Consequently, be aware of the environment and avoid exercise in high humidity.

ACSM Guidelines for Those With Hypertension

Hypertensive individuals are stratified into one of the three risk groups based on blood pressure and the presence of other CVD risk factors. Normal blood pressure is defined as a systolic pressure less than 120 mm Hg *and* a diastolic pressure less than 80 mm Hg; prehypertensive is a systolic pressure of 120 to 139 mm Hg *or* a diastolic pressure of 80 to 89 mm Hg; stage 1 hypertension is a systolic pressure of 140 to 159 mm Hg *or* a diastolic pressure of 90 to 99 mm Hg; and stage 2 hypertension is a systolic pressure ≥160 mm Hg *or* a diastolic pressure ≥ 100 mm Hg. Exercise recommendations vary depending upon the group to which the exerciser belongs.

Exercise Testing

- All hypertensive individuals should obtain a medical clearance prior to participating in exercise testing.
- If vigorous exercise (≥60% VO_{2R}) is the goal, clients should have a medically supervised symptom-limited exercise test.
- A symptom-limited graded exercise test might not be needed for asymptomatic clients with blood pressure measures less than 180/110 mm Hg who want to participate in light or very light activity (<40% VO_{2R}). Anyone with stage 2 hypertension should have an exercise test prior to participating in moderate-intensity activity but not for light or very light activity.
- Gradually stop exercise if systolic blood pressure exceeds 250 mm Hg or if diastolic blood pressure exceeds 115 mm Hg.

QUICK REFERENCE
Exercise is contraindicated for those with a resting blood pressure greater than 200/110 mm Hg.[21]

Exercise Prescription

- Begin each exercise session with at least 10 minutes of limbering movements to prepare the cardiovascular system for the upcoming challenge. In addition, end each exercise session with at least 10 minutes of a cooldown. The warm-up and cooldown are slightly longer than with the general population.
- Progression is much slower than with traditional clients.
- Focus on cardiovascular exercise that engages large muscle groups. Exercise aerobically on most, if not all, days of the week at a moderate intensity of 40% to 60% VO_{2R}. Duration should be 30 to 60 minutes of continuous or intermittent exercise during each session.
- In general, resistance training is not recommended as the major mode of exercise since it is associated with drastic acute increases in blood pressure, especially in those who hold their breath during exertion. In conjunction with aerobic training, however, resistance work using lightweights and higher repetitions seems safe for developing muscle strength and endurance. Emphasize normal breathing throughout execution of the exercise. Perform resistance training on 2 to 3 days per week at 60% to 80% of 1-RM. Do at least one set of 8 to 12 repetitions of 8 to 10 different exercises that target major muscle groups.
- If resting systolic pressure exceeds 200 mm Hg, or if resting diastolic pressure exceeds 110 mm Hg, do not exercise. If systolic pressure rises above 220 mm Hg or diastolic pressure rises above 105 mm Hg during activity, stop the activity.
- The effects of hypertensive medications interfere with monitoring techniques. For instance, beta-blockers, designed to lower heart rate and blood pressure, can decrease exercise capacity. They, along with diuretics, can lead to dehydration—a condition that impairs body temperature regulation and causes hypokalemia and dysrhythmias. These two drugs can also cause hypoglycemia in some individuals.
- Medications such as alpha-blockers, vasodilators, and calcium channel blockers make exercising clients prone to postexercise hypotension, hence the slower and longer cooldown recommended earlier.
- Overall, exercise can result in long-term decreases in blood pressure, which might reduce the required doses of medication.

ACSM Guidelines for Those With Peripheral Artery Disease

Peripheral artery disease occurs as plaque builds up in systemic arteries. This impairs blood flow to body tissues, which results in inadequate oxygen delivery, or ischemia, to affected areas. If blood flow is not restored, tissues die. This often necessitates amputations.

- Exercise testing should only be conducted in the presence of a qualified medical team that is prepared to administer emergency care since these patients are at high risk. See ACSM's Guidelines for Exercise Testing and Prescription, 8th Ed. for specific protocols.
- After leaving a cardiac rehabilitation program, those with PAD may begin independent exercise.

- Warm-up for at least 5 to 10 minutes to prepare the heart and muscles for activity. Include limbering movements and mild stretching. Cooldown for at least 5 to 10 minutes to return the heart to a normal resting rate of contraction. The cooldown also ensures adequate return of blood to the heart as the heart rate adjusts to decreasing demands.
- Walking, a low-impact, weight-bearing activity, is the most effective form of exercise for this population. In the long term, it reduces the symptoms associated with claudication (discussed earlier). Cycling is good for warming up, but it should not be the primary mode of exercise.
- Frequency of aerobic training should be three to five times per week at a moderate intensity (40% to 60% VO_{2R}). Aerobic exercise should initially be intermittent in nature because of the pattern of pain associated with claudication. The pain of claudication increases with exertion and decreases with rest; therefore, a training program needs to work around this pattern. In other words, the client should undergo a series of exercise/rest/exercise/rest segments that are compatible with the pattern of pain. The overall goal is to work up to a longer period of continuous exercise without pain (up to 30 to 60 minutes of uninterrupted activity).
- Exercise in cold environments sometimes aggravates intermittent claudication. Increase length of warm-up if exercising in the cold.
- Clients who participate in at least 5 to 6 months of training typically experience improvements. In fact, the duration of pain-free walking and absolute walking both increase significantly.
- Be careful during progression. Symptoms of cardiac stress might appear as intensity levels increase. Watch for these and be prepared to stop the exercise.
- Resistance exercise can be safe for this population. Perform resistance training at least 2 days per week and follow guidelines for the general population.

SAMPLE EXERCISES

For reasons specified earlier, cardiac patients benefit most from cardiovascular training, so the exercise program should emphasize aerobic exercise. The best exercises in which to participate are those that have minimal impact such as walking, bicycling, or rowing; however, individuals should choose activities they enjoy and can tolerate.

Resistance training is safe for most cardiovascular patients. They must maintain neutral alignment, avoid holding their breath, and use relatively light resistance. Elastic resistance bands work well for this group. These clients need a well-rounded exercise routine that includes upper and lower body strengthening that targets the chest, back, shoulders, biceps, triceps, quadriceps femoris group, hamstrings group, and gluteals. Avoid isometric exercises that excessively increase blood pressure. Overall, cardiovascular patients can perform most standard exercises. Just consider other risk factors such as obesity, diabetes, and joint problems when designing a program.

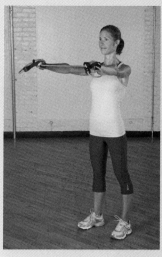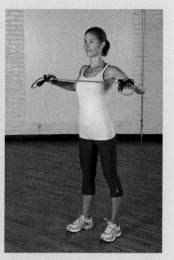

Row Using Elastic Tubing (Fig. 7.7)

Hold one handle of elastic tubing in each hand. Grasp tubing toward the center to create resistance. The farther the hands are apart, the less resistance created. Palms should point down, and arms should be out toward the front at or slightly below shoulder level. Pull both elbows back until hands are at or just in front of chest. Keep elbows below shoulder level. Pause and return to start. Repeat 8 to 10 times. Alternatively, wrap elastic tubing around a sturdy post. Face post and stand with feet shoulder width apart. Hold one handle in each hand while flexing shoulders to front. Point thumbs toward ceiling and pull (or row) the handles toward the abdominals. Pause. Slowly return to starting position and repeat 8 to 12 times. Keep back and neck straight.

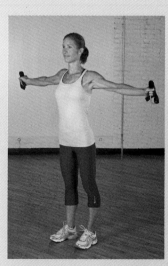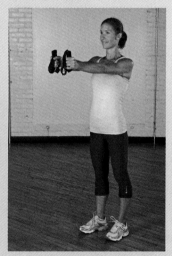

Chest Fly Using Elastic Tubing (Fig. 7.8)

Place tubing around back below shoulder blades. Contract abdominals and maintain neutral spine. Keep shoulders down and relaxed, feet shoulder width apart. Hold one handle in each hand. Grasp tubing toward center to create resistance. Raise arms out to sides, palms facing each other. Pull arms to the front without bending elbows until hands meet at chest level. Pause. Return to start. Repeat 8 to 12 times.

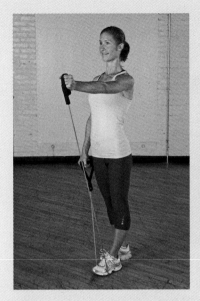
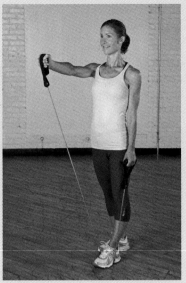

Front Shoulder Raises Using Elastic Tubing (Fig. 7.9)

This exercise works one shoulder at a time. Hold one handle in each hand. Stand on tubing with right foot. Make sure tubing is secure under the foot. Arms should be at side, palms facing inward. With elbow straight but not locked, lift right arm to front while flexing at shoulder. Lift to 70 degrees. Pause. Return to start. Repeat for 8 to 12 repetitions with right arm. Perform on left side.

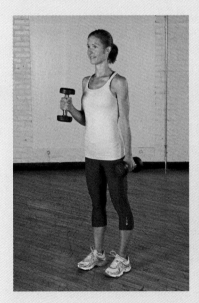
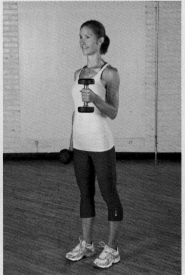

Hammer Curls with Light Dumbbells (Fig. 7.10)

Stand with feet shoulder width apart, abdominals contracted, spine neutral. Hold one light dumbbell in each hand with palms facing each other. Alternate flexing at elbows, one forearm at a time, while palms continue facing each other. Repeat 8 to 12 times.

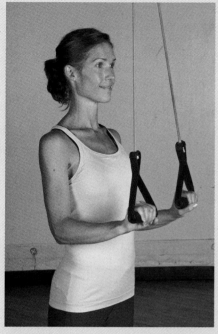
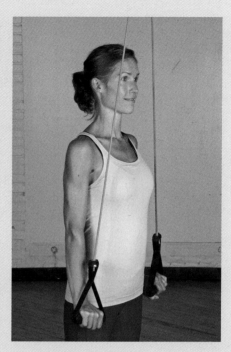

Triceps Press Down (Fig. 7.11)

Attach tube to overhead post or hook. Hold handles, palms facing down, with elbows flexed at 90 degrees. Make sure there is tension in the tube. Extend the elbows while pressing handles down. Pause. Repeat 8 to 12 times.

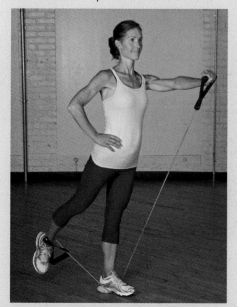

Hip Extension Using Elastic Tubing (Fig. 7.12)

Make a loop with elastic tubing. Place loop securely around right ankle. Hold the other handle in left hand. Step on tubing with left foot. Keep left knee slightly bent. Extend hip. Pause. Then return to start. To make this more difficult, add a left front shoulder raise. Perform 8 to 12 repetitions, and then repeat on left side. Alternatively, attach elastic tubing to a secure object at ankle level. Stand facing the object and loop handle around ankle. Extend at hip while contracting the gluteals and hamstrings. Leg should lift behind the body while knee remains straight. Pause. Slowly return to start. Repeat 8 to 12 times.

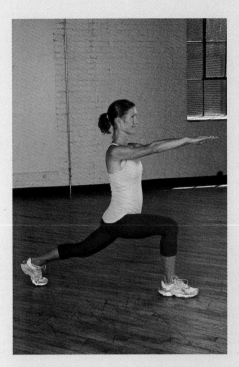

Lunges (Fig. 7.13)

Stand with feet shoulder width apart. Step forward with right leg, landing on heel first. Knee should be at 90 degrees and directly above toes. Slightly drop knee down toward floor (as in lunging). Pause. Pushing through heel, return to starting position. Repeat on left side. Do 8 to 12 repetition on each side.

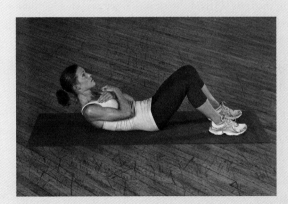

Abdominal Crunches (Fig. 7.14)

Lie on the floor with hands crossed in front of chest. Bend knees and place feet flat on floor. Maintain a neutral spine while contracting abdominals and lifting shoulder blades, head, and neck from floor. Pause. Return to start. Repeat for 8 to 12 repetitions.

QUICK REFERENCE

Safety tips for using elastic tubing:

- Choose resistance based on level of conditioning. Resistance is indicated by the color of the tube. In most cases, resistance increases in the following order: yellow, green, red, blue, and black.
- Make sure tubing is not damaged. Check for tears or cuts.
- Grip handles firmly, but not too tightly.
- Avoid wrapping the tubing around the hands or wrists. Instead, grasp the tubing toward the center to increase resistance.
- Perform tubing exercises on carpeting, wood floors, or grass—not on asphalt or cement because these types of surfaces can damage the tubing.
- Wear comfortable athletic shoes.
- Make sure tubing is secured (either under the feet or to an anchor) before beginning an exercise.

NUTRITIONAL CONSIDERATIONS

Numerous risk factors for CVD relate to dietary intake. Since people have control over what they consume, they can effectively reduce their heart disease risk by making some relatively simple dietary changes. This holds true for those who are currently free from heart disease as well as those with preexisting heart disease.

DIET AND THE RISK FOR CVD

Substantial evidence suggests that certain dietary practices reduce the risk of developing CVD.[49-55] According to the U.S. Food and Drug Administration, Americans can minimize their risk by reducing their intake of *saturated fat, trans fat, cholesterol, salt*, and *total kilocalories*, while increasing their intake of fiber, monounsaturated fats, omega-3 fatty acids, fruits, and vegetables.

Saturated Fats and Trans Fats

Saturated fat increases the risk for heart disease because it elevates blood LDL levels. In fact, the risk for heart disease increases by 2% for every 1% increase in dietary saturated fat intake. To take this one step further, people can actually experience a 2% *reduction in risk* for every 1% reduction in dietary saturated fat intake. The major sources of saturated in the diet include fatty meats, whole fat dairy products, and tropical oils (palm oil, palm kernel oil, and coconut oil). Simply choosing leaner cuts of meat, such as rounds and loins; switching from whole-fat dairy products to low-or-no fat dairy products; and avoiding "hidden" fats can dramatically reduce total saturated fat intake. Hidden fats are the fats found in marbled meats, cheese, and even avocados (though the fat in avocados is the healthier monounsaturated fat).

Trans fats also increase CVD risk by increasing LDL levels, so people should limit trans fat intake as well. Moreover, a high intake of trans fats seems to lower HDL levels, further contributing to a poor blood lipid profile. Trans fats are usually created during the hydrogenation of unsaturated fatty acids. Hydrogenation is a process that alters the structure of unsaturated fatty acids. More specifically, it adds hydrogen atoms to unsaturated fats to make them more like saturated fats. Why do manufacturers do this? First of all, hydrogenated fats do not spoil as quickly as unsaturated fats, so manufacturers can prolong shelf life through hydrogenation. Secondly, hydrogenation can convert liquid vegetable oils into spreadable margarines. The major problem with trans fats is that the body treats them as if they were saturated fats; therefore, they have the same deleterious effects on the body as their saturated counterparts. Trans fats are found abundantly in products such as crackers, doughnuts, cookies, and fried foods. For heart health, limit the intake of trans fats and saturated fats to less than 10% of total daily kilocalories.

Cholesterol

Generally speaking, people should limit their dietary intake to no more than 300 mg of *cholesterol* per day. This is more important to those who are sensitive to dietary cholesterol; however, not everyone responds to changes in cholesterol intake. Be aware that the liver makes 800 to 1,500 mg of cholesterol per day, so genetics play a much more significant role in total cholesterol levels than diet. Dietary cholesterol is only found in animal-based products; it is not found in plant-based products. Eggs, meat, chicken, and certain fish contain large amount of cholesterol and should be limited. About a third of the total cholesterol found in the American diet is contributed by eggs.

Salt

About 60% of Americans are salt-sensitive, which simply means that their blood pressure rises significantly with an increased intake of *salt* (sodium chloride). These individuals need to be especially careful about their sodium chloride intake. Salt sensitivity is likely in those who have a family history of hypertension, those with kidney disease or diabetes, those over the age of 50, those who are obese, and those of African-American descent. Even generally healthy individuals who have normal blood pressures, however, should limit their intake of salt because a salt-restricted diet seems to reduce an already low blood pressure. A major source of salt is processed foods, which are loaded with salt. Salt also occurs naturally in many foods, and it is a component of some medications. According to the AHA and the 2005 Dietary Guidelines, people should limit *salt* intake to no more than 2,300 mg per day; this is the equivalent of about 1 tsp of table salt. To achieve this goal, choose fresh, frozen, and canned foods without added salt; limit the intake of salty snacks; select low salt broths, cheeses, and canned products; and use spices other than salt for seasoning. The "Adequate Intake" suggested by the Dietary Reference Intake Committee says that lower daily intakes meet body requirements. They recommend the following: 1,500 mg per day for 19 to 50 year olds; 1,300 mg per day for 51 to 70 year olds; and 1,200 mg per day for those over 70 years old. Again, the upper limit is 2,300 mg per day. Salt-sensitive individuals who habitually consume amounts in excess of this tend to develop hypertension. Those diagnosed with hypertension might need to severely limit intake. See the section below about the DASH diet for further information.

Energy Intake

Moderate *energy intake* often results in weight loss, and weight loss decreases the risk for CVD. Remember that excess weight, particularly weight stored in the abdominal area, is an independent risk factor for CVD because it increases blood pressure, elevates triglycerides, reduces HDL levels, and enhances insulin resistance. It also influences blood clotting and can promote atherosclerosis. Losing weight, therefore, can decrease risk for CVD. In addition to decreasing the heart's workload and blood pressure, weight loss improves circulation, reduces the risk for diabetes, and lowers LDL and triglyceride levels. All of these factors improve the CVD risk profile.

Fiber

As mentioned, an increased intake of *fiber, monounsaturated fats, omega-3 fatty acids*, and *fruits* and *vegetables* decreases the risk for CVD. Diets high in *fiber*, especially those rich in whole grains, are associated with a reduced risk for heart disease and stroke. Researchers are uncertain whether this benefit derives from the fiber itself or whether it occurs because high fiber diets also tend to be low in saturated fat and cholesterol. Several studies, however, have shown that high fiber diets actually decrease heart disease risk independent of fat intake. Perhaps high fiber diets are healthy because they emphasize consuming fruits and vegetables, which are high in phytochemicals, components also associated with a reduced risk for heart disease. Indeed, researchers are studying the specific effects of certain phytochemicals on heart disease development and progression, and many of these phytochemicals hold promise for reducing overall CVD risk. Overall, research confirms the risk-reducing effect of soluble fibers, such as those found in legumes, oats, and barley. In the digestive tract, these fibers form a gel that binds with dietary cholesterol and prevents absorption. They also trap cholesterol released in bile and prevent it from being reabsorbed. In this way, soluble fibers directly reduce the amount of cholesterol that enters the blood. Overall, people should strive for 20 to 35 g of fiber per day.

Monounsaturated Fats

Monounsaturated fats, such as those found in olive oil, canola oil, peanuts, and avocados, actually decrease the risk for CVD. Monounsaturated fats work by lowering total cholesterol and LDL levels without lowering HDL levels; they decrease triglycerides; they prevent oxidation of LDL (which can reduce plaque buildup on arterial walls); they provide heart healthy phytochemicals; and they seem to lower blood pressure. People should, therefore, *replace* saturated and trans fats with monounsaturated fats.

Monounsaturated fats, like all fats, contain 9 kcal per gram, so people need to be careful if trying to lose or maintain weight. The key for solving this is to *replace* other fats with monounsaturated fats, not supplement other fats with monounsaturated fats. Overall, people should strive to limit fat intake to 20% to 35% of total kilocalorie intake.

Omega-3 Fatty Acids

Omega-3 fatty acids appear to protect against heart disease by reducing blood triglyceride levels, preventing blood clotting, protecting against dysrhythmias, lowering blood pressure, and limiting systemic inflammation, factors that not only help prevent heart disease, but also benefit those who have already experienced a heart attack. Consequently, everyone should increase their intake of omega-3 fatty acids by consuming more fish, flaxseeds, flaxseed oil, and nuts (particularly walnuts). Most experts suggest increasing *dietary sources* of omega-3 fatty acids and avoiding *fish oil supplements* since not all studies show positive results from fish oil supplements. In addition, fish oil supplements often contain dangerous levels of environmental contaminants, which can cause other problems. Unfortunately, research shows that it takes abnormally large doses of fish oil supplements—at least 3,000 to 4,000 mg per day—for maximal effect. Sadly, this amount can cause gastrointestinal tract problems and excessive bleeding.[56,57] Overall, the AHA recommends consuming two 3-oz servings of fatty fish per week to obtain an adequate intake of omega-3 fatty acids. Herring, mackerel, salmon, and tuna are particularly good sources. The Dietary Reference Intake Committee suggests 1.6 g per day for men and 1.1 g per day for women.

Fruits and Vegetables

Fruits and *vegetables* contain several substances thought to combat heart disease. They are packed with antioxidant vitamins and minerals including vitamin C, beta carotene, and selenium. They contain phytochemicals, many of which act as antioxidants as well. In addition, they contain a healthy dose of fiber and large amounts of water. Their fiber content often makes them more satiating than low fiber alternatives, so including them in the diet might decrease total kilocalorie intake, which in turn promotes weight loss or weight maintenance in those striving to control their weight.

ADDITIONAL DIETARY CONSIDERATIONS

Soy

An increased intake of plant sterols and soy products also reduces the risk for CVD. Plant sterols, extracted from soybeans, are sometimes added to products such as margarine and cheese because they seem to lower blood LDL and total cholesterol levels. They do this by binding with cholesterol, from both dietary sources as well as bile, in the small intestine and preventing their absorption. According to the National Cholesterol Education Program, 2 g of plant sterols per day can lower LDL levels by 6% to 15%. This occurs without negatively affecting HDL levels! A daily intake of 25 g seems to be the minimal amount necessary to exert this effect.

Alcohol

For years, *moderate* alcohol consumption has been associated with a reduced risk for heart disease; however, an alcohol intake exceeding 1 drink per day for the average woman and 2 drinks per day for the average man actually increases risk for death.

(A drink is defined as 12 oz of beer, 5 oz of wine, or 1½ oz of 80-proof liquor.) Interestingly, the benefits of alcohol consumption only occur in men over 45 years old and women over 55 years old; alcohol has no beneficial effect on younger drinkers. How does alcohol exert its effects? It lowers total blood cholesterol levels, increases HDL, and minimizes inflammation, blood clotting, and atherosclerosis, factors that reduce the risk for heart disease.

Folate, Vitamin B$_{12}$, and Vitamin B$_6$

An earlier section addressed the relationship between elevated homocysteine levels and heart disease and emphasized that those with abnormally high homocysteine levels are at increased risk. As mentioned, high homocysteine levels are related to low intakes of folate, vitamin B$_{12}$, and vitamin B$_6$, so it would be easy to assume that supplements of these vitamins could reduce risk by decreasing blood homocysteine levels. Supplements of these vitamins do indeed decrease homocysteine, but studies have not confirmed that this translates into a reduced risk for CVD.

Antioxidants

Many people take antioxidant supplements to limit free radical damage. Since free radicals are oxidants, it sounds reasonable that *anti*oxidants can disable them. In fact, antioxidants work wonders by limiting free radical formation, interfering with their ability to destroy cell structures, and repairing oxidative damage. Produced from normal metabolic processes, contact with pollutants, and exposure to UV radiation, free radicals oxidize LDL and its cholesterol thereby contributing significantly to plaque buildup in arterial walls. Thus, free radicals are associated with an increased risk for heart disease.

Epidemiological studies show that people who consume diets rich in antioxidants, including vitamin C, vitamin E, beta carotene, and selenium, seem to have some protection against heart disease. Therefore, researchers are enthusiastically investigating the effects of antioxidant supplements. Currently, however, evidence on the efficacy and safety of antioxidant megadoses is conflicting, so there are no general recommendations for using dietary supplements. General dietary recommendations for antioxidant nutrients are listed in Table 7.12.

TABLE 7-12	RECOMMENDED INTAKE OF SELECTED ANTIOXIDANTS	
Antioxidant	**Recommended Intake**	**Upper Level**
Vitamin C	Men: 90 mg/day	2,000 mg/day
	Women: 75 mg/day	
	Smokers: +35 mg/day	
Vitamin E	Adults: 15 mg/day	1,000 mg/day
Selenium	Adults: 55 μg/day	400 μg/day

THERAPEUTIC LIFESTYLE CHANGES FROM THE NATIONAL CHOLESTEROL EDUCATION PROGRAM

The National Cholesterol Education Program (NCEP), developed by The National Heart, Lung, and Blood Institute (NHLBI), was established to reduce coronary artery disease incidence and prevalence by addressing blood cholesterol levels. Accordingly, "the NCEP aims to raise awareness and understanding [among professionals and the general public] about high blood cholesterol as a risk factor for CHD and the benefits of lowering cholesterol levels as a means of preventing CHD." In an effort to do this, they developed a set of guidelines called "Therapeutic Lifestyle Changes" (TLC) that focuses on diet, physical activity, and weight management. By strictly adhering to these guidelines, participants can expect significant progress by the end of 6 weeks. Essentially, TLC makes the following suggestions:

- Limit saturated fat intake to less than 7% of total daily kilocalories and total fat intake to 25% to 35% of total daily kilocalories (for an 8% to 10% drop in blood cholesterol)
- Consume less than 200 mg of cholesterol per day (for a 3% to 5% drop in blood cholesterol)
- Lose weight if necessary (a 10-lb weight-loss results in a 5% to 8% drop in blood cholesterol)
- Add 5 to 10 g of soluble fiber to the diet (for a 3% to 5% drop in blood cholesterol)
- Add 2 g of plant sterols to the daily diet (for a 5% to 15% drop in blood cholesterol)
- In addition, TLC recommendations suggest accumulating at least 30 minutes of moderate-intensity physical activity each day. This promotes weight-loss and maintenance and can also increase HDL levels.

THE DASH DIET (DIETARY APPROACHES TO STOP HYPERTENSION)

According to the National Heart, Lung, and Blood Institute, the DASH diet significantly lowers blood pressure in those with hypertension and prehypertension. It essentially consists of two diet plans: one limits sodium intake to 1,500 mg per day, while the other limits sodium intake to 2,300 mg per day. The 1,500 mg per day diet is associated with dramatic reductions in blood pressure and is recommended by the Institute of Medicine for everyone.

QUICK REFERENCE
Currently, the average sodium intake is 4,200 mg per day for men and 3,300 mg per day for women—far above the recommended amount of 1,500 mg per day.

Medical and health care professionals began recommending the DASH diet after seeing the results of two landmark studies that indicated that diets low in saturated fat, cholesterol, and total fat and high in fruits, vegetables, and fat-free or low-fat milk products significantly lowered resting blood pressure. The diet also included liberal intakes of whole grain products, fish, poultry, and nuts. It limited intake of red meats, desserts, added sugars, sugar-containing beverages, saturated fats, and cholesterol. Overall, compared to the

TABLE 7-13	DASH DIET RECOMMENDATIONS*	
Total fat	27% of kilocalories	
Saturated fat	6% of kilocalories	
Protein	18% of kilocalories	
Carbohydrates	55% of kilocalories	
Cholesterol	150 mg	
Sodium	2,300 mg (limiting intake to 1,500 mg has an even greater effect on blood pressure)	
Potassium	4,700 mg	
Calcium	1,250 mg	
Magnesium	500 mg	
Fiber	30 g	

*Based on a daily intake of 2,100 kcal.

TABLE 7-14	CONTROLLING HIGH BLOOD PRESSURE

- Achieve and maintain a healthy weight
- Participate in daily moderate-intensity physical activity
- Consume healthy foods low in sodium
- Drink alcohol in moderation, if at all
- Take prescribed medications for hypertension as directed by a physician

Source: National Heart, Lung, and Blood Institute. www.nhlbi.nih.gov.

typical American diet, the DASH diet is rich in potassium, magnesium, calcium, and fiber. Researchers noticed a slight decrease in blood pressure within 2 weeks, but by the end of just 8 weeks, they saw an average drop of 11.4 mm Hg in systolic blood pressure![10,58] Table 7.13 provides general recommendations based on a 2,100 kcal diet.

For additional information and more specific suggestions on how to follow the DASH diet, please visit the NHBLI Web site at www.nhlbi.nih.gov/health/public/heart/hbp/dash/new. In addition, see Table 7.14 for suggestions on controlling high blood pressure.

SUMMARY

Exercise for many high-risk cardiovascular patients was once discouraged. In fact, treatment often involved complete bed rest with minimal activity. Current research, however, shows that exercise provides substantial benefits for this population, just as it does for other populations, provided the patient is stable and symptoms are controlled; however, because the heart and/or blood vessels are already compromised, exercise can be risky. Essentially, exercise places a greater demand on the heart and blood vessels, which could possibly promote a cardiac event. That risk can be minimized by following certain guidelines provided by the patient's physician, the AHA, ACSM, and the ACC. In fact, the benefits of exercise far outweigh the risks when safety precautions are followed. Improved circulation, minimized disease-related symptoms, lowered blood pressure, improved survival rates, and decreased number of hospital visits enhance quality of life and self-esteem. Couple a safe exercise regimen with a healthy diet and the cardiac patient can actively reduce the risk of future complications—or at least slow the rate of deterioration.

CASE STUDY

A 68-year-old client asks you to train him after he just finished a 3-month cardiac rehabilitation program. Although he walked 3 miles per day and strength trained two times per week until just a few months ago, he still experienced a heart attack. Fortunately, his physician referred him to a cardiac rehabilitation program soon after his heart attack. Since then, he has felt much better and stronger, but he would like more guidance. He is currently taking a blood thinner.

■ How would you approach this situation?

■ What type of exercise testing and prescription would you recommend?

■ Would you offer any advice on his diet?

THINKING CRITICALLY

1. Explain the difference between atherosclerosis and arteriosclerosis.
2. Discuss the major function(s) of the cardiovascular system. Explain how its three components work together to accomplish these tasks.
3. What is a risk factor? Explain the difference between a modifiable risk factor and a nonmodifiable risk factor. What cardiovascular risk factors are nonmodifiable?
4. List and explain four modifiable risk factors for CVD.
5. What condition causes most of the common forms of CVD? Explain how it develops and increases risk.
6. How does ischemia promote a heart attack or stroke?
7. List and explain four benefits of exercise in this population.
8. Why is it important to know what heart medications a client is taking?
9. Explain how diet affects heart health.
10. Discuss the role of antioxidants in the prevention of heart disease.

REFERENCES

1. Schnyder G. Homocysteine-lowering therapy with folic acid, vitamin B_{12}, and vitamin B_6 on clinical outcome after percutaneous coronary intervention. The Swiss Heart Study: a randomized controlled trial. JAMA 2002;288:973–979.

2. Tanne D. Prospective study of serum homocysteine and risk of ischemic stroke among patients with preexisting coronary heart disease. Stroke 2003; 34:632–636.

3. Verhoef P. Plasma total homocysteine, B vitamins, and risk of coronary atherosclerosis. Arterioscler Thromb Vasc Biol 1997;17:989–995.

4. Ridker P, Hennekens C, Buring J, et al. C-Reactive protein and other markers of inflammation in the prediction of cardiovascular disease in women. N Engl J Med 2000;342(12):836–843.

5. Ernst E. Fibrinogen as a cardiovascular risk factor—interrelationship with infections and inflammation. Eur Heart J 1993;14(K):82–87.

6. Stec J, Silbershatz H, Tofler G, et al. Association of fibrinogen with cardiovascular risk factors and cardiovascular disease in the Framingham offspring population. Circulation 2000;102:1634.

7. Lauer M. Inflammation and infection in coronary artery disease. Preventive Cardiology: Strategies for the Prevention and Treatment of Coronary Artery Disease. Totowa, NJ: Human Press. 2001: 47–66.

8. American Heart Association. www.americanheart.org

9. Laughlin MH, Newcomer SC, Bender SB. Importance of hemodynamic forces as signals for exercise-induced changes in endothelial cell phenotype. J Appl Physiol 2008;104:588–600.

10. National Heart, Lung, and Blood Institute. www.nhlbi.nih.gov

11. Opie L, Commerford P, Gersh B. Controversies in stable coronary artery disease. Lancet 2006;367: 69–78.

12. Vita JA, Keaney JF. Endothelial function: a barometer for cardiovascular risk? Circulation 2002; 106:640–642.

13. Libby P. Changing concepts of atherogenesis. J Int Med 2000;247:349–358.

14. Texas Heart Institute Heart Information Center. www.texasheartinstitute.org

15. Gatti J. Exercise-based rehabilitation for coronary heart disease. Am Fam Physician 2004;70(3):485–486.

16. Cobb S, Brown D, Davis L. Effective interventions for lifestyle change after myocardial infarction or coronary artery revascularization. J Am Acad Nurse Pract 2006;18:31–39.

17. Reis S, Holubkov R, Smith J. Coronary microvascular dysfunction is highly prevalent in women with chest pain in the absence of coronary artery disease: results from the NHLBI WISE Study. Am Heart J 2001;141(5):735–741.

18. Harvard Women's Health Watch. New view of heart disease in women. February 2007. www.health.harvard.edu/newsweek/New-view-of-heart-disease-in-women.htm

19. Camici P, Crea F. Coronary microvascular dysfunction. N Engl J Med 2007;356:830–840.

20. Arroyo-Espliguero R, Mollichelli N, et al. Chronic inflammation and increased arterial stiffness in patients with cardiac syndrome X. Eur Heart J 2003;24(22):2006–2011.

21. American College of Sports Medicine. ACSM's Guidelines for Exercise Testing and Prescription. 8th Ed. Philadelphia: Lippincott Williams & Wilkins, 2010:229–231.

22. American Stroke Association. www.american-stroke.org

23. Nedeltchev K, der Mar T, Georgiadis D, et al. Ischemic stroke in young adults: predictors of outcome and recurrence. J Neurol Neurosurg Psychiatry 2005;76:191–195.

24. National Institute of Neurological Disorders and Stroke. www.ninds.nih.gov

25. Oka R, Altman M, Giacomini J, et al. Exercise patterns and cardiovascular fitness of patients with peripheral arterial disease. J Vasc Nurs 2004;22(4): 109–114.

26. Leng G, Fowler B, Ernst E. Exercise for intermittent claudication. The Cochrane Library, Issue 1. 2004. Available at: http://212.49.218.202/abstracts; ab000990.htm

27. Federman D, Bravata D, Kirsner R. Peripheral artery disease: a systemic disease extending beyond the affected extremity. Geriatrics 2004; 59(4): 26–36.

28. Myers J. Exercise and cardiovascular health. Circulation 2003;107:e2.

29. Tsai J, Yang H, Wang W, et al. The beneficial effect of regular endurance exercise training on blood pressure and quality of life in patients with hypertension. Clin Exp Hypertens 2004;36(3):255–265.

30. Lifefitness. www.us.commercial.lifefitness.com

31. Meyer K, Foster C. Nontraditional exercise training for patients with cardiovascular disease. Am J Med Sci 2004;March/April:78–81.

32. Meyer K. Resistance exercise in chronic heart failure—landmark studies and implications for practice. Clin Invest Med 2006;29(3):166–169.

33. Albert C, Mittleman M, Chae C, et al. Triggering of sudden death from cardiac causes by vigorous exertion. N Engl J Med 2000;343:1355–1361.

34. Thompson P, Buchner D, Pina IL, et al. Exercise and physical activity in the prevention and treatment of atherosclerotic cardiovascular disease: a statement from the Council on Clinical Cardiology (Subcommittee on Exercise, Rehabilitation,

and Prevention) and the Council on Nutrition, Physical Activity, and Metabolism (Subcommittee on Physical Activity). Circulation 2003;107:3109–3116.

35. Thompson P, Franklin B, Balady G, et al. Exercise and acute cardiovascular events. Circulation 2007; 115:2358–2368.

36. American Diabetes Association. www.diabetes.org

37. Reybrouck T. Gas exchange kinetics in patients with cardiovascular disease. Chest 2000;118:285–286.

38. Hambrecht R, Walther C, Mobius-Winkler S, et al. Percutaneous coronary angioplasty compared with exercise training in patients with stable coronary artery disease: a randomized trial. Circulation 2004;109:1371–1378.

39. Al-Khalili F, Janszky I, Andersson A, et al. Physical activity and exercise performance predict long-term prognosis in middle-aged women surviving acute coronary syndrome. J Int Med 2006;261:178–187.

40. Fletcher G, Balady F, Amsterdam E, et al. American Heart Association exercise standards for testing and training: a statement for healthcare professionals. Circulation 2001;104:1694–1740.

41. Miller T. Exercise and its role in the prevention and rehabilitation of cardiovascular disease. Ann Behav Med 1997;3:220–229.

42. Fagard R. Exercise characteristics and the blood pressure response to dynamic physical training. Med Sci Sports Exerc 2001;33:S484–S492.

43. National Cholesterol Education Program. www.nhlbi.nih.gov/about/ncep/

44. Herd A. Clinical Cardiac Rehabilitation: A Cardiologist's Guide: Book Review. Circulation 2000; 102:e48.

45. Fletcher B, Gulanic M, Braun L. Physical activity and exercise for elders with cardiovascular disease. Medsurg Nurs 2005;14(2):101–110.

46. Jolliffe J, Rees K, Taylor R, et al. Exercise-based rehabilitation for coronary heart disease. Cochrane Database Syst Rev 2001;1:CD001800.

47. Gibbons RJ, Balady GJ, Bricker JT, et al. ACC/AHA 2002 guideline update for exercise testing: a report of the American College of Cardiology/American Heart Association Task Force on Practice Guidelines (Committee on Exercise Testing). 2002. American College of Cardiology. www.acc.org/clinical/guidelines/exercise/dirIndex.htm

48. American College of Cardiology. www.acc.org

49. Fung T, Chiuve S, McCullough M, et al. Adherence to a Dash-style Diet and risk of coronary heart disease and stroke in women. Circulation 2007; 116:II 519.

50. He K, Song Y, Daviglus M, et al. Accumulated evidence on fish consumption and coronary heart disease mortality: a meta-analysis of cohort studies. Circulation 2004;109:2705–2711.

51. Kromhout D, Menotti A, Kesteloot H, Sans S. Prevention of coronary heart disease by diet and lifestyle: evidence from prospective cross-cultural, cohort, and intervention studies. Circulation 2002;105:893–898.

52. Lichtenstein A, Appel L, Brands M, et al. Diet and lifestyle recommendations revision 2006: a scientific statement from the American Heart Association Nutrition Committee. Circulation 2006;114: 82–96.

53. Mozaffarian D, Ascherio A, Hu F, et al. Interplay between different polyunsaturated fatty acids and risk of coronary heart disease in men. Circulation 2005;111:157–164.

54. Pietinen P, Rimm E, Korhonen P, et al. Intake of dietary fiber and risk of coronary heart disease in a cohort of Finnish men: the alpha-tocopherol, beta-carotene cancer prevention study. Circulation 1996;94:2720–2727.

55. Robertson RM, Smaha L. Can a Mediterranean-style diet reduce heart disease? Circulation 2001;103:1821–1822.

56. Eritsland J. Safety considerations of polyunsaturated fatty acids. Am J Clin Nutr 2000;71:197S–201S.

57. Hendler S, Rorvik D. PDR for Nutritional Supplements. USA: Medical Economics Company/Thomson Healthcare, 2001:148–150.

58. Centers for Disease Control and Prevention. www.cdc.gov

SUGGESTED READINGS

Aronow W, Fleg J, eds. Cardiovascular Disease in the Elderly. 3rd Ed. NY: Marcel Dekker. 2004.

American Heart Association. www.aha.com

Skinner J. Exercise Testing and Exercise Prescription for Special Cases. 3rd Ed. Baltimore: Lippincott Williams & Wilkins, 2005.

Stein R. Outliving Heart Disease. The 10 New Rules for Prevention and Treatment. NY: Newmarket Press, 2006.

Woolf-May K. Exercise Prescription: Physiological Foundations. UK: Churchill Livingstone Elsevier, 2006.

EXERCISE FOR THOSE WITH DISORDERS OF THE SKELETAL SYSTEM

8

The skeletal system is composed of bones, joints, cartilage, and ligaments. It offers structural support to the body; provides attachment points for muscles and tendons; protects internal organs; acts as a lever system in movement; serves as a calcium reservoir; and houses red bone marrow, the site of blood cell formation. Numerous factors hasten the deterioration of this system and promote chronic disorders. Some of the more common bone and joint disorders include osteoporosis, osteoarthritis, and rheumatoid arthritis.

OSTEOPOROSIS

Osteoporosis results as bone tissue deteriorates and loses mass. It currently affects an estimated 10 million Americans, 80% of whom are women. An additional 34 million people have osteopenia, a condition of lower-than-normal bone mass that is not quite low enough to be classified as osteoporosis. Those with osteopenia have a high risk of developing osteoporosis.

Although risk for development usually increases with age, osteoporosis can affect anyone. White women and women of Asian descent tend to have the greatest risk, but it is beginning to become more common in other ethnic groups as well, particularly Hispanic women. Osteoporosis is dangerous because it results in weak, fragile bones that break easily. Consequently, it is responsible for several debilitating fractures, particularly in seniors. Fractures tend to occur in the pelvic (hip) bones, vertebrae (spine), and wrist, but any bone is susceptible. According to the National Osteoporosis Foundation, 50% of all women and 25% of all men over the age of 50 can expect to have an osteoporosis-related fracture during their lifetimes. In fact, in 2005, there were 2 million osteoporosis-related fractures, which were associated with a cost of $19 billion. By the year 2025, the total number of fractures is expected to climb to 3 million; imagine the associated costs![1]

Hip fracture is one of the most devastating and debilitating consequences of osteoporosis. Women tend to have a two to three times greater risk for hip fracture than men. In addition, their risk for a second hip fracture is four times greater. Unfortunately, 24% of those who suffer from hip fractures die within one year, with many more requiring long-term care following treatment.[1]

ARTHRITIS

The word "arthritis" literally means inflammation at a joint. Statistics from the Centers for Disease Control indicate that 46.4 million American adults have doctor-diagnosed arthritis, and out of this total an estimated 18.9 million experience arthritis-related limited activity. By the year 2030, arthritis is expected to affect over 67 million Americans.

More than 100 different forms of arthritis exist, but the most common type is osteoarthritis. According to the Arthritis Foundation, osteoarthritis affects over 27 million people in the United States alone. Also known as "wear and tear" arthritis or "degenerative arthritis," osteoarthritis develops as the **articular cartilage** thins after years of repeated use. The deterioration of this layer increases friction between the two bones that form the joint, which results in pain and limited range of motion. Osteoarthritis can affect any joint including the hands, feet, spine, hips, and knees.

Rheumatoid arthritis is an **autoimmune disease** that affects approximately 2 million people in the United States.[2] It is three times more common in women than in men, and although it can develop at any age, its onset is typically between the ages of 40 and 60. In rheumatoid arthritis, the immune system attacks the **synovial membrane** at joints. As the synovial membrane degenerates, it begins producing a grainy fluid that destroys the joint cartilage and interferes with joint movements. In a sense, the grainy synovial fluid acts like a piece of sandpaper that wears away the cartilage at the ends of the bones. Over time, bone deteriorates along with the cartilage. Rheumatoid arthritis often affects small joints bilaterally such as those of the hands and wrists. This makes activities of daily living difficult to perform. The resulting limited movement then causes muscle atrophy, joint deformity, and possibly complete loss of function.

Undiagnosed and untreated rheumatoid arthritis affects other body organs (such as the heart and lungs), so it can have widespread effects. According to the Arthritis Foundation, early diagnosis and aggressive treatment are, therefore, necessary to limit damage and improve the likelihood of living a productive life.

ANATOMICAL AND PHYSIOLOGICAL CHANGES IN THE SKELETAL SYSTEM

To understand the impact of osteoporosis, osteoarthritis, and rheumatoid arthritis on the skeletal system, consider the structure of bones and joints.

BONE TISSUE

Bone is actually not completely solid. In fact, it contains numerous spaces and is classified as either compact bone or spongy bone depending upon the amount of space inside (Fig. 8.1). Compact bone contains a relatively small amount of space compared to spongy bone. Compact bone constitutes 80% of total skeletal mass and is the major type of bone tissue in the femur, tibia, humerus, radius, and other long bones of the appendicular skeleton. It also forms the outermost layer of all bones. Spongy bone makes up the remaining 20% of total skeletal mass and is the predominant type of bone tissue in the axial skeleton, which includes the head, neck, and torso. It is called "spongy" because it has relatively large spaces surrounding **trabeculae**. The greater amount of space in spongy bone makes it lighter in weight than compact bone.

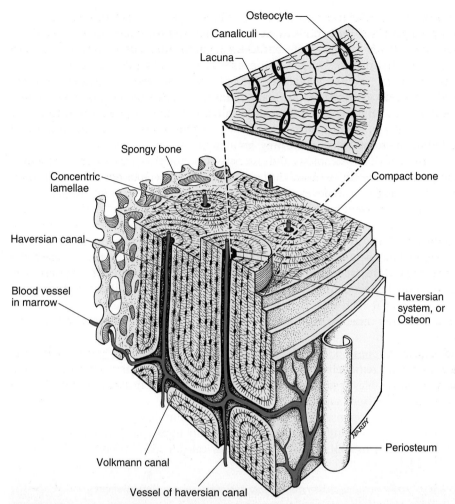

FIGURE 8.1 ■ Structure of bone. (From Stedman's Medical Dictionary. 27th Ed. Baltimore: Lippincott Williams & Wilkins, 2000.)

Articular cartilage—the hyaline cartilage layer that covers the ends of bones in a joint. It reduces friction during joint movements and provides shock absorption during impact.

Autoimmune disease—a disease that results when the immune system attacks body cells.

Synovial membrane—a connective tissue membrane that lines the joint capsule at moveable joints. It produces synovial fluid, nourishes local cartilage, and removes cellular debris.

Trabeculae—branches of bone tissue surrounded by relatively large cavities containing red bone marrow. The structural foundation of spongy bone.

Bone Remodeling

Bone is a dynamic tissue that undergoes a continual process of remodeling that replaces old bone tissue with new bone tissue. To facilitate remodeling, bone has a huge network of blood vessels that delivers oxygen and nutrients to its cells, while it removes waste products from them. The two major types of cells involved with remodeling are osteoblasts and osteoclasts. **Osteoblasts** are bone-builders that deposit bone tissue in response to demands placed on bone. Osteoblasts also initiate calcification, or the hardening of bone, as mineral salts are deposited. **Osteoclasts** are bone-destroyers that attack and break down bone tissue to clear the way for new bone growth. Obviously, a balance between the activities of osteoblasts and osteoclasts is crucial if bone mass is to remain stable. Overall, most spongy bones in the body are completely replaced every 3 to 4 years; whereas, it takes nearly 10 years to replace most compact bone. The rate of remodeling, however, varies in different bones.

Osteoclast activity allows bone to serve as a calcium reservoir that ensures appropriate blood calcium levels. Thus, if dietary calcium intake is inadequate and blood calcium levels drop, the body actually sacrifices bone tissue to replenish it. This is because other than serving as an integral component of bone tissue, calcium is necessary for nerve cell functioning, muscle fiber contraction, and blood clotting, processes that are much more important to survival than maintaining bone structure. Consequently, it is imperative that people regularly consume foods high in calcium to preserve bone tissue.

The Effects of Hormones on Bone Remodeling. Numerous hormones influence the rate and extent of bone remodeling (Table 8.1). Calcitonin and parathyroid hormone, for example, are responsible for maintaining blood calcium levels, but as they work to ensure an adequate blood calcium supply, they indirectly affect bone density. The thyroid gland releases calcitonin in response to an elevated blood calcium level that results from consuming foods high in calcium. Among its various functions, calcitonin inhibits osteoclasts and stimulates osteoblasts, which increases calcium deposition in bone. When

TABLE 8-1 HORMONES THAT INFLUENCE BONE REMODELING

Hormone	Action
Estrogen and testosterone	Inhibit apoptosis of osteoblasts and stimulate osteoblast activity thus increasing calcium deposition in bone; enhance apoptosis of osteoclasts and thereby inhibit osteoclast activity
Human Growth Hormone	Stimulates the lengthening of long bones by acting on the epiphyseal plate
Thyroxine	Stimulates release of additional hGH from pituitary gland, so it indirectly promotes bone lengthening. Nevertheless, since thyroxine stimulates epiphyseal plate ossification, it ultimately halts growth in length
Calcitonin and Parathyroid hormone	Primary function is to maintain normal blood calcium levels. Indirect effect on bone tissue. Calcitonin is released when blood calcium levels increase. Among its numerous functions, calcitonin stimulates osteoblasts. Parathyroid hormone is released when blood calcium decreases. Among its various functions, it stimulates osteoclasts and inhibits osteoblasts.

blood calcium levels drop, the parathyroid gland releases parathyroid hormone to stimulate osteoclasts and inhibit osteoblasts. Parathyroid hormone also slows down the loss of calcium via urine, while it stimulates the kidneys to activate vitamin D. Vitamin D then increases calcium absorption in the digestive tract.

Estrogen and testosterone also affect remodeling and **peak bone mass**. Nearly 95% of the peak bone mass achieved during childhood and adolescence occurs under the influence of these two sex hormones. Estrogen and testosterone inhibit **apoptosis** of osteoblasts and stimulate osteoblast activity, thereby facilitating calcium deposition. Furthermore, they enhance apoptosis of osteoclasts, which limits the osteoclast's destructive activity.[3–5] Overall, achieving peak bone mass during the bone-building years of adolescence is crucial in preventing osteoporosis.[6]

Human growth hormone, a hormone produced by the pituitary gland, promotes bone growth in length through its action on the **epiphyseal plate**. As the epiphyseal plate thickens, the bone lengthens. Thyroxine from the thyroid gland stimulates the pituitary gland to release increasing amounts of hGH, so thyroxine indirectly stimulates bone lengthening as well. Nevertheless, since thyroxine also stimulates ossification of the epiphyseal plate (discussed next), it ultimately halts growth in length.

Bones continue to grow in length as long as the epiphyseal plates remain. These cartilage plates typically **ossify** between the ages of 19 to 25 in most people, and as soon as they ossify, bones can no longer grow in length. Theoretically, bones can grow in width as long as mechanical stress is applied, osteoblasts are present, and minerals are available for deposition.

The Effect of Dietary Intake and Exercise on Bone Remodeling. Dietary intake and exercise affect the quality of bone remodeling. Healthy bone tissue forms when appropriate forces are applied to the bone and adequate calcium, vitamin D, protein, and other nutrients are present. Weight-bearing exercises, including walking, running, and resistance training, stimulate osteoblast activity along lines of mechanical stress. Osteoblasts ultimately deposit bone tissue to withstand the new forces applied. To form this new bone

---

Osteoblasts—bone-building cells that secrete the matrix in which calcium salts are deposited.

Osteoclasts—bone-destroyers that release acid and enzymes to dissolve bone matrix.

Peak bone mass—the amount of bone mass present at the end of skeletal maturity; depends upon bone size and density.[57]

Apoptosis—a process in which body cells self-destruct; it occurs naturally and is genetically programmed in certain cells. It can also be triggered by hormones, toxins, or radiation.

Epiphyseal plate—also known as the growth plate. Consists of a layer of hyaline cartilage found at the ends of long bones (such as the femur and humerus). Bone continues to grow in length as long as the epiphyseal plate is present. Bone ceases to grow in length when this cartilage layer ossifies into the epiphyseal line. Ossification is the process by which bone tissue replaces the cartilage layer.

Ossify—to form bone.

tissue, protein, calcium, and additional salts must be available. With inadequate nutritional intake and minimal mechanical stress, bone tissue breaks down faster than it is deposited.

The Impact of Aging on Bones

Aging dramatically affects the skeletal system and often promotes bone and joint disorders. During childhood and adolescence, osteoblast activity outpaces osteoclast activity. This results in longer, stronger, and denser bones and typically continues until the ages of 20 to 30. In early adulthood, the activity of the bone-builders slows slightly until osteoblast activity equals osteoclast activity. By middle age, osteoclast activity outpaces osteoblast activity, resulting in a net loss of bone tissue that predisposes bone to osteoporosis. As the amount of bone tissue decreases and osteoporosis progresses, the risk for fracture increases. In some instances, bone structure becomes so fragile that a slight impact can completely fracture the affected bone. To make matters worse, the number and activity of osteoblasts decrease with age, while the relative proportion of osteoclasts increases, so bone repair in the elderly is quite slow.

QUICK REFERENCE

Interestingly, by the age of 70, the rate of bone loss in men and women is approximately the same.

Women begin to lose bone mass at a much earlier age and at a much more rapid rate than men. Not until men reach the age of 60 do they lose 3% of their bone mass every decade. Compare this to women who begin losing approximately 8% of their bone mass every decade once they reach age 45. These differences are largely because of two factors: (1) men usually have a greater peak bone mass than women and (2) women experience a dramatic drop in estrogen production postmenopause (whereas men experience a less dramatic drop in testosterone production much later in life). The sudden drop in estrogen significantly interferes with bone remodeling by enhancing bone resorption. Ultimately, bone loses density in the absence of adequate estrogen as calcium is stripped from it. Furthermore, bone becomes brittle as a result of decreased **collagen** synthesis (collagen is a protein essential to the structure of bone tissue). Spongy bone succumbs to the effects of osteoporosis more rapidly and more significantly than compact bone, but both deteriorate as the disease progresses (Fig. 8.2).

Within 5 to 10 years after menopause, women lose spongy and compact bone at a rate three to four times that of men or premenopausal women. Osteoporosis is therefore quite common among senior females. Since osteoporotic bone is more likely to fracture during a fall, and since fractures tend to immobilize the elderly, what seems like a "simple" fracture can promote deterioration in other body systems as the affected individual is forced into bed rest. With limited activity, people tend to lose range of motion, muscle mass, and cardiovascular endurance.

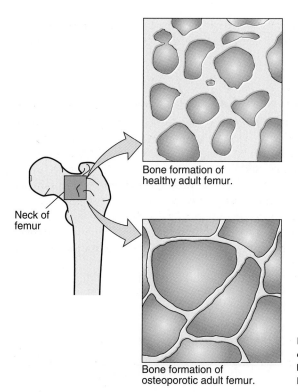

Bone formation of
healthy adult femur.

Neck of
femur

Bone formation of
osteoporotic adult femur.

FIGURE 8.2 ■ Healthy spongy bone versus osteoporotic bone. (From Kamen G. Foundations of Exercise Science. Baltimore: Lippincott Williams & Wilkins, 2001.)

QUICK REFERENCE

Osteopenia is a condition thought to precede full-blown osteoporosis. It occurs when bone mass is less than optimal but not low enough to meet the criteria for osteoporosis. Because bone with osteopenia is not as dense as it could be, it has a greater likelihood of becoming osteoporotic in future years.

Both men and women typically lose height after the age of 30 at an average rate of 1/16 of an inch per year. The loss of vertebral bone mass coupled with bone fracture and deterioration of **intervertebral discs** account for this decrease in height. Moreover, as bone density decreases and discs wear away, abnormal spinal curvatures tend to develop.

Collagen—a protein found in numerous body tissues, in this case bone. It provides bone with tensile strength and flexibility.

Intervertebral discs—fibrocartilage discs found in between vertebrae in the spinal column. Provide cushioning and shock absorption for vertebrae.

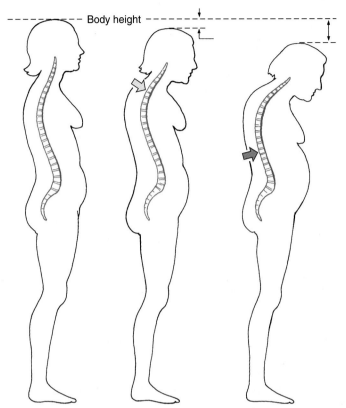

FIGURE 8.3 ■ Osteoporosis with aging. Osteoporosis results in the loss of height over time. (LifeART image copyright © 2009 Lippincott Williams & Wilkins. All rights reserved.)

Kyphosis, also referred to as "hunchback," is an excessive thoracic curvature of the spine common in elderly people, particularly women (Figs. 8.3 and 8.4).

JOINTS

Joints exist wherever two bones meet. Although the body has immoveable, slightly moveable, and freely moveable joints, this section focuses on freely moveable joints since they are the most prone to deterioration and disorder. Moveable joints are called synovial joints (Fig. 2.1).

Joint Structure and Stability

The ends of two articulating bones are covered by articular cartilage, a slippery layer of hyaline cartilage that essentially protects bone ends from abrasion and shock during impact. Moveable joints are held together by a double-layered joint capsule. The joint capsule, also called the synovial capsule, consists of two layers. The outermost fibrous

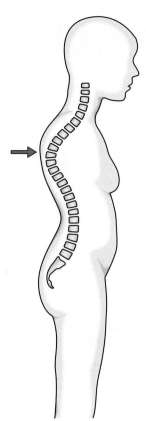

FIGURE 8.4 ■ Kyphosis ("hunchback") is the excessive curvature of the thoracic spine.

capsule is strong enough to resist pulling forces yet flexible enough to maintain structure. The innermost synovial membrane produces synovial fluid. Synovial fluid not only reduces friction between two bone ends but also supplies nutrients to the articular cartilage and contains cells that eliminate debris found in the synovial cavity. Synovial fluid has a consistency similar to an egg white; it is clear and somewhat viscous. When joints are immobile, synovial fluid becomes almost gel-like, which can limit joint mobility. Anyone who has experienced stiff joints in the morning upon getting out of bed knows what this feels like! With activity, synovial fluid thins and joint mobility returns.

Additional structures found at or near joints provide stability to joints. They include tendons, ligaments, menisci, bursae, and tendon sheaths. *Tendons*, which are technically a part of the muscular system, attach bones to muscles. Muscles maintain low-level contractions, called muscle tone, that contribute significantly to strength and stability at

Kyphosis—an excessive thoracic curvature of the spine common in the elderly. Also called "hunchback."

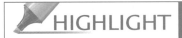

HIGHLIGHT   Cartilage

Cartilage is a special type of connective tissue composed of cells surrounded by matrix. Matrix includes both ground substance and fibers. The ground substance consists of water and varying amounts glycosaminoglycans, proteoglycans, and glycoproteins—substances that determine the consistency of the matrix and preserve the water content of cartilage. About 85% of the cartilage in children, adolescents, and young adults is made up of water. With advancing age, the proportion of water decreases to 70%—a factor that interferes with cartilage functioning.

Each of the three major types of cartilage—hyaline cartilage, elastic cartilage, and fibrocartilage—contains one of the two main fiber types: collagen or elastin.

Collagen fibers provide support, tensile strength, and flexibility to tissues. They are often bundled together much like the fibers of a rope. Collagen is the major fiber type in hyaline cartilage and fibrocartilage. Hyaline cartilage, the most abundant form of cartilage in the body, forms the articular cartilage at the ends of long bones, the costal cartilages, the nose, the epiphyseal plates, and most of the larynx.

Fibrocartilage, the strongest type of cartilage, forms the intervertebral discs, the menisci in the knees, and the symphysis pubis—areas subjected to tremendous compressive forces.

Elastic fibers allow for stretch and recoil; thus, they are found in areas subjected to mechanical stretching. Elastic fibers are the major fibers found in elastic cartilage, which is located in the ear and epiglottis.

moveable joints. *Ligaments* unite bones to bones and provide additional stability to the joint. *Menisci* are pads of cartilage found between the articulating surfaces of some bones. The menisci in the knee, for example, increase stability by creating a better fit between the femur of the thigh and the tibia of the leg. *Bursae* are simply bags of lubricant that act as ball bearings to reduce friction at joints such as the shoulder and the knee. They are similar in structure and function to joint capsules. *Tendon sheaths* are similar to bursae and joint capsules; however, they wrap around tendons in areas that are prone to stress, such as the wrist and ankle.

"Range of motion," or the flexibility permitted by a joint, is the degree of movement that can occur at a joint. Flexibility and stability tend to be inversely related. As stability increases, flexibility tends to decrease; as stability decreases, flexibility tends to increase. Factors that affect range of motion at a joint include the structure or shape of the articulating surfaces, the tension of the ligaments holding two bones together, tension in the muscles acting on the joint, and the amount of joint usage.

Stability and Shape of the Articulating Surfaces. As mentioned, two bones that fit closely together are stable but not very flexible. Compare the hip joint to the shoulder joint. Both are ball-and-socket joints, but the hip joint is much more stable because of how closely the head of the femur fits into the acetabulum of the hip bone. It is, however, much less flexible than the shoulder joint for the same reason.

Stability and Tension of Ligaments. If two bones are held together by tight ligaments, they are more stable but less flexible. The actual amount of tension on the ligament varies depending upon the position of the joint. For example, during knee flexion, tension on the posterior cruciate ligament limits posterior movement of the tibia relative to the femur; whereas, when the knee is extended, tension on the anterior cruciate ligament limits anterior movement of the tibia in relation to the femur.[7]

Tension in Surrounding Muscles. Increased muscle tension restricts the flexibility of a joint. For example, contraction of the hamstrings muscle group limits flexion of the thigh when the knee is extended. Flexing the knee, however, allows the thigh to be lifted higher.

Joint Use. The more a joint is used and moved through its full range of motion, the more mobile it remains. This is because activity maintains pliability of the supporting structures such as ligaments, tendons, and muscles. Activity also stimulates synovial fluid production, which further promotes and preserves range of motion.

The Impact of Aging on Joints

The age-related changes in joints are usually apparent by age 40, sometimes sooner. With age, total water content in the body diminishes, a condition that pulls water out of the cartilage pads found in between the vertebrae in the spine. This decreases flexibility and eventually stiffens the spine. Synovial joint function is also affected, often as early as age 30. The articular cartilage in between two articulating bones begins wearing away, so bones lose cushioning during impact. Joint mobility decreases as the collagen fibers in ligaments shorten and change orientation; this decreases the flexibility and movement permitted by the ligaments. Capillary supply to the synovial membrane drops as well, so less synovial fluid is made (synovial fluid, like most body fluids, derives from blood). A decrease in synovial fluid further promotes joint stiffness and immobility. In addition, debris and microbes accumulate in the synovial cavity as less synovial fluid is made, and this further impairs mobility.

Sprains and Bursitis

Whenever cartilage, ligaments, or tendons are overstretched, the joint is said to be *sprained*. Consider a ligament as an example. A ligament is like a piece of taffy. It resists stretching up to a certain point but will rip if the force is excessive. If the force is not quite intense enough to rip it, the ligament can actually stretch to some degree, but it will never return to its original length—even after the force is removed. Unfortunately, once a joint is sprained, that joint is more susceptible to future injuries. A sprained joint exhibits swelling, pain, and reduced range of motion in the short term. Most sprains respond well to rest, ice, compression, and elevation, but more serious sprains require medical attention. Active seniors seem to sprain ankles and wrists more frequently than younger people in part because of their impaired balance, diminished muscle mass, weakened joints, and shorter and tighter ligaments.

Bursitis refers to inflammation of the bursa sacs associated with joints. Often the result of overuse, bursitis is a chronic condition treated with rest, ice, compression, elevation, and sometimes steroid injections. Bursitis of the shoulder, elbow, or heel is common in the elderly. Seniors with bursitis must be careful since overusing an affected joint results in extreme tenderness, pain, and immobility.

Osteoarthritis

As mentioned earlier, osteoarthritis (OA), the most common form of arthritis, occurs over time as joints are repeatedly used. It affects the small joints of the fingers, feet, and spine as well as weight-bearing joints such as the hips and knees. It is less common in the wrists, elbows, and shoulders. Although 90% of individuals show x-ray evidence of OA by the age of 40, most do not experience symptoms until much later.

In osteoarthritis, the articular cartilage thins as it loses water and collagen (Fig. 8.5). Unfortunately, cartilage does not regenerate once it deteriorates. Therefore, degeneration is permanent and makes the underlying bone vulnerable. In some extreme cases, the articular cartilage completely wears away causing bone to rub directly against bone. This promotes local inflammation, ligament weakening, and muscle atrophy. Furthermore, the bone thickens, **bone spurs** form, and **loose bodies** fill the synovial cavity—factors that further impair joint functioning. Overall, discomfort develops gradually over years and the sufferer experiences varying degrees of pain whenever the affected joints are used. The exact symptoms vary depending upon the joint involved. Table 8.2 shows the common symptoms of osteoarthritis.

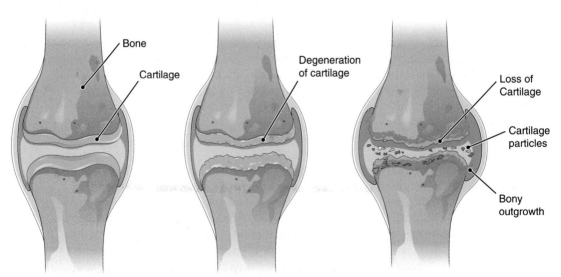

FIGURE 8.5 ■ Development of osteoarthritis. (From Cohen BJ. Medical Terminology. 4th Ed. Philadelphia: Lippincott Williams & Wilkins, 2003.)

TABLE 8-2 SYMPTOMS OF OSTEOARTHRITIS

- Aching in a joint that worsens with increased activity and decreases with rest
- Stiffness in joints for up to 30 minutes following long periods of immobility
- Pain that occurs in waves with periods of bad pain followed by periods of relief
- A crackling noise in the knee, particularly upon movement
- Loss of range of motion around an affected joint
- Affects a joint on only one side of the body (unlike rheumatoid arthritis)

TABLE 8-3 RISK FACTORS FOR OSTEOARTHRITIS (OA)	
Factor	**Risk**
Gender	Men over the age of 45 are at greater risk; women over the age of 55 are at greater risk
Ethnicity	Compared to white men and women, black men and women have an elevated risk for OA of the knee and hip. Those of Asian descent have a higher risk of OA of the knee than whites but a lower risk of OA of the hip.
Obesity	Increases the risk of OA because of the excess burden on joints. OA is about 4–5 times more prevalent in obese women and men than it is in healthy weight women and men.
Working conditions	Those required to kneel or squat at work have an increased risk for OA of the knee.
Genetics and heredity	Those with a family history of OA are at increased risk
Anatomic abnormalities	Some factors such as unequal leg length, abnormal spinal curvatures, or misaligned knees and/or feet are associated with an increased risk of OA.
Former joint injuries	Those who have injured a joint are at an increased risk for OA in the affected joint.

Although the exact causes are unknown, osteoarthritis seems to run in families. In addition, factors such as aging, obesity, diabetes, and joint trauma increase the likelihood of developing osteoarthritis. Table 8.3 provides a summary of the risk factors related to osteoarthritis.

The goal of treatment for osteoarthritis is to reduce the severity of symptoms, improve range of motion, and slow deterioration. Physicians typically prescribe non-steroidal anti-inflammatory drugs to provide relief from pain and inflammation. Heat and cold therapy also alleviate short-term discomfort. For long-term management, they suggest weight loss for those who are overweight or obese and encourage exercise to

Bone spurs—abnormal, bony growths often found at the ends of long bones in those with osteoarthritis.

Loose bodies—fragments of tissue found in the joint (synovial) cavity. May consist of bone or cartilage.

improve balance, coordination, and functional ability. Flexibility exercise, in particular, increases range of motion and maintains joint function. Isometric exercises are beneficial because they can increase strength around targeted joints without actually moving the joint—something that many arthritis sufferers need since even the slightest movements can sometimes cause severe pain. Unfortunately, isometric contractions only minimally increase muscular strength. Aerobic exercise such as swimming improves cardiorespiratory functioning without excessively stressing joints. Using orthotics while walking can improve balance and minimize stress. For those who have severe degeneration, doctors might suggest surgery to realign the bones at a joint, remove excess debris from the joint, permanently fuse the joint to prevent motion, or replace the joint with a new one.

Rheumatoid Arthritis

Rheumatoid arthritis (RA) is an autoimmune disease that usually affects multiple joints (unlike OA, which can be isolated to a single location). It develops earlier than OA with symptoms typically appearing between the ages of 30 and 40. In rheumatoid arthritis, cells of the immune system attack a joint's synovial membrane. The precise stimulus for this attack is unknown, but as the synovial membrane degenerates, it begins producing a grainy synovial fluid that interferes with joint movements. This causes the articular surfaces of the two articulating bones to wear away from friction (Fig. 8.6).

The symptoms of rheumatoid arthritis are not consistently present; instead, they come and go. In other words, rheumatoid arthritis has an *active phase* during which the body relapses and experiences inflammation, pain, limited range of motion, and fatigue, and an *inactive phase* during which the body is in remission. Rheumatoid arthritis often affects small joints bilaterally; in other words, it attacks the same joints on both sides of the body. Inflammation is common and makes the affected joints appear swollen and red. If inflammation is chronic, bone and cartilage deteriorate rapidly, range of motion

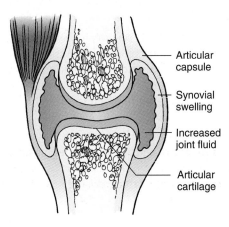

Articular
capsule

Synovial
swelling

Increased
joint fluid

Articular
cartilage

FIGURE 8.6 ■ Rheumatoid arthritis. This illustration shows a joint structure with synovial swelling and fluid accumulation in joint. (From Nettina SM. The Lippincott Manual of Nursing Practice. 7th Ed. Lippincott Williams & Wilkins, 2001.)

decreases, muscles atrophy, joints deform, and function is lost. Stiffness develops after periods of rest and tends to last for hours; this makes activities of daily living difficult, if not impossible. In most instances, however, stiffness lessens with activity. Generalized fatigue, weight loss, and fever are typical, and symptoms progress rapidly. Rheumatoid arthritis is also characterized by widespread inflammation that often interferes with cardiorespiratory functioning.

As with osteoarthritis, there is currently no cure for rheumatoid arthritis. The goal, therefore, is to manage pain, reduce inflammation, and prevent further deterioration and joint deformity. Early, aggressive treatment is recommended to preserve functioning. Drugs such as aspirin and nonsteroidal anti-inflammatories quickly reduce inflammation and eliminate pain, but unfortunately, they do nothing to slow deterioration. Fortunately, additional drugs are available to prevent joint destruction and promote disease remission. Symptom severity varies significantly among different people, but no matter how extreme the symptoms, rest is important during the active phase. In fact, rest should be continued until acute symptoms cease. Regular exercise during the inactive phase is also now recognized as an important component for preserving joint functioning because it improves range of motion, muscle strength, and the ability to produce synovial fluid.[8,9] As with OA, swimming seems to be the safest mode because it minimizes stress on joints, while it works them through a full range of motion. In cases of severe joint deformity, surgery is an option. During these procedures, surgeons may choose to remove excess debris, repair damaged tissue, or totally replace the joint.

PRECAUTIONS DURING EXERCISE

AVOID HIGH-IMPACT ACTIVITIES

Though high-impact activities such as jogging and high-impact aerobics stimulate bone growth, they are generally not recommended for this special population.[10] Those suffering from osteoporosis have weak, frail bones that may break during minimal impact—imagine what could happen during high impact. Those with arthritis have vulnerable, degenerating joints that are often inflamed and sore; high-impact activities tend to aggravate these symptoms and accelerate progression.[11] Thus, encourage low-impact or no-impact activities such as walking or bicycle riding for those with bone and joint problems. Try to attain a balance between intensity and impact that preserves bone mass and joint mobility, while it minimizes risk for fracture.

AVOID EXPLOSIVE OR TWISTING MOVEMENTS

Explosive and twisting movements significantly stress the skeletal system. Because the muscles surrounding degenerating bones and joints are often emaciated, these joints might not be able to withstand rapid direction changes. The knee, hip, and shoulder joints are especially vulnerable. Additionally, osteoporotic bone can actually fracture with abrupt direction changes or explosive movements—even in the absence of a fall.

TABLE 8-4   SIGNS OF OVERTRAINING FOR THOSE WITH ARTHRITIS
■ Excessive joint swelling accompanied by decreased joint mobility
■ Increased weakness
■ Persistent fatigue
■ Prolonged pain following exercise

BALANCE PROBLEMS

Because their muscles are often weak, those suffering from bone and joint disorders frequently experience balance problems, and unfortunately, imbalance can result in falls. Thus, emphasize care on exercise equipment. Avoid free weights since free weights require more stability than machines. Make sure clients wear shoes with appropriate tread to minimize the risk of falling. In addition, ensure adequate cushioning to reduce the load on joints.

Balance problems might result from postural imbalances such as kyphosis, or hunchback. Kyphosis can develop in response to chronic slouching, osteoporosis, degenerating discs, weak back muscles, or tight chest muscles. Kyphosis not only interferes with body mechanics during strength training but also impedes functioning of the diaphragm, intercostal muscles, and lungs, thus interfering with cardiovascular exercise as well.

BE AWARE OF COMORBIDITIES

Many people with bone and joint disorders suffer from additional conditions that interfere with exercise ability. Osteoporosis, for instance, is common in seniors, cigarette smokers, excessive alcohol users, the sedentary, and those who have inadequate diets—risk factors that also hinder exercise ability. As with all populations, assess coexisting risk factors, and identify all chronic conditions before permitting clients with osteoporosis or arthritis to exercise.

AVOID HEAVY WEIGHT LIFTING

Lifting heavy weights puts excessive stress on osteoporotic bone and arthritic joints. This can further damage the already compromised skeletal system. Lightweights, resistance bands, and resistance equipment using light resistance are much safer for this special population and do not appear to exacerbate the condition in most RA sufferers. Table 8.4 provides signs of overtraining in those with arthritis.

BENEFITS OF EXERCISE

Exercise is the lifestyle behavior that offers the most promise for preserving and improving bone integrity and joint functioning. Overall, exercise benefits the skeletal system by decreasing the rate of bone loss, maintaining joint functioning, preserving muscle strength, improving cardiorespiratory functioning, controlling weight, reducing arthritis pain, and improving mood.

DECREASES RATE OF BONE LOSS AND INCREASES BONE MASS

As mentioned, osteoblast activity decreases when bones are not challenged and increases when bones are subjected to mechanical stress. Several studies show that this occurs even in those with preexisting osteoporosis. For example, researchers investigated the effects of exercise on postmenopausal women with low bone mass and found significant increases in bone mass by the end of 1 year.[12,13] Additionally, regular activity prevents the risk of second fractures in those who have already experienced a fracture.[14] This suggests that weak bone, like healthy bone, responds to increased workloads.

MAINTAINS AND INCREASES JOINT FUNCTION

Most research agrees that a combination of cardiovascular and strength training promotes synovial fluid production, maintains and improves flexibility, and contributes to balance.[11,15–17] Producing adequate synovial fluid helps preserve pain-free joint mobility; normal joint flexibility reduces the risk of acute joint injury; while improved balance decreases the risk of falling. This is true for those with and without preexisting osteoporosis or arthritis.

It is only fair to mention that some researchers have found that exercise does *not* improve joint functioning in those with arthritis.[18,19] In fact, they find no benefits to joints at all, but they agree that exercise does not exacerbate existing arthritis symptoms either.

PRESERVES AND INCREASES MUSCLE STRENGTH

Muscle strength often diminishes as activity levels decline and muscles atrophy. Research has demonstrated that, at the very least, exercise slows the age-related loss in strength by preserving muscle mass. Moreover, it likely increases muscle mass and thus contributes to strength gains. Since strength of the muscles surrounding a joint is the greatest contributor to joint stability, those who are physically active likely have better stability and functional capacity.[15,17,20]

IMPROVES CARDIORESPIRATORY FUNCTIONING

Exercise clearly improves coordination between the cardiovascular system and the respiratory system by improving heart functioning, VO_{2max}, oxygen availability, blood lipid levels, and various other factors discussed in Chapter 7. Overall, exercisers experience a lower blood pressure, lower total blood cholesterol, lower triglycerides, higher red blood cell count, improved tidal volume, and improved maximal oxygen uptake—factors that reduce the heart's overall workload and the risk for conditions such as heart disease and stroke.[17]

WEIGHT CONTROL

The maintenance of a healthy weight not only reduces the heart's workload but also lessens the burden on weight-bearing joints.[21] Since exercise, accompanied with a healthy diet, often results in weight loss, overweight individuals suffering from joint problems can improve their condition by increasing daily activity. Increased activity coupled with weight loss prevents further joint deterioration, minimizes pain, and improves range of motion around targeted joints.

REDUCES PAIN FROM ARTHRITIS

Most studies show that exercise reduces the intensity and frequency of pain experienced by those with arthritis. In fact, exercise is the only nonpharmaceutical core treatment shown to be effective against pain.[22–24] This might be because continued use of a joint encourages blood flow to the area, which in turn promotes synovial fluid production. Increased synovial fluid then reduces friction between bone ends and prevents the buildup of waste products—factors that can minimize pain.

IMPROVES MOOD

Exercise is associated with an elevated mood in every population studied, including the elderly, the obese, those with cardiovascular disease, those with disorders of the skeletal system, and the clinically depressed. Studies suggest that a dose response exists; in other words, the more consistent an exercise program, the greater the effect on mood.[25–29] Perhaps this is because exercise promotes the release of brain chemicals associated with improved mood. Or maybe it results from the improved functional capacity and increased self-efficacy that accompany consistent exercise training. Whatever the cause, exercise seems to improve the mental and emotional well-being of all participants.

RECOMMENDATIONS FOR EXERCISE FOR THOSE WITH OSTEOPOROSIS

EXERCISE TESTING

According to the American College of Sports Medicine, exercise testing guidelines for those with osteoporosis are the same as the guidelines for the general population. Clients with severe osteoporosis in the vertebral column should participate in the cycle ergometer test rather than the traditional treadmill test if walking causes pain.[30] If using the treadmill test, verify that clients are wearing sturdy shoes with nonskid rubber soles to ensure safe movement and to minimize the risk of falling. Be aware that some medications cause dizziness or lightheadedness that increase the risk for falls.[2,31]

Many osteoporosis sufferers have abnormal spinal curvatures as a result of compressed vertebrae. Kyphosis, or an excessive thoracic curvature, is common and might offset the center of balance and increase the risk for falls. It can also reduce ventilatory capacity and hamper test results.[30] Tests for balance, muscular strength, and gait can also be performed, but avoid spinal flexion and be prepared to stop exercise testing if pain results. In addition, avoid maximal strength testing in those with severe osteoporosis since fragile bones can fracture when forced to overcome excessive forces.[30]

EXERCISE PRESCRIPTION

ACSM suggests that the population of individuals with osteoporosis be subdivided into two groups: those with one or more risk factors for developing osteoporosis and those currently diagnosed with osteoporosis. Therefore, the following section is separated into two parts.

Guidelines for Those at Risk of Developing Osteoporosis

- Begin all exercise sessions with an 8 to 15 minute warm-up that includes mild stretching. This increases blood flow and warms up muscles. Follow each exercise session with an 8-minute cooldown to return the body to a resting state.[32]
- Weight-bearing cardiovascular activities such as walking, tennis, stair climbing, volleyball, and basketball are beneficial for this population and should be done on 3 to 5 days per week. Resistance training at a moderate (60% to 80% of 1-RM for 8 to 12 repetitions) to high intensity (80% to 90% of 1-RM for 5 to 6 repetitions) helps preserve bone mass and should be performed on 2 to 3 days per week.[30] Weight machines, elastic bands, and calisthenics are all effective and safe options. Free weights can also be safe, but they are riskier because they require balance. Nonweight-bearing activities, such as swimming and water aerobics, are beneficial for the cardiorespiratory system, but they do not stimulate osteoblast activity. Therefore, they will not slow mineral loss.[33] Overall exercise sessions should include 30 to 60 minutes of weight-bearing aerobic exercise combined with resistance training.[30]

Guidelines for Those Diagnosed with Osteoporosis

- Weight-bearing cardiovascular activities such as walking or stair climbing should be performed on 3 to 5 days per week at a moderate intensity of 40% to 60% VO_{2R}. Resistance training should be performed on 2 to 3 days per week at a moderate intensity of 60% to 80% of 1-RM for 8 to 12 repetitions. Increase load as tolerated. Overall duration should be 30 to 60 minutes of weight-bearing aerobic exercise combined with resistance training.[30]
- Flexibility exercises help preserve and improve joint functioning, which often diminishes as a result of osteoporosis. Clients should perform stretching exercises as recommended to the general population. Stretches should be gentle and slow. To minimize the risk of compression fracture, avoid stretches that require spinal flexion. Chest and shoulder stretches are particularly important in restoring neutral posture.
- Functional activities, such as stair climbing or the chair sit-and-stand, help improve normal activities of daily living. These functional exercises, therefore, should be performed on 2 to 5 days per week. Additionally, balance activities, such as standing on one leg with or without the eyes closed, walking backward, walking on the tip toes, or walking on the heels, can help reduce the risk for falls.

QUICK REFERENCE

Those suffering from osteoporosis should avoid high-impact activities and explosive movements since these excessively stress bones and can result in fracture. In addition, do not participate in activities that require trunk flexion and rotation because these movements generate compressive forces that might fracture vertebrae (Table 8.5).[30]

TABLE 8-5   THOSE WITH OSTEOPOROSIS SHOULD AVOID

- Jumping
- Jogging
- Rowing machines
- Sit-ups
- Golfing
- Bowling
- Certain yoga poses

SAMPLE EXERCISES

Those suffering from osteoporosis can perform various activities. It is crucial to participate in weight-bearing aerobic activity that improves bone density in the spine and lower extremities. Although walking is the safest mode of exercise, it actually preserves only a modest amount of vertebral bone mass.[34] This is because a positive correlation exists between impact and bone building, so it seems that a higher impact and greater resistance result in greater osteoblast activity. In fact, an intensity above 70% of 1 RM is most effective at preserving bone mass. Nevertheless, since this intensity can be dangerous for those with osteoporosis, it should only be performed under close supervision—if at all.[35] Swimming, cycling, and water aerobics are also safe choices that train and improve cardiorespiratory system functioning; however, they insufficiently stress the bones and do not increase bone mass or preserve existing bone tissue. Dancing and stepping activities are better osteoblast stimulators.

Strength training should target the chest, back, arms, shoulders, and legs. For beginners, start with resistance bands or elastic tubing to develop basic strength and joint mobility. Gradually advance to resistance machines and be sure to use lightweights. Because those with osteoporosis often have postural problems, they typically have weak back muscles and tight chest muscles. Avoid free weights until these problems are corrected.

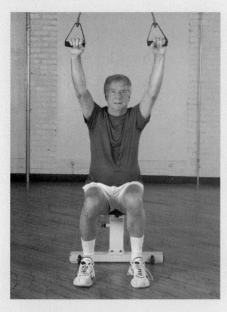
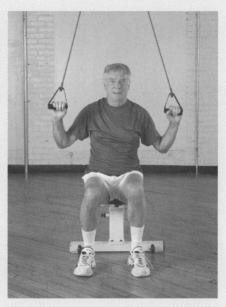

■ Lateral Pull Down (Fig. 8.7)

To strengthen the muscles of the back and the bones of the vertebral column, perform the lat pull down either with elastic bands, elastic tubing, or a lat pull down machine using a light-weight. Maintain a neutral spine, contract abdominals, and breathe normally. Avoid the row since it requires spinal flexion, which can result in compression fractures.

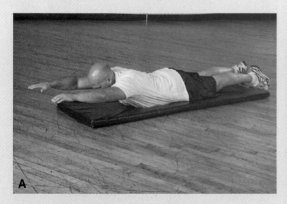
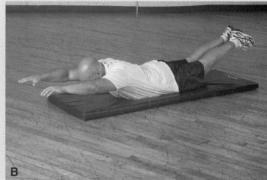

■ Back Extension (Fig. 8.8)

Back extension exercises, performed slowly and in neutral alignment, strengthen the vertebrae as well as the muscles along the spine. This can improve posture and balance. Lie on the stomach with forehead on floor. Extend arms overhead. As a unit, raise the head and arms a few inches off the floor as in **A**. Hold for 8 seconds and return to floor. Repeat. Perform 1 to 2 sets of 8 to 10 repetitions. A more advanced alternative involves lifting the arms, head, and legs for 8 seconds as in **B**.

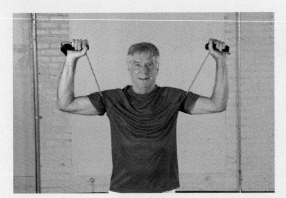
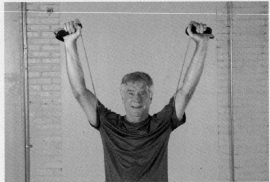

■ Shoulder Press Using Elastic Tubing (Fig. 8.9)

The shoulder press works shoulder and arm muscles and improves the capacity to lift items such as groceries. Place tubing around the back just below the shoulder blades. Hold one handle in each hand. Grasp tubing toward center to increase resistance. Bring hands to ear level. Push arms up toward ceiling. Pause. Slowly return to start and repeat. Palms should face forward.

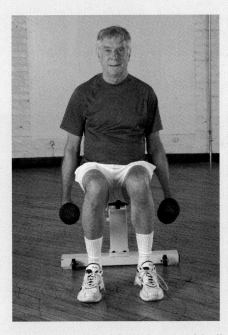
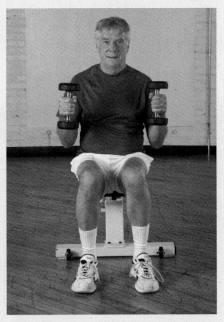

■ Biceps Curl with Light Dumbbells (Fig. 8.10)

Sit on a bench with a lightweight dumbbell in each hand, elbows extended, palms toward the midline. Slowly flex both elbows while lifting weight. Keep elbows in but not pressed to sides. Pause at the top of the movement. Then lower the weight. Repeat 8 to 12 times.

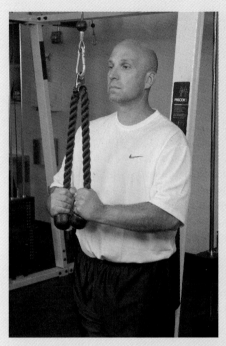 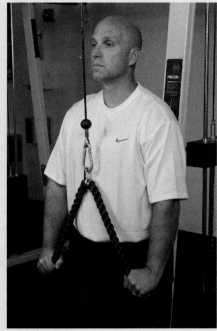

■ Triceps Extension Using Cable Rope (Fig. 8.11)

Stand facing a rope at a cable machine. Spine should be neutral and abdominals contracted. Grasp the rope with both hands. Slowly press the rope down. At end of movement, move hands laterally. Pause. Return to start and repeat 8 to 12 times.

To train the lower body, perform leg extensions and leg curls on resistance machines. Strong leg muscles often improve posture and balance.

Because of the postural problems so common in this special population, individuals often experience tight chests and upper backs. Emphasize stretches that target these areas, but avoid any stretch that requires forward flexion.

Additional activities for this special population include the chair sit-and-stand, heel-toe walking, walking on tiptoes, standing on one leg, or simply balancing on a stability ball. These improve functional capacity and balance and reduce the risk for falls. Clients who have been sedentary for a long time might need to begin by using only their body weight for resistance. Moving their joints through a full range of motion can be adequate as they begin their training program. Progress to elastic bands, elastic tubing, or weight machines later.

EXERCISE RECOMMENDATIONS FOR THOSE WITH ARTHRITIS

EXERCISE TESTING

The American College of Sports Medicine suggests exercise testing for those with arthritis to assess cardiorespiratory capacity, neuromuscular status, and joint flexibility. They say that most patients are able to perform graded tests without eliciting major symptoms, but because clients with arthritis experience such diverse functional capacities and limitations, be prepared to modify or stop testing if pain or fatigue develops. Testing is contraindicated during acute inflammation. The treadmill test is acceptable for evaluating cardiovascular condition in those who can tolerate it, but the cycle ergometer is usually less painful. Make sure that participants warm up prior to testing and monitor pain level throughout the test. Some arthritis sufferers tolerate 1-RM testing, but they might be limited by pain in affected joints.[30]

EXERCISE PRESCRIPTION

The goals for those with arthritis are to restore range of motion around affected joints, increase muscular strength to stabilize joints, and improve cardiovascular conditioning to reduce the risk for heart disease.[30,36]

QUICK REFERENCE

Those with arthritis should avoid exercise during flare-ups and acute inflammation.[30]

Specific suggestions include the following:

- Obtain clearance from a physician since arthritis sufferers often have comorbidities.
- Avoid exercise during arthritis flare-ups since exercise during this time can be painful and promote inflammation and joint damage.
- Be aware of the medications clients are taking. Some nonsteroidal anti-inflammatories cause digestive tract bleeding that predisposes clients to anemia. Anemia causes severe fatigue and muscle weakness and can interfere with a client's ability to discern musculoskeletal pain.
- Begin each exercise session with a 5 to 10 minute warm-up and follow it with a 5 to 10 minute cooldown.
- Ease into exercise and progress gradually. Arthritis sufferers have often been sedentary for a long time; therefore, they are likely functioning at a lower fitness level than average clients.
- Ask about and check for misaligned or unstable joints. Pay close attention to these joints during activity. Watch for pronation or supination; if excessive, orthotics might be necessary.

> ### QUICK REFERENCE
> As improvements are made, focus on increasing duration rather than increasing intensity.

- Perform flexibility activities first, resistance exercise second, and cardiovascular training third.
- Flexibility training decreases stiffness, increases joint mobility, and protects surrounding tissues. It should be performed daily for optimal improvements. Sessions may occur once or twice daily. Use a pain-free range of motion and static stretch all major muscle groups. Hold each stretch for 15 to 60 seconds. Repeat four times. Muscles should feel tight when stretching, but there should be no pain. Avoid overstretching or hypermobility exercises.
- Resistance training to strengthen the muscles around joints should be done 2 to 3 days per week. Include resistance machines, elastic bands or tubing, isometric exercises, or free weights. Initially, use a resistance equal to 10% of 1-RM and progress at a maximum of 10% per week as tolerated. Complete one or more sets of 10 to 15 repetitions per set.[30]
- Initially perform low-impact cardiovascular exercise, including walking, water exercise, or cycling, in 5- to 10-minute bouts to accumulate 20 to 30 minutes of activity on 3 to 5 days per week. Gradually increase duration of bouts by 5-minute increments until 30 minutes is reached (for a total of 150 minutes of weekly activity). To protect joints, avoid high-impact activities, rapid changes in direction, and excessive repetitions of any given movement. Walking at high speeds can severely stress joints; be cautious of walking speed and make sure it is tolerable to the client. Water aerobics is particularly beneficial for this group because water buoyancy reduces stress to joints but allows movement through a full range of motion.[37] In addition, water temperatures kept at 83°F to 88°F make exercise more tolerable and less painful. Suggestions for intensity are the same as those for the general population.[30]
- Include daily activities that focus on functional abilities including sit-and-stand and stair climbing.
- Cross-training is important in this group to avoid overstressing individual joints.
- Upon waking, those with rheumatoid arthritis often experience joint stiffness that lasts for hours. Morning training, therefore, should probably be avoided. Create a training schedule compatible with medication intake.
- Rest is as important as the actual exercise session, so allow at least 48 hours in between training sessions. Be aware of limitations and have clients pay attention to their bodies.
- Choose stable shoes that absorb shock to reduce impact at joints
- See Table 8.6 for conditions that suggest a client stop exercising.

TABLE 8-6   STOP EXERCISE IF YOU EXPERIENCE ANY OF THE FOLLOWING

- Unusual fatigue
- Excessive weakness
- Decreased range of motion
- Increased joint inflammation
- Pain following exercise that lasts for more than 1 hour

QUICK REFERENCE

Joint discomfort following exercise is perfectly normal. If pain persists for 2 hours following exercise, reduce the duration and/or intensity of the following exercise session.[30]

SAMPLE EXERCISES

To preserve and restore range of motion around affected joints, clients with arthritis should participate in flexibility training. Most people can perform typical flexibility exercises according to guidelines for the healthy population. Stretch all major joints including the knee, hip, ankle, shoulder, wrist, and neck. Avoid hyperextension and any movements that cause pain.

During strength exercises, train all muscles but emphasize those surrounding the affected joint(s). For example, if someone has osteoarthritis of the knee, train the thigh muscles. Have clients perform leg extensions and leg curls with lightweights or resistance bands. If the hips are affected, train the thighs and gluteals. This strengthens and stabilizes the area around the hip joint and improves flexibility. Overall, this population can perform most traditional resistance exercises with minor adjustments in intensity and modifications for joint limitations. Emphasize neutral body alignment and movement through a full range of *pain-free* motion.

As mentioned, water exercise is recommended for people with arthritis, especially if they have affected hips or knees. The water's buoyancy and warm temperature make it possible to gently work joints through their full range of motion without excessive stress. Water exercise, however, does not adequately stimulate osteoblast activity, so bone mass is not preserved with aquatics.

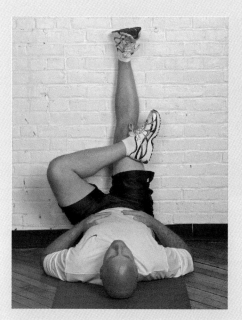

■ Gluteal Stretch on a Wall (Fig. 8.12)

Lie on the floor perpendicular to a wall with right leg extended up the wall. Right leg should be flat against the wall. The part of the back at the base of the spine should be flat on floor. Cross the left leg over the right leg (left ankle rests on right knee). Adjust the position of the ankle and the distance between the torso and the wall to increase or decrease the intensity of the buttocks stretch. Hold the stretch. Switch sides.

Pilates Kingdom. *www.pilateskingdom.com/content/view/57/42/*

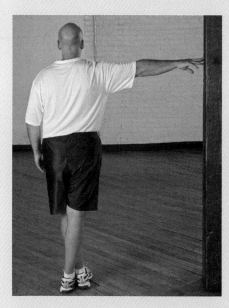 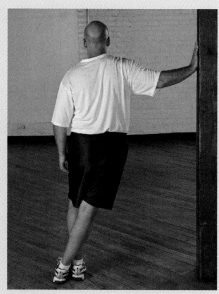

■ Outer Thigh Stretch (Fig. 8.13)

Stand at arm's length away from a wall with right leg closest to wall and right hand on wall. Cross the right leg behind the left leg. Flex right elbow and lean into the wall while putting all weight on the right leg. A stretch should be felt through the right hip. Switch sides.

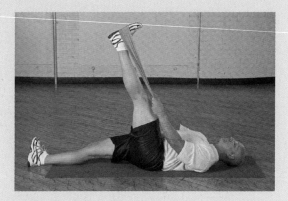

■ Hamstring Stretch Using Elastic Band (Fig. 8.14)

Lie supine on the ground. Wrap an elastic band around bottom of left foot and grasp with both hands. Flex at the hip so that left leg is perpendicular to ground with bottom of foot toward ceiling. Keep knee straight but not locked while pulling on band. Stretch is felt in hamstring. Repeat on right leg.

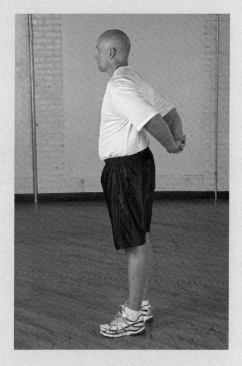

■ Chest, Shoulder, and Biceps Stretch (Fig. 8.15)

Stand with feet shoulder width apart, spine in neutral position, abdominals contracted. Interlace fingers behind the back while straightening arms. Gently lift arms up while keeping shoulders down away from ears. Feel the stretch in the chest, shoulders, and biceps.

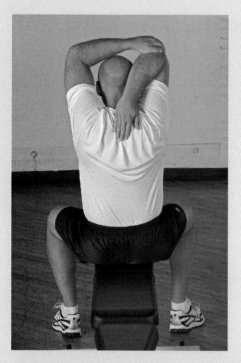

■ Triceps Stretch (Fig. 8.16)

Sit on a bench with spine neutral, abdominals contracted, feet flat on floor. Bring right arm up toward ceiling. Flex at elbow and let forearm drop toward floor. Elbow should point toward ceiling. Take left hand and place on right elbow. Gently pull on elbow to feel stretch in right triceps. Repeat on left triceps.

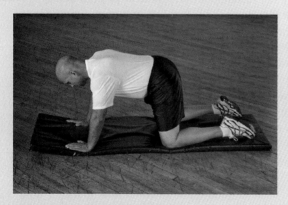 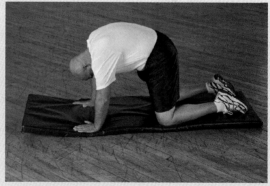

■ Back Stretch (Fig. 8.17)

Get onto hands and knees with hands shoulder width apart, knees hip width apart, abdominals contracted, and spine in neutral. Contract abdominals as if pulling the naval toward the vertebral column while rounding the back toward the ceiling. Allow head and neck to fall naturally between arms. Hold. Return to start.

NUTRITIONAL CONSIDERATIONS

According to the Johns Hopkins Arthritis Center, little scientific evidence confirms a relationship between diet and the development or management of arthritis. In fact, this organization claims that scientists are "no closer to knowing whether food components cause or cure arthritis than [they] were seventy years ago." Most research has investigated the influence of dietary manipulations on rheumatoid arthritis rather than on other forms of arthritis. Based on current evidence, it appears that a balanced, varied diet—appropriate for the general population—is also appropriate for those with RA. Specifically, RA sufferers should balance kilocalorie intake with energy expenditure to maintain a healthy weight; include fruits, vegetables, and whole grains, which contain antioxidants that help fight inflammation; choose low fat, low saturated fat, and low cholesterol products to maintain healthy blood lipids; consume moderate amounts of sugar to avoid weight gain; and drink alcohol in moderation, if at all.[31,38]

QUICK REFERENCE

High dietary protein intake, particularly from red meat, is associated with an increased risk of developing RA.[39]

Dietary evaluations suggest that many RA sufferers are deficient in protein and energy. The reason for this is not clear. Perhaps it is because chronic inflammation elevates metabolic rate, so sufferers actually need more energy in general. Increasing both kilocalorie and plant-based protein intake can solve this problem.

Another nutritional problem results from arthritis medication. Some medications interfere with vitamin and/or mineral absorption and handling, so RA sufferers taking long-term prescriptions should inquire about nutrient/drug interactions. The most common deficiencies occur with folic acid, vitamin C, vitamin D, vitamin E, vitamin B_6, vitamin B_{12}, calcium, magnesium, zinc, and selenium; therefore, those with RA are often encouraged to take a multivitamin/mineral supplement to prevent these deficiencies.[38,40] Of course, food sources are always best, but in instances where intake falls below need, a supplement providing 100% of daily requirements is safe and effective.[38]

Researchers are investigating the effects of omega-3 fatty acids on RA since these fatty acids act as anti-inflammatories. Although *dietary* sources appear to help control systemic inflammation, the effect of *supplements* is not yet clear. In addition, some fatty acid supplements are dangerous because they derive from fish skin and might contain hazardous amounts of mercury. Another problem with taking supplemental omega-3 is that excesses prolong bleeding time. Consequently, current evidence suggests that people try to obtain omega-3 fatty acids from dietary sources only. Good dietary sources include fatty fish, flaxseeds, flaxseed oil, canola oil, walnuts, and soy products.[41]

RA sufferers with food hypersensitivities should avoid any food that exacerbates symptoms. To determine which foods promote flare-ups, totally eliminate a suspicious food and gradually reintroduce it back into the diet to discover if it elicits symptoms.[38]

An abundance of research supports the idea that diet prevents and helps manage osteoporosis. The remainder of this section, therefore, discusses dietary strategies for preserving bone tissue and slowing the rate of bone loss.

VITAMINS AND MINERALS

Several vitamins and minerals are necessary for normal bone remodeling. These include calcium; potassium; magnesium; copper; zinc; and vitamins D, K, A, and C. This section explores those that contribute the greatest to bone health.

Calcium and Vitamin D

Calcium is the key to healthy bone development because it is the major constituent of bone matrix. Calcium absorption from the digestive tract requires vitamin D because vitamin D stimulates the formation of calcium receptors in the small intestinal wall. Without receptors, dietary calcium cannot be absorbed and is therefore unavailable to the body. This is why calcium and vitamin D are often discussed together. It is also the reason why most high-calcium foods are fortified with vitamin D.

Some research suggests that maternal intake of calcium and vitamin D during fetal development affects the offspring's peak bone mass potential. In fact, a calcium and vitamin D deficiency during gestation positively correlates with low bone mass and increased bone deterioration later in the offspring's life, despite the offspring's intake.[42]

All studies agree that adequate dietary calcium and vitamin D intake during the peak bone-building years of childhood and adolescence is essential for achieving optimal peak bone mass. By achieving optimal peak bone mass, the progressive age-related loss of bone is less detrimental. Those who do not obtain an adequate intake during peak bone building years do not develop a healthy skeleton and are predisposed to a lower-than-normal bone mass as adults.[42–44]

Adequate calcium and vitamin D intake *after* the peak-bone-building years is still important to preserve existing bone tissue and slow osteoporosis development. If dietary intake is low, the body catabolizes bone tissue to ensure that blood levels remain within normal limits (remember the significance of blood calcium). Table 8.7 provides recommended intake levels of calcium and vitamin D.

Calcium is found abundantly in milk, milk products, sardines with bones, broccoli, legumes, and tofu. Vitamin D, on the other hand, is naturally found in very few foods. It is added to milk and fortified cereal and is naturally found in salmon, tuna, and mackerel. Smaller amounts are in liver, cheese, and egg yolk. Although the body cannot make calcium, it *can* make vitamin D when exposed to UV radiation from the sun. As little as 5 to 30 minutes of sun exposure on 2 to 3 days per week stimulates the production of enough vitamin D to meet needs.[45] Be aware that sunblock not only protects the skin from UV damage, but it also limits the body's ability to activate vitamin D. Therefore, exposure must be in the absence of sunblock, which also increases the risk for sunburn and skin cancer.

Age	Recommended Intake for Calcium (AI; mg/day)	Recommended Intake for Vitamin D (AI; μg/day)
1–3	500	5
4–8	800	5
9–18	1,300	5
19–50	1,000	5
51–70	1,200	10
>70	1,200	15
Pregnant women	1,000	5

TABLE 8-7 CALCIUM AND VITAMIN D RECOMMENDATIONS

Women rarely meet their needs for calcium and vitamin D, and since they tend to have a lower peak bone mass than men, they are at an increased risk for developing weak bones. Some authorities, therefore, recommend 1,500 mg per day of calcium for post-menopausal women who are not on hormone replacement therapy.

QUICK REFERENCE

The tolerable upper intake level for calcium is 2,500 mg per day. Intakes above this tend to promote constipation and the formation of urinary stones. They also interfere with the absorption of other minerals. The tolerable upper intake level for vitamin D is 50 μg per day. Symptoms of excessive intake include elevated blood calcium levels, calcification of soft tissues, and frequent urination.

Approximately 70% of the population develops lactose intolerance with age. Lactose intolerance occurs when a person produces insufficient lactase, the enzyme required to break down the primary carbohydrate in dairy products. The average lactose intolerant person produces only 5% to 10% of the amount of lactase produced by the average person. Without lactase, lactose remains in the small intestine where it attracts water. As the small intestine fills with excess water, cramping and bloating develop. In addition, bacteria in the GI tract digest the milk sugar and produce gas and acid as by-products. Gas buildup causes more cramping and frequent episodes of flatulence, both of which can become uncomfortable.

Besides the physical discomfort associated with lactose intolerance, sufferers also often become deficient in calcium and vitamin D since they tend to avoid dairy products altogether. Since dairy products are the major sources of calcium and vitamin D, a lactose intolerant person can quickly lose bone mass as a result of insufficient dietary intake of calcium. Remember: maintenance of blood calcium is critical, so if a dietary source is lacking, the body breaks down bone to replenish blood supplies. This increases the risk for osteoporosis.

Potassium and Magnesium

Studies show that an appropriate level of blood potassium promotes calcium retention by the kidneys. Therefore, potassium indirectly affects bone mass by limiting calcium excretion. If blood levels are normal, the parathyroid glands release minimal parathyroid hormone, which in turn controls osteoclast activity.[44]

Although it does not contribute as significantly to bone structure as calcium, magnesium is a component of the bone matrix as well. In fact, 60% of the body's total magnesium supply is stored in bone. Therefore, those with insufficient dietary magnesium intake tend to have less bone mass than those with a normal magnesium intake. Magnesium also helps transport both calcium and potassium across cell membranes, so it balances intracellular and extracellular levels of these ions. In addition, the pituitary gland, a gland that controls many other glands in the body, requires magnesium to function properly. Without magnesium, the pituitary loses some of its control over other glands, which indirectly causes greater bone resorption.[1,44]

Vitamin C

Among its many functions, vitamin C is necessary for collagen synthesis. Collagen is a structural protein that makes up about 25% of bone tissue. Without adequate collagen, bones become weak, malformed, and painful, and the risk for fracture increases.

Sodium

It seems plausible that a high dietary sodium intake indirectly contributes to bone loss because as sodium intake increases, calcium excretion by the kidneys increases. As more and more calcium escapes through urine—and if calcium is not replaced through the diet—blood calcium levels drop. If calcium levels drop, hormones are released to stimulate osteoclast activity and inhibit osteoblast activity in an effort to restore blood levels.

A few studies indicate that high salt diets do not affect blood calcium levels in healthy adults *as long as calcium intake is adequate*. In other words, though calcium excretion increases on high salt diets, this increase does not affect bone structure if adequate dietary intake replaces lost calcium.[46] On the other hand, a large-scale study in which postmenopausal women were put on high sodium diets found an increased calcium excretion followed by a greater bone turnover rate. This suggests that high dietary sodium promotes bone loss. (This study did not mention whether or not dietary calcium intake was adequate.)[44]

Overall, the actual relationship between sodium intake and bone loss is still controversial.[44,47,48] One consistent finding is that a high salt intake coupled with an increased potassium intake from fruits and vegetables limits bone breakdown and calcium excretion, so perhaps potassium supplements can slow the rate of bone loss associated with high salt diets.[44,48]

Vitamin A

Vitamin A is necessary for osteoclasts to break down bone tissue.[44] Keep in mind that bone resorption is essential for remodeling because old bone tissue must be removed to make way for new, healthier bone tissue. The RDA for vitamin A differs in men and women. Men require 900 μg per day, while women require 700 μg per day. Excessive intakes might promote bone loss by overstimulating osteoclasts. Therefore, an upper level of 3,000 μg per day is suggested to avoid this and other symptoms of a vitamin A toxicity.

PROTEINS, CARBOHYDRATES, AND FATS

Proteins have such diverse functions that the body could not operate optimally without a continual and adequate supply. Proteins form structures, act as enzymes, regulate fluid and acid/base balance, and participate in transport.

The protein collagen forms the foundation of bone tissue. As mentioned, bone becomes weak, brittle, and susceptible to fracture when collagen is deficient. Therefore, adequate dietary protein is necessary to ensure adequate collagen availability during bone remodeling.

Enzymes, which are catalysts that facilitate chemical reactions, are also necessary for each step of the remodeling process. With inadequate protein supplies, enzyme availability decreases and reactions slow. Additionally, there also seems to be a direct interaction between dietary protein and calcium; however, whether or not protein enhances or hinders the handling of calcium is still uncertain.

Protein availability also indirectly affects bone mass. If dietary protein intake falls, the body sacrifices muscle to ensure an adequate supply. As muscle mass diminishes, participation in physical activity decreases, so bones are no longer subjected to the mechanical stresses they need to remain healthy and strong. Ultimately, this impairs bone deposition, enhances bone resorption, and promotes bone loss.

The RDA for protein is listed in Table 8.8. Another means of calculating the daily requirement for protein is to multiply weight in kilograms by 0.8 g of PRO per day. This intake is sufficient to meet the needs of most adults.

Research is currently investigating the effects of varying amounts of protein on the integrity of bone tissue. Short-term studies have shown a positive correlation between *excessive* protein intake and an increased calcium excretion of up to 50%. They have also implicated high protein diets with diminished bone mass. Other studies suggest a positive correlation between *low* protein intake and the risk for bone loss and fracture in various

TABLE 8-8 RDA FOR PROTEIN	
Age	RDA for Protein (g/day)
Men > 19	56
Women > 19	46
Pregnant women	+25

groups, so too little protein negatively affects bone structure as well. Additionally, the *source* of protein also seems to affect bone health. Several studies found animal sources of protein to be negatively correlated with bone fracture.[44,49,50] Weikert et al., however, found that plant sources of protein preserve bone tissue more than animal sources. Apparently, the precise effect of abnormal protein intake on healthy bone formation varies depending upon the actual intake level and source, so further research is needed before drawing conclusions. Ensure an adequate intake of protein, particularly in seniors who are often deficient in this nutrient.

The effects of carbohydrates and fats on bone tissue have not been thoroughly investigated; therefore, it is suggested that those with bone and joint disorders follow recommendations for the general population. Carbohydrates should constitute 45% to 65% of total daily kilocalorie intake. The RDA suggests a *minimum* of 130 g per day to meet basic needs. Fats should comprise 20% to 35% of total daily kilocalorie intake with a maximum of 10% from saturated and trans fats. The result of one study showed a positive correlation between dietary saturated fat intake and low bone mass—particularly in men—so complying with the general guidelines can prevent bone loss.[51]

SMOKING AND ALCOHOL

Neither cigarettes nor alcohol are nutrients; however, smoking and excessive alcohol consumption damage bone tissue, so they are worthy of mention.[52,53] Across all age groups and physical activity levels, smokers have a lower bone mass than nonsmokers. Why? First of all, smokers are typically vitamin D–deficient, a factor that diminishes calcium absorption in the GI tract. Additionally, blood levels of cysteine, an amino acid necessary for collagen synthesis, are low, so the rate of new bone formation drops since collagen is not available for structure. Homocysteine levels of smokers are also elevated. High levels of this amino acid appear to stimulate osteoclast activity, which further decreases bone mass.[52] Furthermore, women who smoke have a 40% to 50% increased risk for hip fracture, and since hip fracture, particularly in the elderly, is associated with increased morbidity and mortality, smoking should be avoided. Overall, the components of cigarettes deprive body cells—including bone cells—of the oxygen required for normal cell functioning, growth, repair, and division; therefore, they detrimentally affect all cells in the body. Fortunately, the body is resilient, so most of the damage incurred from tobacco use is reversed when smoking is stopped.

Moderate alcohol consumption—defined as 1 to 2 alcoholic beverages per day—has no detrimental effect on bone.[44,54,55] In fact, studies show that moderate alcohol consumption is associated with a lower rate of bone loss, perhaps because of its positive influence on the rate of bone remodeling.[44] Excessive alcohol intake, however, correlates with poor bone health for various reasons. First, it increases the risk of falling because it impairs balance and control centers in the brain. This increases the likelihood of fractures, especially in those with low bone mass. Secondly, alcohol acts as a diuretic and increases fluid loss. Accompanying the lost fluid are various electrolytes, including calcium. Additionally, alcohol interferes with the liver's ability to produce enzymes necessary for vitamin D activation. Without vitamin D, the GI tract cannot absorb dietary calcium. Since calcium is a major component of the bone matrix, a deficiency results in insufficient bone mass. Alcohol can also damage the pancreas, an organ that produces most of the enzymes necessary for digestion in the small intestine. Without these enzymes, food is not broken down completely, so nutrients are not accessible. Furthermore, alcohol inhibits osteoblast activity, so the rate of bone deposition slows. It also enhances osteoclast activity, so bone breakdown accelerates. Lastly, excessive alcohol consumption interferes with normal hormone levels in such a way that bone loss is favored. For instance, it increases levels of parathyroid hormone, a hormone that stimulates osteoclast activity and inhibits osteoblast activity. Alcohol also lowers blood concentrations of testosterone and estrogen in men and women, respectively. An earlier section explained how low levels of these hormones detrimentally affect bone health. Excessive alcohol consumption also correlates positively with cortisol levels, a hormone that slows osteoblast activity and increases osteoclast activity. High cortisol levels, therefore, increase the rate of bone loss, which promotes osteoporosis development.[45,56]

SUPPLEMENTS

As with most other populations, those with bone and joint disorders should strive to obtain adequate nutrition from dietary sources rather than from supplements. For those who cannot consume enough calcium-rich foods to meet daily requirements, however, supplements (500 to 1,200 mg per day) might be necessary. An individual calcium supplement, as opposed to a multivitamin/mineral, is preferable because multivitamin/minerals contain very little calcium. Most individual calcium supplements contain between 250 and 1,000 mg of calcium per dose, but read the label to be sure. Antacids and caramel chewables contain calcium carbonate, but calcium carbonate is actually only 40% calcium. Other sources might contain calcium citrate, but calcium citrate is only 21% calcium. If the source is lactate, only 13% is calcium. It is best to take smaller dosages several times per day rather than an entire day's worth at once because the digestive tract handles and absorbs amounts ≤500 mg at a time better than it does larger doses. Smaller doses also decrease the risk of constipation, gas, and bloating that often accompany larger doses.

Some calcium supplements are made from oyster shells, limestone, or bone meal. Be careful with these because they often contain lead, a heavy metal that accumulates in the blood and body cells and can cause irreversible neurological damage, heart problems, and kidney disease.

Because vitamin D is found in very few foods, vitamin D supplements are sometimes advised for seniors and anyone else who does not get regular sun exposure. Low vitamin D intake is associated with hip fracture, but supplemental vitamin D (up to 800 IU per day) coupled with calcium supplements significantly reduces this risk in elderly individuals.[44] The National Institutes of Health suggests supplementing the diet with 700 to 800 IU of vitamin D and 500 to 1,200 mg of calcium to decrease the risk of fractures and bone loss in those over the age of 62. See Table 8.9 for tips on how to increase dietary intake of vitamin D.

TABLE 8-9 TIPS FOR INCREASING DIETARY INTAKE OF VITAMIN D

- Consume various fruits, vegetables, and whole grains for overall health
- Include vitamin D–fortified cereals in the diet
- Consume vitamin D–fortified fat-free or low-fat milk
- Add vitamin D–fortified yogurt and orange juice to the diet
- Increase dietary intake of fish such as salmon, tuna, and mackerel; they are naturally rich in vitamin D
- Include an occasional serving of liver or eggs in the diet; they naturally have small amounts of vitamin D
- Use a vitamin D–fortified margarine instead of butter

Source: National Institutes of Health. www.nih.gov

SUMMARY

Although formerly thought to be detrimental for those with preexisting osteoporosis or arthritis, exercise is now recognized as a safe and beneficial adjunct to traditional therapies. For those with osteoporosis, exercise prevents further bone loss and might even build bone mass if intensity is adequate. Even if bone mass does not increase, exercise reduces the overall risk for heart disease, stroke, diabetes, high blood pressure, and various other diseases. For those with arthritis, exercise preserves or restores normal joint functioning and thereby increases functional capacity. Furthermore, it reduces inflammation, improves joint stability, and reduces pain. In fact, exercise is the only mode of treatment for osteoarthritis that offers as much pain relief as medications.

CASE STUDY

A 65-year-old overweight woman with mild osteoporosis and osteoarthritis in her left wrist would like to begin an exercise program. She has no other arthritic joints.

- How would you approach this client?
- What information would you need before beginning?
- What are some realistic expectations and goals for this client?
- What nutritional advice would you offer?

THINKING CRITICALLY

1. Which hormones affect bone remodeling? Discuss their actions.
2. How do diet and exercise affect bone mass?

3. List and explain some of the age-related changes in bone.
4. What are some factors that determine the range of motion permitted by a joint? Explain.
5. Describe the development of osteoarthritis. What factors contribute to it? What can be done to prevent it?
6. Describe rheumatoid arthritis. What factors contribute to it? What can be done to reduce the symptoms?
7. What are some precautions necessary when working with this special population? List several benefits of exercise.
8. Explain why calcium intake is still necessary for those beyond their bone-building years. Describe the role of vitamin D in this process.
9. How does cigarette smoking affect bone integrity?
10. Explain protein's role in bone structure.

REFERENCES

1. National Osteoporosis Foundation. www.nof.org
2. Centers for Disease Control. www.cdc.gov
3. Falahati-Nini A, Riggs B, Atkinson E, et al. Relative contributions of testosterone and estrogen in regulating bone resorption and formation in normal elderly men. J Clin Invest 2000;106:1553–1560.
4. Leder B, LeBlanc K, Schoenfeld D, Eastell R, Finkelstein J. Differential effects of androgens and estrogens on bone turnover in normal men. J Clin Endocrinol Metab 2003;88:204–210.
5. Szulc P, Marchand F, Duboeuf F, Delmas P. Cross-sectional assessment of age-related bone loss in men: the MINOS study. Bone 2000;26:123–129.
6. Bass S, Pearce G, Bradney M, et al. Exercise before puberty may confer residual benefits in bone density in adulthood: studies in active prepubertal and retired gymnasts. J Bone Miner Res 1998;13(3):500–507.
7. Hamell J, Knutzen K. Biomechanical Basis of Human Movement. 2nd Ed. Baltimore: Lippincott Williams & Wilkins, 2003.
8. Pool A, Axford J. The effects of exercise on the hormonal and immune systems in rheumatoid arthritis. Rheumatology 2001;40:610–614.
9. Stenstrom C, Minor M. Evidence for the benefit of aerobic and strengthening exercise in rheumatoid arthritis. Arthritis Rheum 2003;49(3):428–434.
10. Kettunen J, Kujala U. Exercise therapy for people with rheumatoid arthritis and osteoarthritis. Scand J Med Sci Sports 2004;14(3):138–142.
11. Hughes S, Seymour R, Campbell R, et al. Impact of the fit and strong intervention on older adults with osteoarthritis. Gerontologist 2004;44(2):217–228.
12. Bergstrom I, Landgren B, Brinck J, Freyschuss B. Physical training preserves bone mineral density in postmenopausal women with forearm fractures and low bone mineral density. Osteoporos Int 2008;19(2):177–183.
13. Zechnacker C, Bemis-Dougherty A. Effect of weighted exercises on bone mineral density in post menopausal women: a systematic review. J Geriatr Phys Ther 2007;30(2):79–88.
14. Huntoon E, Schmidt C, Mehrsheed S. Significantly fewer refractures after vertebroplasty in patients who engage in back-extensor-strengthening exercises. Mayo Clin Proc Rochester 2008;83(1): 54–57.
15. Jan M, Lin J, Liau J, et al. Investigation of clinical effects of high- and low-resistance training for patients with knee osteoarthritis: a randomized controlled trial. Phys Ther 2008;88(4):427–436.
16. Metsios G, Stavropoulos-Kalinoglou A, Veldhuijzen van Zanten J, et al. Rheumatoid arthritis, cardiovascular disease and physical exercise: a systematic review. Rheumatology 2008;47(3):239–248.
17. Resnick B. Managing arthritis with exercise. Geriatr Nurs 2001;22(3):143–150.
18. Christie A, Jamtvedt G, Thuve Dahm K, et al. Effectiveness of nonpharmacological and nonsurgical interventions for patients with rheumatoid arthritis: an overview of systematic reviews. Phys Ther 2007;87(12):1697–2013.
19. Moe R, Haavardsholm E, Christie A, et al. Effectiveness of nonpharmacological and nonsurgical

interventions for hip osteoarthritis: an umbrella review of high-quality systematic reviews. Phys Ther 2007;87(12):1716–1713.

20. Young C, Weeks B, Bech B. Simple, novel physical activity maintains proximal femur bone mineral density, and improves muscle strength and balance in sedentary, postmenopausal Caucasian women. Osteoporos Int New York. 2007;1(10):1379–1387.

21. Koster A, Patel K, Visser M, et al. Joint effects of adiposity and physical activity on incident mobility limitation in older adults. J Am Geriatr Soc 2008; 56(4):636.

22. Dalbeth N, Arroll B. Commentary: controversies in NICE guidance on osteoarthritis. Br Med J 2008;336:504.

23. de Jong O, Hopman-Rock M, Tak E, et al. An implementation study of two evidence-based exercise and health education programs for older adults with osteoarthritis of the knee and hip. Health Educ Res 2004;19(3):316–325.

24. Jamtvedt G, Dahm K, Christie A, et al. Physical therapy interventions for patients with osteoarthritis of the knee: an overview of systematic reviews. Phys Ther 2008;88(1):123–131.

25. Cox R, Thomas T, Hinton P, et al. Effects of acute bouts of aerobic exercise of varied intensity on subjective mood experiences in women of different age groups across time. J Sport Behav 2006;29(1):40–58.

26. Elavsky S, McAuley E. Physical activity and mental health outcomes during menopause: a randomized controlled trial. Ann Behav Med 2007; 33(2):132.

27. Knubben K, Reischies F, Adli M, et al. A randomised, controlled study on the effects of a short-term endurance training programme in patients with major depression. Br J Sports Med 2007;41(1):29.

28. Lee M, Pittler M, Ernst E. Tai chi for rheumatoid arthritis: systematic review. Rheumatology 2007; 46(11):1648–1651.

29. Sarsan A, Ardic F, Ozgen M, et al. The effects of aerobic and resistance exercises in obese women. Clin Rehabil 2006;20(9):773.

30. American College of Sports Medicine. ACSM's Guidelines for Exercise Testing and Prescription. 8th Ed. Philadelphia: Lippincott Williams & Wilkins, 2010:225–228,256–258.

31. Arthritis Foundation. www.arthritis.org

32. Ashe M. Exercise prescription. J Am Acad Orthop Surg 2004;12(1):21–27.

33. Mayo Clinic. www.mayoclinic.com

34. Brooke-Wavell K, Jones P, Hardman AE, et al. Commencing, continuing, and stopping brisk walking: effects on bone mineral density, quantitative ultrasound of bone and markers of bone metabolism in postmenopausal women. Osteoporos Int 2001;12:581–587.

35. Nelson M, Fiatarone M, Morganti C, et al. Effects of high-intensity strength training on multiple risk factors for osteoporosis fractures: a randomized controlled trial. J Am Med Assoc 1994;272:1909–1914.

36. Ettinger W, Burns R, Messier S, et al. A randomized trial comparing aerobic exercise and resistance exercise with a health education program in older adults with knee osteoarthritis. The Fitness Arthritis and Seniors Trial (FAST). J Am Med Assoc 1997;277(1):25–31.

37. Minor M, Hewett J, Webel R, et al. Efficacy of physical conditioning exercise in patients with rheumatoid arthritis and osteoarthritis. Arthritis Rheum 1989;32(11):1396–1405.

38. The Johns Hopkins Arthritis Center. www.hopkins-arthritis.org

39. Tufts University. Cut the red meat to reduce Rheumatoid Arthritis risk. Tufts Univ Health Nutr Letter 2005;23(1):8.

40. Bae S, Kim S, Sung M, et al. Inadequate antioxidant nutrient intake and altered plasma antioxidant status of rheumatoid arthritis patients. J Am Coll Nutr 2003;22:311–315.

41. Tufts University. Anti-inflammatory eating. Tufts Univ Health Nutr Letter 2004;21(12):4–6.

42. Cooper C, Westlake S, Harvey N, et al. Review: developmental origins of osteoporotic fracture. Osteoporos Int 2006;17(3):337.

43. Swanenburg J, Douwe de Bruin E, Stauffacher M, et al. Effects of exercise and nutrition on postural balance and risk fo falling in elderly people with decreased bone mineral density: randomized controlled trial pilot study. Clin Rehabil 2007; 21(6):523–534.

44. Tucker K. Dietary intake and bone status with aging. Curr Pharm Des 2003;9(32):2687.

45. National Institutes of Health. www.nih.gov

46. Natri A, Karkkainen M, Ruusunen M, et al. A 7-week reduction in salt intake does not contribute to markers of bone metabolism inyoung healthy subjects. Eur J Clin Nutr 2005;59(3):311–313.

47. Atkinson S, Ward W. Clinical nutrition: 2. The role of nutrition in the prevention and treatment of adult osteoporosis. Can Med Assoc 2001;165(11):1511–1514.

48. Burger H, Grobbee D, Drueke T. Osteoporosis and salt intake. Nutr Metab Cardiovasc Dis 2000; 10(1):46–53.
49. Budek A, Hoppe C, Ingstrup H, et al. Dietary protein intake and bone mineral content in adolescents—The Copenhagen Cohort Study. Osteoporos Int 2007;18(12):1661–1667.
50. Weikert C, Walter D, Hoffmann K, et al. The relation between dietary protein, calcium and bone health in women: results from the EPIC-potsdam cohort. Ann Nutr Metab 2005;49(5):312.
51. Corwin R, Hartman T, Maczuga S, et al. Dietary saturated fat intake is inversely associated with bone density in humans: analysis of NHANES III1,2. J Nutr 2006;136(1):159–164.
52. Baines M, Kredan M, Davison A, et al. The association between cysteine, bone turnover, and low bone mass. Calcif Tissue Int 2007;81(6): 450–454.
53. Naves M, Diaz-Lopez J, Gomez C, et al. Prevalence of osteoporosis in men and determinants of changes in bone mass in a non-selected Spanish population. Osteoporos Int 2005;16(6):603.
54. McClung B. Reducing your risk of osteoporosis. Nurs Manag 2001;April, Suppl.:4–5,8.
55. Williams F. The effect of moderate alcohol consumption on bone mineral density: a study of female twins. Ann Rheum Dis 2004. Doi:10.1136/ard.2004.022269.
56. National Institute on Alcohol Abuse and Alcoholism. www.niaaa.nih.gov
57. Bonjour J, Theintz G, Law F, et al. Peak bone mass. Osteoporos Int 1994;4(Suppl 1):7–13.

SUGGESTED READINGS

Arthritis Foundation website. www.arthritis.org
Fischer H, Yu W. What to do When the Doctor Says it's Rheumatoid Arthritis. MA: Fair Winds, 2005.
Lane, N. The Osteoporosis Book: A Guide for Patients and Their Families. NY: Oxford University Press, 2001.
National Institute of Arthritis and Musculoskeletal and Skin Disease. www.niams.nih.gov
Sanson, G. The Myth of Osteoporosis. Ann Arbor, MI: MCD Century Publications, 2003.

EXERCISE FOR PEOPLE WITH DIABETES

9

According to statistics from the American Diabetes Association (ADA), 7% of the American population, which includes 20.8 million adults and children, suffer from diabetes. Because certain ethnic groups have an increased risk for developing diabetes, they must be aware of indications (Table 9.1). Diagnosis is the first crucial step in preventing many diabetes-associated complications, but, sadly, only 14.6 million sufferers know that they have this condition. The remaining 6.2 million victims are completely oblivious and are therefore at an increased risk for developing long-term organ system damage. A condition called "prediabetes" affects an additional 54 million people in the United States and is associated with an increased risk for heart disease and stroke. Also known as impaired glucose tolerance, prediabetes exists when a person does not specifically meet the criteria for diabetes but experiences higher than normal blood glucose levels. Those classified with prediabetes tend to develop type 2 diabetes within 10 years.

Physicians typically use one of three tests to diagnose diabetes.[1,2] The fasting plasma glucose (FPG) test is the easiest to administer. It requires that the patient abstain from eating for at least 8 hours after which blood glucose is measured. A normal value for blood glucose under these conditions is ≤99 mg/dL. A reading of 100 to 125 mg/dL suggests prediabetes, while a measure of 126 mg/dL indicates diabetes. A physician usually performs this test at least two times before confirming a diagnosis.

The oral glucose tolerance test (OGT) is not as convenient as the FPG, but it is much more reliable. Like the FPG, it requires 8 hours of fasting followed by a blood glucose measurement. After this initial assessment, the patient must consume a liquid containing 75 g of glucose. The physician then measures blood glucose levels again 2 hours after ingestion to determine if diabetes or prediabetes exists. A normal value for blood glucose 2 hours after consuming the glucose drink is ≤139 mg/dL. A reading of 140 to 199 mg/dL suggests prediabetes, while a measure of ≥200 mg/dL indicates diabetes. As with the FPG test, a physician performs this test at least two times before confirming diabetes.

TABLE 9-1	PREVALENCE OF DIABETES ACROSS ETHNIC GROUPS, 2005
Alaska Natives/American Indians	17.9%
Non-Hispanic African Americans	15.4%
Hispanic Americans	13.8%
Non-Hispanic Caucasians	8.7%

Source: American Diabetic Association. www.diabetes.org

   The random plasma glucose test (RPG), which is effective in determining diabetes but not as reliable for prediabetes, measures blood glucose levels without requiring a fasting period. A reading of ≥200 mg/dL suggests diabetes if the patient also complains of frequent urination, excessive thirst, and unexplained weight loss. To confirm the diagnosis, a physician usually follows the RPG test with an FPG or OGT.

   Those who are diagnosed with diabetes must stay alert for diabetes-associated complications such as high blood pressure, heart disease, stroke, liver damage, **retinopathy**, **neuropathy**, **nephropathy**, and poor circulatory problems that often necessitate amputation. Furthermore, those suffering from diabetes are frequently more susceptible to rheumatoid arthritis as well as respiratory illnesses such as influenza and pneumonia.[2,3] Because of the devastating system-wide effects of diabetes, early diagnosis and treatment that slows deterioration are critical. Managing diabetes requires careful planning to ensure a long and healthy life. This chapter addresses how exercise and diet improve the outcome of living with diabetes.

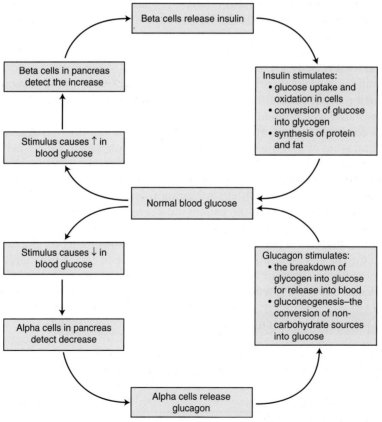

FIGURE 9.1 ■ Negative feedback loop for insulin and glucagon.

ANATOMICAL AND PHYSIOLOGICAL CHANGES

The pancreas is composed of two different types of tissues. The *exocrine* cells, arranged in clusters called acini, play an important role in digestion; they produce most of the enzymes necessary to break down carbohydrates, proteins, and fats prior to absorption. In addition, they release bicarbonate to neutralize the acidic contents moving into the small intestine from the stomach since pancreatic enzymes cannot function effectively in a low-pH environment.

The *endocrine* cells, arranged in islets of Langerhans, produce hormones that maintain blood glucose levels at **homeostasis**. Blood glucose levels are kept within narrow limits to ensure that body cells receive a continuous supply. The islets of Langerhans, which make up only 1% to 2% of the total number of cells in the pancreas, closely monitor and regulate blood glucose through a process called **negative feedback** (Fig. 9.1). Blood glucose levels are critical because most body cells prefer to use glucose for fuel. The islets of Langerhans within the pancreas contain various cell types that enable it to accomplish this task. The two most important pancreatic cells are the α cells and the β cells. α cells produce the hormone **glucagon**, while β cells produce the hormone **insulin**. The α cells release glucagon when blood glucose levels drop as occurs in between meals. Glucagon then travels to the liver, the only organ with glucagon receptors, where it sets into motion a series of events that returns

---

Retinopathy—a condition that affects the retina of the eye. Occurs as elevated blood glucose damages small blood vessels like those serving the eye. This damage can ultimately result in blindness. Retinopathy affects up to 80% of those who have had diabetes for 15 years or more.

Neuropathy—any disease of the nervous system. Symptoms include tingling, numbness, pain, swelling, or weakness—typically in the extremities.

Nephropathy—a progressive kidney disorder that damages the structural units of the kidneys.

Homeostasis—a state that exists when the internal environment of the body is maintained at optimal conditions for functioning. Chronic homeostatic imbalances cause illness. Through negative feedback, the body has the ability to maintain relatively constant internal conditions despite an ever-changing external environment. Blood glucose levels, body temperature, blood pH levels, and blood pressure are examples of conditions maintained at homeostasis.

Negative feedback—a mechanism used to maintain homeostasis that involves receptors, a control center, and effectors. Receptors continuously monitor internal conditions and relay information to the control center. The control center establishes a set point for any given condition. This set point is the range at which the body functions optimally. If the control center detects a deviation from the set point, it activates effectors to restore normal conditions. As soon as conditions are normal, the effectors are inhibited.

Glucagon—a hormone produced by α cells in the pancreas. It stimulates the liver to release glucose into the blood.

Insulin—a hormone produced by β cells in the pancreas that facilitates the movement of glucose into liver and muscle cells.

blood glucose levels to normal. These events include **glycogenolysis**, **gluconeogenesis**, **lipolysis**, amino acid uptake into liver cells, and ketone body formation. Glycogenolysis and gluconeogenesis directly increase blood glucose concentrations. Glycogenolysis occurs as the liver breaks down and releases its stored glucose into the blood for use by other body cells. Simultaneously, the liver converts certain amino acids into glucose whenever its **glycogen** supply dwindles. As the demand for glucose continues, more and more amino acids move into the liver so that the liver can continue gluconeogenesis. The synthesis and release of ketone bodies into the blood actually has a glucose-sparing effect. When energy needs are

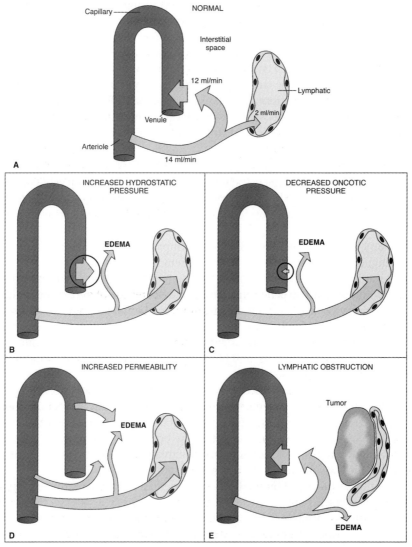

FIGURE 9.2 ■ Mechanisms of edema formation. (Image from Rubin E, Farber JL. Pathology. 3rd Ed. Philadelphia: Lippincott Williams & Wilkins, 1999.)

high, both skeletal and cardiac muscles easily use ketone bodies for fuel. By supplying these muscle cells with an alternative to glucose, the liver frees up circulating glucose for cells that rely solely on glucose (such as neurons).

β cells in the pancreas produce and release insulin in response to an increase in blood glucose. Glucose levels typically rise relatively rapidly after a meal. As the digestive system breaks down carbohydrates into smaller subunits—many of which are glucose molecules—glucose enters the blood and travels to the liver and other organs. Essentially, β cells in the pancreas detect rising blood glucose levels and release insulin in response. Insulin levels typically peak within 10 minutes following a meal.[4] Circulating insulin then binds to receptors on liver and muscle cells thereby opening channels that permit glucose entry. If energy demands are high, cells immediately convert glucose into a usable form of energy (**adenosine triphosphate [ATP]**) and use that energy to fuel cellular processes. If energy demands are low, the cells store glucose as glycogen through the process of **glycogenesis**. As blood glucose levels normalize, typically between 2 and 4 hours after a meal, the β cells respond by slowing their insulin release. A problem arises, however, if insulin is unable to bind to its receptors or if insufficient insulin is present. In these cases, blood glucose levels reach dangerously high levels because glucose cannot enter most body cells without insulin's action. Nerve cells and liver cells are exceptions; they do not require insulin to access glucose. In cases where blood glucose levels soar despite the presence of insulin, the pancreas continues to produce and release insulin in an attempt to correct the ever-increasing blood glucose levels. Eventually, this results in excess levels of insulin in the blood. Excess insulin promotes the development of insulin resistance, high blood pressure, increased sodium retention with subsequent **edema** (Fig. 9.2), elevated **homocysteine** levels, and possibly osteoporosis.

Glycogenolysis—breakdown of glycogen and subsequent release of glucose into blood.

Gluconeogenesis—the formation of glucose from noncarbohydrate sources such as amino acids, lactic acid, glycerol, and pyruvate.

Lipolysis—breakdown of fats and release of fatty acids into the blood.

Glycogen—the storage form of glucose. The liver converts its glycogen back into glucose to maintain normal blood glucose levels in between meals.

Adenosine triphosphate (ATP)—a high-energy molecule used for most cellular processes. Although glucose is the ultimate fuel for the body, the energy stored within its bonds is not usable until converted into ATP.

Glycogenesis—formation of glycogen in muscle and liver cells.

Edema—fluid accumulation in the spaces in between cells. Results in swelling accompanied by pain, reduced range-of-motion, and discomfort.

Homocysteine—an amino acid that floats freely in the blood. Formed from the amino acid methionine when methionine loses a methyl group. The body usually reconverts homocysteine back into methionine, or it alters it to form the amino acid cysteine. The blood normally contains low levels of homocysteine. High levels are associated with an increased risk of heart disease, stroke, and birth defects.

TABLE 9-2   EFFECTS OF INSULIN ON MUSCLE, LIVER, AND FAT CELLS

Stimulates glucose uptake in muscle cells and adipocytes

Stimulates **glycogenesis** in liver and muscle cells

Inhibits glycogenolysis in liver and muscle cells

Stimulates amino acid uptake into muscle cells

Stimulates fatty acid transport and triglyceride formation in adipocytes and liver cells

Stimulates protein synthesis in all cells while simultaneously inhibiting protein break down

Inhibits lipolysis

Enhances glucose use in cellular respiration by stimulating glycolytic enzymes

Interestingly, stimuli other than blood glucose fluctuations promote glucagon and insulin release. For example, β cells release insulin in response to increasing blood fatty acid levels; the presence of certain small intestine hormones during digestion; and the ingestion of large quantities of the amino acid arginine. The α cells release glucagon when blood levels of fatty acids drop and when large amounts of arginine are consumed in the absence of sufficient carbohydrates. Why would the pancreas release both insulin *and* glucagon in response to the presence of arginine? Consider a situation where a person consumes a high-protein, low-carbohydrate meal and remember that one of insulin's actions is to stimulate protein synthesis. A high-protein meal supplies amino acids for protein synthesis, so insulin is released to support this process. Arginine, in particular, elicits a huge release of insulin. Nevertheless, since insulin simultaneously stimulates glucose uptake, dangerously low blood glucose levels can quickly develop when dietary intake is insufficient. α Cells, therefore, release glucagon to encourage the liver to normalize blood glucose levels with its own supply. Table 9.2 provides a summary of insulin's effects on muscle, liver, and fat cells.

QUICK REFERENCE

The monosaccharide glucose is the preferred source of energy for most body cells. In fact, it is the only source that certain nerve cells use. It can be used to create energy both aerobically and anaerobically and is required for the body to efficiently burn fats. When inadequate glucose is available, the body incompletely breaks down fatty acids and produces ketone bodies as by-products. Excess ketone bodies interrupt normal metabolism as discussed in the next Highlight box.

In general, diabetes occurs when blood glucose levels in the body are chronically elevated, a condition called **hyperglycemia**. Glucose typically accumulates in the blood from either inadequate insulin production or insensitivity to insulin's action. In either case, blood glucose levels rise to dangerous levels.

The two major forms of diabetes are type 1 and type 2 diabetes mellitus. Type 1 diabetes, the less common type, is an autoimmune disorder in which the body's immune

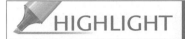
HIGHLIGHT   Hyperglycemia

Hyperglycemia occurs when blood glucose levels remain elevated. It results when the body either produces insufficient insulin or is resistant to insulin's effects. Although uncommon in nondiabetics, it *can* develop in those without diabetes under certain conditions. Mild symptoms of hyperglycemia include sweating, trembling, rapid heart rate, hunger, frequent urination, and increased thirst. Increased urine output and excessive thirst result from the large volume of water lost as the kidneys filter increasing amounts of glucose. Normally, the kidney tubules reabsorb 100% of the filtered glucose; however, when excessive amounts enter the filtrate, the tubules are unable to keep up. Consequently, glucose becomes a component of urine, a condition called glucosuria. A higher glucose concentration in the filtrate and urine creates an osmotic pressure that pulls water out of the kidney's blood vessels. This increases both the volume and frequency of urination. It also results in dehydration and chronic thirst. In addition to these mild symptoms, severe hyperglycemia causes neurological symptoms such as confusion, disorientation, and weakness. Extreme cases might even cause seizure, coma, or death.[4]

In diabetics, hyperglycemia can result in ketoacidosis. Ketoacidosis develops in the following manner: (1) blood glucose levels rise after a meal; (2) insulin release is either insufficient or ineffective; (3) body cells cannot access glucose for fuel, so glucose accumulates in the blood; and (4) body cells are forced to use fatty acids for fuel. During fatty acid oxidation, ketone bodies form. The body can handle normal levels of ketone bodies since many cells use them for energy. As production exceeds elimination, however, problems develop. First of all, the kidneys excrete excess ketone bodies in urine, and these ketone bodies often pull ions such as sodium and potassium along with them. Excess and chronic loss of these ions can promote life-threatening electrolyte imbalances. Second, some ketone bodies are ketoacids. Uncontrolled buildup of ketoacids in the blood lowers blood pH. If blood pH is too low, chemical reactions essential for life do not occur at an appropriate rate. Additionally, a low pH destroys the structure of many proteins, and since structure determines function, physically altered proteins are unable to perform their jobs. Shortness of breath, a fruity odor to the

(continued)

Hyperglycemia—a condition defined by chronically elevated blood glucose levels, even during fasting states. Occasional incidences of hyperglycemia in the absence of a formal diagnosis of diabetes typically suggest the onset of diabetes.

Ketoacidosis—a condition that results when the body is forced to use fatty acids for fuel when glucose is unavailable. By-products of fatty acid oxidation are ketone bodies, many of which are ketoacids. Normally, blood levels of ketoacids are low since the kidneys filter most ketoacids. When produced in excess, as happens when the body must rely on fatty acids for fuel, ketoacids build up in the blood and lower pH. This condition dramatically interferes with metabolism.

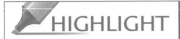 **HIGHLIGHT**   Hyperglycemia (*continued*)

breath, dry mouth, and nausea are symptoms of ketoacidosis.

According to the ADA, common causes of hyperglycemia in the diabetic include inadequate insulin injection prior to a meal or insufficient food intake. Additionally, diabetics exposed to the flu virus or other infections often suffer from excess ketoacids in the blood. Anyone suspecting ketoacidosis should seek immediate medical care.

system destroys β cells in the pancreas. As β cells continue to die, insulin production slows and ultimately ceases. This results in excess blood glucose and the starvation of body cells. Symptoms include extreme feelings of hunger despite normal consumption, severe and systemic weakness, and weight loss. Because of damage to β cells, type 1 diabetics must take **exogenous** insulin in order for their cells to access glucose.

Type 2 diabetes, which accounts for approximately 90% of all diabetes cases, is still not as well understood as type 1 diabetes. The pancreas of a type 2 diabetic usually continues to produce insulin. In fact, it often produces larger-than-normal quantities of insulin. Sometimes, however, the insulin supply is inadequate to meet demands. In either case, liver and muscle cells do not respond to the insulin as expected. Consequently, blood glucose levels rise and force cells to seek other fuel sources.

The first step in the development of type 2 diabetes is insulin resistance. Insulin resistance results when insulin binding does not permit glucose entry into cells or when insulin cannot physically bind to its receptors at all. As glucose accumulates in the blood, the β cells compensate by producing and releasing larger and larger quantities of insulin—to no avail. Glucose continues to build up, thereby causing hyperglycemia. Eventually, the high demand placed on β cells can actually destroy them, so the type 2 diabetic might

TABLE 9-3 RISK FACTORS FOR DIABETES	
Risk Factors for Type I Diabetes	**Risk Factors for Type II Diabetes**
Family history of type 1 diabetes; a child with a parent or sibling with type I diabetes has a 2% to 6% risk for diabetes	Family history of diabetes (either a parent or sibling)
Personal or family history of autoimmune diseases such as celiac disease	Being overweight or obese; 85% of all type 2 diabetics carry excess weight
Exposure to cow's milk before the age of 1	History of gestational diabetes or delivery of a baby weighing ≥9 lb
Cessation of breastfeeding before three months of age	HDL < 35 mg/dL or triglycerides > 250 mg/dL
Early exposure to certain viruses including rubella, Epstein-Barr, and coxsackie B	Blood pressure of 140/90 mm Hg or higher

Sources: Pi-Sunyer, F. How effective are lifestyle changes in the prevention of type 2 diabetes mellitus? Nutr Rev 2007;65(3):101–110; Wyatt L, Ferrance R. The musculoskeletal effects of diabetes mellitus. J Can Chiropractic Assoc 2006;50(1):43–50.

ultimately have to rely on exogenous insulin. Table 9.3 shows risk factors associated with type 1 and type 2 diabetes.

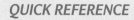

QUICK REFERENCE

According to the International Diabetes Federation, those with metabolic syndrome have a five times greater risk of developing diabetes than those without the syndrome. See Chapters 6 and 7 for further information on metabolic syndrome.

As mentioned earlier, diabetes is associated with additional complications, which include high blood pressure, heart disease, stroke, liver damage, retinopathy, neuropathy, nephropathy, and poor circulation that often result in amputations (Table 9.4). Most of these result from the vascular changes experienced by diabetics as their blood vessel linings are damaged.

High blood pressure develops as elevated blood glucose levels destroy blood vessel walls. Damaged vessels then develop plaques that eventually harden, a condition called atherosclerosis. This triggers a cycle of events that sustain high blood pressure since hardened arteries have narrow passageways that are under increasing pressure from the heart's pumping action. Chronic hypertension then increases the risk for coronary artery disease, heart failure, stroke, and peripheral vascular disease. Peripheral vascular disease, or hardening of the arteries in the lower extremities, restricts blood flow to the legs and thus places extreme demands on the heart. This burden further increases blood pressure. High blood pressure can then rupture inflexible blood vessels supplying the heart or brain. Additionally, poor circulation in the lower extremities might eventually necessitate amputation as cells and tissues die in the absence of adequate nutrient and oxygen supply.

TABLE 9-4 COMPLICATIONS ASSOCIATED WITH DIABETES
Heart disease, stroke, and hypertension
Blindness
Nervous system disorders
Amputation
Pregnancy problems
Respiratory infection
Gum disease

Data available from the Centers for Disease Control website on diabetes, www.cdc.gov/diabetes.

Exogenous—originating from outside the body.

TABLE 9-5   FUNCTIONS OF THE LIVER
Stores excess glucose as glycogen
Releases glucose into the blood when blood levels decline
Undergoes gluconeogenesis
Stores fat
Converts ammonia to urea
Detoxifies harmful substances such as drugs and alcohol
Stores vitamins (such as A, D, E, K, and B$_{12}$) and minerals (such as iron and copper)
Makes bile for the emulsification of fats

According to the ADA, diabetics have a risk for heart disease and stroke that is twice that of nondiabetics. The number of deaths as a result of heart disease in diabetic women has increased by 23% over the past 30 years, even though the rate among nondiabetic women dropped by 27%. Although the rate of heart-disease-related deaths in diabetic men has actually decreased by 13% over the past three decades, this rate of decline does not match the 36% decline experienced by nondiabetic men. Not only do high blood glucose levels damage blood vessels, but they also damage cardiac muscle cells. This often results in irregular heartbeats, tissue swelling, and severe fatigue since the heart cannot perform its job effectively. If vessels supplying either the heart or brain weaken or burst, a heart attack or stroke occurs.

Diabetes increases the risk for nonalcoholic fatty liver, a condition characterized by fat accumulation in liver tissue. The mild type of nonalcoholic fatty liver does not seem to impair liver functioning; however, the more advanced form can cause chronic inflammation, fibrous tissue formation, or even cirrhosis. Although rare, the advanced type can be life threatening given the various functions performed by the liver (Table 9.5). Researchers do not quite understand the exact relationship between diabetes and liver problems. Does diabetes precede liver disease, or does liver disease promote diabetes? At least one study shows that high blood insulin levels interfere with fatty acid oxidation in liver cells. This promotes an accumulation of triglycerides in these cells which then triggers inflammation and subsequent fibrosis.[5] Researchers are also uncertain about the role of diabetes in the development of liver cancer; although some studies have noted a relationship between the two.[6-8]

Retinopathy, neuropathy, and nephropathy are additional concerns for the diabetic. Why? Because high blood glucose levels damage small blood vessels, so the vessels supplying the eyes, nerves, and kidneys are vulnerable. **Angiopathy** is a general term that refers to diseases of blood vessels. The two forms of angiopathy are **macroangiopathy** and **microangiopathy**. In *macroangiopathy*, fat deposits and blood clots adhere to blood vessel walls thereby restricting blood flow. In *microangiopathy*, smaller blood vessel walls weaken and lose proteins to the surrounding space. This slows blood transport to body cells and deprives them of necessary oxygen and nutrients.

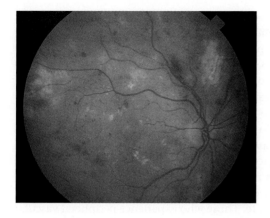

FIGURE 9.3 ■ Retinal hemorrhage with background diabetic retinopathy. (From Tasman W, Jaeger E. The Wills Eye Hospital Atlas of Clinical Ophthalmology, 2e. Philadelphia: Lippincott Williams & Wilkins, 2001.)

Retinopathy, which occurs as lesions develop in the small blood vessels that supply the retina of the eye, results in blindness in many diabetics (Fig. 9.3). Blood seeps from these leaky vessels and accumulates around the fragile retina. As blood supply to the cells of the retina is interrupted, new blood vessels often develop to try to compensate. These new vessels often stimulate scar tissue formation on the retina surface—a condition that promotes retinal detachment. Unfortunately, the new vessels become leaky just like the preexisting vessels, so pressure from accumulating fluid eventually kills cells and impairs vision.[9] Fifty percent of people who have had diabetes for at least 10 years develop some degree of retinopathy. That percentage increases to 80% in those who have had diabetes for at least 15 years.

According to the National Diabetes Information Clearinghouse, more than 50% of diabetics have some form of neuropathy, even in the absence of symptoms. A neuropathy is a nerve disorder that often results in pain; numbness; tingling; weakness; muscle atrophy; and loss of sensation in the hands, arms, feet, and legs. In fact, nearly 30% of diabetics over the age of 40 lack at least some sensation in their feet. The causes of neuropathy are likely chronic high blood glucose levels, low insulin levels, abnormal blood lipid levels, damage to blood vessels supplying nerves, and autoimmune disorders that target nerves. The damage occurs slowly and often without overt symptoms, so neuropathies frequently seem to develop out of nowhere. When present, the actual symptoms vary depending upon which nerves are affected. Treatment involves tight blood glucose control, stringent foot care to check for lingering wounds, smoking cessation since smoking exacerbates foot problems, and pain relievers to manage discomfort.

Angiopathy—damage or disease of arteries, capillaries, or veins.
Macroangiopathy—affects larger blood vessels. Fat and blood clots accumulate on the walls of larger vessels and restrict blood flow.
Microangiopathy—damage to very small blood vessels. Typically results when the walls of capillaries thicken and become leaky.

The two forms of neuropathy are **peripheral neuropathy** and **autonomic neuropathy**. Those suffering from peripheral neuropathy tend to have significant foot problems. Consequently, they must wear protective footwear with appropriate support and cushioning. The selection of a seamless, supportive sock is crucial. Seams often cause friction on the skin that promotes blisters or pressure ulcers, two conditions the diabetic needs to avoid because of poor wound healing. In addition, a good diabetic sock often extends up to the knee to prevent blood pooling in the leg and to assist in venous return to the heart. Socks should be absorbent to protect against fungal growth and warm to encourage circulation. Diabetics with peripheral neuropathy must also perform regular, daily foot-checks to inspect for injuries. Since they frequently lose sensations in their feet, diabetics are at risk of developing severe infections from minor but undetected blisters, cuts, or bruises. The degree of peripheral neuropathy determines the type of activity in which the diabetic client can safely participate. Those who experience peripheral vascular disease along with peripheral neuropathy might exhibit **intermittent claudication** during activity. If this occurs, stop the activity or change to a lower impact activity until the pain subsides.

Autonomic neuropathy damages nerves supplying internal organs such as those of the urinary, digestive, cardiovascular, and reproductive systems. If the nerves innervating the heart are affected, blood pressure and heart rate are altered. Thus, sufferers often experience both hypertension and hypotension. In addition, thermoregulation is impaired as radiative cooling becomes less effective; consequently, proper hydration is crucial. The specific symptoms of autonomic neuropathy depend upon the nerves affected, but they often include dizziness, constipation, diarrhea, impotence, and incontinence.

The ADA estimates that 20% to 30% of diabetics suffer to some extent from nephropathy. Nephropathy is a progressive condition that slowly destroys blood vessels supplying the kidneys (Fig. 9.4). It often results in end-stage renal disease (ESRD). In 2002, 44% of all cases of kidney failure was attributed to diabetes.[10]

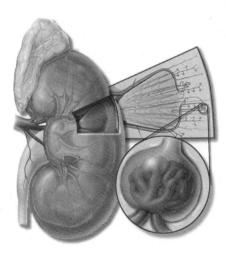

FIGURE 9.4 ■ Nephropathy is a progressive condition that slowly destroys blood vessels supplying the kidneys. (Asset provided by Anatomical Chart Co.)

Nephropathy results in damage to the microscopic nephrons found in the kidneys. To understand how devastating this condition is, consider basic kidney functioning. Each kidney contains over a million filtering and processing centers called **nephrons**. A nephron consists of a renal corpuscle and a renal tubule. Ultimately, nephrons remove waste products and excess water and salts from the blood by three main processes. Blood is **filtered** in the region of the nephron called the renal corpuscle. The renal corpuscle consists of the glomerulus and the glomerular capsule. The renal artery divides many times after it enters the kidney and ultimately branches into an individual afferent arteriole for each nephron in each kidney. The afferent arteriole then forms the glomerulus, a capillary bed through which blood is filtered. Because of the proximity of the afferent arterioles to the aorta, blood pressure within these vessels is high. This high pressure forces, or more accurately filters, the smaller components of blood plasma from the glomerulus into a space called the glomerular capsule. The resulting fluid is filtrate. Because proteins are large, they are never filtered by a healthy kidney; therefore, urine normally contains no traces of protein.

The proximal convoluted tubule, the Loop of Henle, and the distal convoluted tubule are the three segments of the renal tubule. The distal convoluted tubules of many nephrons empty into a collecting duct that ultimately empties into a structure called the renal pelvis. From the renal pelvis, urine passes through a ureter into the urinary bladder. The filtrate that enters the proximal convoluted tubule is different in composition from the urine that enters the renal pelvis. This difference exists because of the processes of **reabsorption** and **secretion**, which occur along the tubule. Reabsorption returns water, salts, glucose, amino

---

Peripheral neuropathy—damage typically occurs to nerves supplying the extremities. Effects, therefore, often develop in the feet. Very painful in the initial stages. Ultimately results in the loss of sensation in the affected areas.

Autonomic neuropathy—damage to the nerves that control cardiac and smooth muscle. Results from chronic hyperglycemia. Often causes blood pressure problems, digestive tract motility difficulties, and sexual impotence.

Intermittent claudication—a condition that results from poor circulation in the legs. Consists of a cramping or burning feeling in the legs that develops as activity level increases. It resolves as activity level decreases. The discomfort is not continuous; instead, it comes and goes.

Nephron—the microscopic filtering units found in the kidneys. Each kidney has over 1 million nephrons, which process blood to form urine.

Filtration—the process of forcing certain blood components through a series of membranes to form filtrate. Filtration occurs as a result of hydrostatic pressure, forms a fluid called filtrate, and occurs in the renal corpuscle of the nephron.

Reabsorption—a process that returns certain substances such as water, glucose, and salts to blood vessels after these items have been filtered.

Secretion—a process that removes from blood additional wastes including urea, drugs, and hydrogen ions. Removed substances become a part of filtrate (which eventually becomes urine).

TABLE 9-6 ALBUMIN LEVELS IN THE URINE		
	Albumin in Urine (μg/minute)	**Albumin in Urine (μg/day)**
Normal	<20	<30
Microalbuminuria	20–200	30–300
Macroalbuminuria	>200	>300

TABLE 9-7 SYMPTOMS OF KIDNEY DISEASE
Loss of sleep
Poor appetite
Upset stomach
Weakness
Difficulty concentrating

acids, and other useful materials to the blood. Secretion moves additional nitrogenous waste products, excess salts, excess hydrogen ions, drugs, and some toxic materials into the kidney tubule. The composition and quantity of urine varies widely depending on the relative intake of water and salt versus their loss by digestion, respiration, and perspiration.

The kidneys of a person with diabetes are subjected to a tremendous amount of stress. Excess blood glucose often increases blood pressure in renal blood vessels. Since blood pressure is already high in the afferent arterioles, any increase can damage the lining of the glomerulus. A damaged glomerulus becomes leaky and permits filtration of large molecules like proteins and red blood cells. The presence of small amounts of protein in the urine is called **microalbuminuria**; it is the first indication of kidney disease. At this stage, there are several treatment options. Frequently, however, kidney disease is not diagnosed until it reaches the stage of **macroalbuminuria**, a condition that usually results in ESRD. Table 9.6 shows normal and abnormal albumin content in the urine. Once ESRD is present, the kidneys fail and waste products accumulate in the blood. At this point, the only treatment options are dialysis and kidney transplant. Symptoms of kidney disease often do not appear until kidney failure is imminent (Table 9.7). Precise blood glucose control and blood pressure management are the only means of preventing ESRD.

PRECAUTIONS DURING EXERCISE

Treatment for diabetes usually involves diet modification, medication administration, and exercise. Overall, the goal is to decrease the risk of developing diabetes-associated complications such as heart disease and vascular disorders. Although type 1 diabetics always require an external source of insulin, type 2 diabetics often manage their condition by controlling blood glucose through diet and exercise. However, both type 1 and type 2 diabetics seem to benefit from exercise.

People with diabetes must be cautious when participating in physical activity since diabetes-associated complications often increase exercise risk. It is important to remember that the specific precautions vary depending upon how well-controlled the diabetes is. This section explores some issues of particular concern for diabetic exercisers.

INCREASED RISK FOR CARDIOVASCULAR DISEASE

Both type 1 and type 2 diabetes increase the risk for cardiovascular disease through various mechanisms. Diabetics often have plaque build up on their arteries, a condition that interferes with blood flow. As a result, the workload of the heart increases. To meet oxygen demands, respiration rate increases as well. As the heart pumps harder to move blood through narrowed vessels, blood pressure rises. Now add exercise to the mix. Exercise is an additional stressor to the heart, lungs, and blood vessels, so the intensity of both cardiovascular and resistance training must be closely monitored and might even be contraindicated for certain diabetics.

INCREASED RISK OF HYPOGLYCEMIA

In someone without diabetes, insulin release from the pancreas slows during aerobic exercise, but insulin sensitivity improves. Thus, less insulin is necessary to ensure that working muscles receive adequate glucose. As insulin levels decline, the relative amount of glucagon increases to ensure that the liver continues to maintain blood glucose levels as muscles use it up during exertion. Therefore, exercise promotes glucose availability during activity. Furthermore, fat loss usually accompanies consistent exercise, and this loss of fat mass has been shown to enhance insulin sensitivity and improve glucose tolerance in type 2 diabetics. In addition, exercise reduces circulating free fatty acid levels, while it increases muscle mass and vascularity—changes that improve glucose delivery to working cells.[11]

Type 1 diabetics who *inject* insulin, however, have circulating insulin levels that do not respond to exercise. In other words, the pancreas of a type 1 diabetic cannot decrease insulin release during exercise since the pancreas is not the source of insulin. Consequently, type 1 diabetics who inject normal doses of insulin prior to exercise have *relatively* high blood levels during exercise. The problem with this is that cells *still* become more sensitive to insulin during physical activity. Thus, relatively elevated insulin levels combined with improved insulin sensitivity predisposes type 1 diabetics to hypoglycemia since blood glucose levels will drop rapidly during exertion. To avoid hypoglycemia, the type 1 diabetic must carefully plan insulin injections to ensure that insulin levels do not peak during exercise (the higher the insulin level during exercise, the faster blood glucose plummets). Consuming carbohydrates immediately preceding exercise—or even during exercise—can prevent a drastic drop in blood glucose.

Microalbuminuria—when small amounts of the protein albumin leak into the urine.
Macroalbuminuria—when large amounts of the protein albumin leak into the urine.

Some type 1 diabetics reduce their insulin dosage prior to exercise to compensate for the increased insulin sensitivity experienced during exercise. This typically prevents hypoglycemia. However, if the injected amount is too low or if exercise duration is too long, cells cannot obtain adequate glucose from the blood. This significantly stresses and fatigues muscle cells while allowing blood glucose levels to climb as the liver tries to compensate. The result is that the body uses fat for fuel but makes excessive ketone bodies during the process. This increases the likelihood of ketosis.

One additional concern for the diabetic is that for 30 minutes to 48 hours after exercise, skeletal muscle cells often increase their rate of glucose uptake to replenish their dwindling glycogen stores. This means that the type 1 diabetic remains at risk for hypoglycemia for several hours following exercise.

A note of caution: because the effects of exercise are often similar to the symptoms of low blood sugar (sweating, fatigue, muscle weakness, dizziness, etc.), exercise can mask a hypoglycemic attack. The exercising diabetic should be aware of this.

INCREASED RISK OF DEHYDRATION

Proper hydration is essential for all exercisers since inadequate body fluid can result in dangerously high core temperatures and electrolyte imbalances. A diabetic with a high blood glucose level has an increased risk for dehydration since elevated blood glucose increases urine production. In addition, as the blood loses water, the blood glucose level rises even more relative to water content. This could result in increased blood viscosity, abnormal blood pressure, and glucosuria.

INCREASED RISKS ASSOCIATED WITH HIGH-INTENSITY RESISTANCE TRAINING

The Valsalva Maneuver occurs when individuals hold their breath during exercise, particularly during resistance exercise. Not only does this practice impede the return of venous blood to the heart, but it also dangerously increases blood pressure. Consequently, all exercisers should maintain normal breathing during strength training. Proper breathing during resistance training includes breathing out during the exertion phase and breathing in during the return phase. Since they are already at risk for narrowed blood vessels, impaired circulation, and high blood pressure, diabetics should be especially careful to avoid holding their breath during exertion. Additionally, they should avoid high-intensity resistance training. These practices can help prevent excess pressure buildup that might rupture small vessels such as those supplying the retina of the eye.

INCREASED RISK OF INJURY TO THE EXTREMITIES

Diabetics tend to have poor circulation because of occluded arteries, so blood flow to distal capillaries and their tissues is often limited. In fact, the number of blood vessels in the diabetic body actually decreases over time. Neuropathy in the legs, feet, arms, and hands often follows since peripheral nerves are deprived of adequate blood. This neuropathy then results in the loss of sensation, particularly in the feet and legs. Diabetics, therefore, must be careful not to damage their feet during exercise since damage often goes unde-tected. If damage remains undetected for too long, infection follows. Once an infection develops, the immune system struggles to fight it since white blood cells have difficulty accessing the area. Why—because of circulation problems. Therefore, wound healing is impaired as inadequate oxygen and nutrients are supplied to the area.[10,12–14]

BENEFITS OF EXERCISE

IMPROVED INSULIN SENSITIVITY AND GLUCOSE TOLERANCE

Studies show that insulin resistance and glucose tolerance are improved with exercise, even in the absence of weight loss.[15–18] The results of one study suggest that both energy restric-tion and physical activity independently contribute to improved glucose levels and insulin response in previously sedentary overweight type 2 diabetics. However, when these two variables are combined, effects are multiplied.[16,19] Results of the Diabetes Prevention Pro-gram confirm this finding and suggest that exercise, in conjunction with a low fat, low kilocalorie diet, helps regulate blood glucose levels and insulin response in type 2 diabetic patients.

REDUCED RISK FOR CARDIOVASCULAR DISEASE AND IMPROVED WORK CAPACITY

Compared to nondiabetics, both type 1 and type 2 diabetics have a higher risk for cardio-vascular disease. Exercise seems to reduce this risk by improving the lipid profile, blood pressure, body weight, and work capacity. It enhances blood flow, increases vascularity, improves cholesterol levels, improves VO_{2max}, and develops overall heart and lung functioning.

REDUCED NEED FOR MEDICATION

Type 2 diabetics, who are typically overweight and sometimes take oral medications, often manage their condition by incorporating exercise and healthier eating into their lifestyles. Although losing weight dramatically improves a type 2 diabetic's outcome, studies show that exercise and a low-fat, low-energy diet—even in the absence of weight loss—independently help in the management of type 2 diabetes.

IMPROVED MOOD AND WELL-BEING

Diabetics, along with others who have to live with chronic health conditions, sometimes feel helpless when it comes to their health. This feeling can develop into a hopelessness that might ultimately result in bouts of depression.

Exercise is associated with improved mood in all populations.[20] In fact, moderate intensity exercise for a minimum of 20 minutes several days per week elevates mood, enhances sleep, and improves outlook for most participants. Most exercisers feel a sense of control over their own bodies, and this feeling translates into a better overall attitude.

BETTER WEIGHT MANAGEMENT

Exercise promotes weight management across all populations. This is important because excess weight—especially when stored in the midsection—increases the risk for heart disease, certain cancers, and stroke. Interestingly, intraabdominal fat responds well to exercise, so initial weight loss is noticeable in the midsection. As exercise removes abdominal fat, the risk for cardiovascular disease diminishes. Another benefit of weight loss is that type 2 diabetics might be able to significantly reduce—or totally eliminate—the need for oral medications once they achieve and maintain a healthy weight.

RECOMMENDATIONS FOR EXERCISE

Although exercise poses potential risks for individuals with diabetes, it can improve circulation, reduce total cholesterol, lower blood pressure, decrease the risk for heart disease, and possibly improve glucose tolerance; therefore, it should be considered a part of the treatment plan for many diabetic patients.[15,21-23]

EXERCISE TESTING

According to the American College of Sports Medicine (ACSM), diabetics should seek in-depth medical evaluations prior to initiating exercise because of their high risk for cardiovascular, renal, neurological, and visual problems. Asymptomatic diabetics who have less than a 10% chance of having a cardiac event over a 10-year period may begin a low-to-moderate intensity exercise program without exercise testing. Those with higher risks who want to start a vigorous program ($\geq$60% VO_{2R} with a substantial increase in breathing rate and heart rate) need a medically supervised graded exercise test with electrographic monitoring. Some diabetics might need additional testing such as a radionuclide stress test or stress echocardiography, but this should be determined by the medical care provider.[22]

EXERCISE PRESCRIPTION

Although additional research is needed, available information suggests that both strength training and cardiovascular training are safe and beneficial for diabetics if they follow certain guidelines.[12,15,22,24,25] In most cases, young diabetics who have control over their glucose levels can safely participate in most forms of exercise. Diabetics who are middle aged or older also benefit from exercise, but they should only exercise after careful screening. In compliance with existing literature and guidelines from the ACSM and the ADA, the following recommendations are considered safe for diabetics who have already received clearance from a physician.

- Precede all forms of exercise with a 5- to 10-minute warm-up to prepare the heart, lungs, muscles, and joints for activity. The ADA recommends an additional 5 to 10 minutes of stretching during the warm-up to ensure muscle readiness. Each workout session should end with a 5- to 10-minute cooldown to return heart rate to its preexercise level.

- Cardiovascular training should be performed for 20 to 60 minutes per day, 3 to 7 days per week, at a moderate intensity of 50% to 80% of VO_{2R} or **heart rate reserve (HRR)**. This is a 12 to 16 on the rate of perceived exertion scale. The workout sessions can be split into 10-minute sements with a goal of reaching 150 to 300 minutes of activity each week. The type of exercise depends on additional coexisting health problems. In most cases, low-impact activities such as walking, low-impact floor aerobics, water aerobics, and the elliptical trainer are safe and beneficial. If neuropathy exists in the feet and legs, however, nonimpact exercises such as swimming, stationary cycling, and rowing are safer.
- All diabetics should be aware that hypoglycemia can occur during *and* after exercise since metabolic changes occur during exertion that often cause a rapid depletion of blood glucose. Symptoms of hypoglycemia include fainting, profuse sweating, dizziness, fatigue, irritability, headache, nervousness, slurred speech, poor coordination, and heart palpitations.
- Type 2 diabetics should expend at least 2,000 kilocalories per week in moderate exercise to lose weight.
- As mentioned in an earlier section, type 1 diabetics who have poor control over blood glucose levels need to be aware of the symptoms of hyperglycemia. These include weakness, excessive thirst, excessive urination, dry mouth, nausea, vomiting, acetone breath, and abdominal tenderness. If hyperglycemia is suspected but no ketones are present in the blood or urine, diabetics may exercise as long as they refrain from vigorous exercise.
- Resistance training seems safe for diabetics if they do not have retinopathy, recent laser treatments, or any contraindications. Diabetics should strength train on 2 to 3 days per week at an intensity of 60% to 80% of 1 RM. Perform 2 to 3 sets, each consisting of 8 to 12 repetitions, for 8 to 10 multijoint exercises. Include at least 48 hours of rest in between workouts. Because of blood pressure issues, clients should avoid sustained tight gripping, isometric exercises, and the Valsalva Maneuver since each of these dangerously elevate blood pressure. Of particular concern are diabetics with retinopathy; they have an increased risk of retinal detachment, so they might need to avoid strength training altogether. The physician makes the final decision. Diabetics with peripheral neuropathy should not put undue stress on their feet, legs, or other affected limbs since they are often unable to sense injury.
- Clients suffering from neuropathy in the legs and feet might experience balance and gait problems that interfere with their exercise ability. These clients need to avoid exercises that include quick changes in foot patterns.

Heart rate reserve (HRR)—also known as the Karvonen Method. To calculate HRR, subtract resting heart rate from maximal heart rate to obtain HRR. For example, if resting heart rate is 70 bpm and maximal heart rate is 200, HRR = 200 − 70 = 130. To determine intensity for the diabetic client, multiply 130 by 50% and then 80% to find the appropriate target heart rate range.

ADDITIONAL SUGGESTIONS AND CONCERNS ACCORDING TO ACSM AND THE MAYO CLINIC

- Participating in physical activity at the same time each day helps track glucose response to exercise.
- Well-fitting shoes and breathable, comfortable socks are essential for this population since diabetics often experience severe foot problems. Poor circulation coupled with loss of protective sensation in the feet makes the diabetic more susceptible to lower extremity damage. Once a foot is injured or infected, a diabetic suffering from neuropathy must conscientiously inspect the feet several times per day to see if the injury or infection has spread. They cannot rely on feelings of pain or discomfort like nondiabetics. Even a minor blister can wreak havoc on the feet of a diabetic.
- Diabetics should always wear a medical identification bracelet or tag on an easy-to-see place on the body. This helps medical professionals treat them if they go unconscious.
- According to Mayoclinic.com, diabetics should check blood glucose levels closely before exercising. If blood glucose is less than 100 mg/dL, eat a small amount of carbohydrate such as a piece of fruit, a glass of juice, or a few crackers before beginning. A blood glucose reading of 100 to 250 mg/dL is a safe preexercise range. If blood glucose equals or exceeds 250 mg/dL, be careful. Test the urine for ketones. If excess ketones are present, the body is deficient in insulin and exercise should be avoided until ketone level normalizes.
- Diabetics should carry a source of carbohydrates along with them in case of hypoglycemia. This is crucial during long bouts of exercise. If planning to exercise for a long duration, check blood glucose every 30 minutes during the workout. If blood glucose is ≤70 mg/dL, stop exercising and consume something to elevate blood glucose. Options include 2 to 3 glucose tablets, ½ cup of orange juice, 4 oz of non-diet soda, or five pieces of hard candy. Recheck blood glucose 15 minutes later. Repeat until blood glucose exceeds 70 mg/dL. Avoid exercise before bed because of the risk of delayed postexercise hypoglycemia. Furthermore, do not exercise during peak insulin action since this might also cause hypoglycemia. Symptoms of hypoglycemia include weakness, abnormal sweating, nervousness, anxiety, tingling of the mouth or fingers, and hunger. Additionally, some experience headache, visual disturbances, confusion, and seizures.[22] To avoid hypoglycemia, adjust carbohydrate and medication intake based on activity level. If blood glucose levels before or after exercise are less than 100 mg/dL, ingest 20 to 30 g of carbohydrates.
- Do not inject insulin into exercising limbs since this can cause hypoglycemia. Instead, inject insulin into the abdominal area.
- Consume adequate water before, during, and after exercise. The elevated blood glucose levels experienced by diabetics often result in excessive urination. This fluid loss coupled with fluid loss from perspiration during exercise promotes thermoregulatory problems, so monitor for heat illness. Additionally, dehydration itself affects relative blood glucose levels and predisposes the diabetic to hyperglycemia.

- Always exercise with a partner or trainer just in case a hypoglycemic emergency occurs.
- Be aware of the risk for silent ischemic attacks. These occur six times more frequently in diabetics than in nondiabetics.
- Use perceived exertion to determine intensity rather than solely relying on heart rate and blood pressure since response to exercise is sometimes diminished. See Appendix A for rating of perceived exertion scale.
- Clients with nephropathy usually have a reduced overall exercise capacity, so they tend to self-limit their activity level. In any case, avoid high-intensity or strenuous exercise in this group. Low-to-moderate exercise is safe.
- Clients with retinopathy have an increased risk for retinal detachment and vitreous hemorrhage if blood pressure increases too much, so avoid vigorous activity.
- Table 9.8 provides tips for diabetic exercisers and Table 9.9 presents conditions that preclude a diabetic from exercising.

Increasing daily physical activity provides benefits to all populations. The increased activity may be in the form of a regimented exercise routine consisting of aerobic exercise, strength training, and flexibility work, but it may also include simple adjustments to normal daily behaviors. Encourage clients to park their cars in distant parking spaces at work, use the stairs instead of the elevator, and walk over to a coworker's office rather than send an e-mail. All of this extra movement gradually adds up and benefits the body systems. Sedentary diabetics should definitely become more active in their normal activities of daily living as they embark on a healthier lifestyle.

TABLE 9-8 TIPS FOR THE DIABETIC EXERCISER

- Check blood glucose levels before and after a workout
- Wear an identification band that indicates diabetes
- Wear appropriate footwear
- Stay well-hydrated before, during, and after exercise
- Track and record blood glucose response to different activities and intensity levels
- Have a carbohydrate source available for hypoglycemic emergencies

TABLE 9-9 WHEN DIABETICS SHOULD AVOID EXERCISE

- Fasting blood glucose level is >250 mg/dL and ketones are present in the urine; use caution if fasting blood glucose is >300 mg/dL and no ketones are present
- Experiencing shortness of breath
- Experiencing any pain or numbness in the lower extremities
- Insulin levels are peaking

SAMPLE EXERCISES

Before encouraging a diabetic client to exercise, make sure a physician has examined and cleared the client for activity. Once the diabetic has achieved adequate control of blood glucose levels through diet and medication, exercise is both safe and beneficial.

Precede all forms of exercise with a 5 to 10 minute warm-up. Some diabetics require a longer warm-up to avoid ischemia or irregular heart rates. Walking effectively prepares the body for the upcoming workout. Include limbering movements for the upper extremities, but avoid holding hands overhead for an extended period of time since this increases blood pressure. Mild stretching of the shoulder, back, chest, biceps, triceps, hip flexors, quadriceps, hamstrings, and calf is appropriate. Diabetics with foot problems who cannot walk without difficulty might prefer stationary cycling. As always, trainers need to accommodate each individual client.

Encourage aerobic activity that the client enjoys, such as walking, jogging, cycling, swimming, low-impact aerobics, or other activities that engage large muscles of the body. Because they are predisposed to foot and circulation problems, diabetic clients often benefit more from low-impact activities performed at a low-to-moderate intensity for a longer duration than high-intensity, high-impact activities.

Resistance exercise improves blood glucose control, enhances insulin action, and can be safely performed by most diabetics. Diabetics suffering from peripheral vascular disease, retinopathy, nephropathy, and neuropathy need to be careful because of the risks associated with these conditions. Once all comorbidities are identified and accounted for, resistance exercises using free weights, bands, or resistance machines are appropriate. A general program that incorporates traditional exercises that target the back, chest, shoulders, biceps, triceps, and legs provides an effective workout. Although resistance exercises were formerly discouraged in this population because blood pressure increases as muscles strain, it is now recommended for those with controlled diabetes. Diabetics should avoid gripping bars or bands too tightly, use less resistance, and avoid holding their breath. Resistance machines, which require less balance and allow more focus on form, might be best since they do not affect blood pressure as dramatically as free weights.

UPPER BODY EXERCISES

Strengthening the upper body helps maintain posture and improves the ability to perform normal activities of daily living. Maintain neutral body alignment throughout each exercise. Most of these may be done using free weights, resistance bands, or machines, but watch blood pressure. Perform 2 to 3 sets of each with 8 to 12 repetitions each.

Chest Press

A seated chest press machine is preferable to a lying chest press machine since dizziness can result from lying down and getting up too quickly. Use light resistance and ensure a neutral spine. Sit on a seated chest press machine with back against the pad and handles at shoulder level. Push forward without arching the back or grasping the handles too tightly. Pause and return to original position.

Lateral Pull Down

Lightly grasp the bar using a wide grip and sit with back straight. Stabilize the shoulders and lean back slightly. Without jerking, pull the bar to the chest and pause. Return to original position.

Seated Row

Avoid arching the back. Maintain a stable core. Lean forward to grasp the handle with both hands. Sit with back perpendicular to legs and arms extended. Pull arms toward chest or abdomen—avoid leaning back or gripping the handle too tightly. Pause and lower the weight. Do not lean forward when doing this. The hips should remain at a 90° angle. Use light weights and avoid holding the breath.

Shoulder Press

Align the body according to the instructions on the machine and ensure smooth movements. Lightly grasp the handles with both hands and slowly push up until elbows are extended. Pause and return to original position.

Biceps Curl

Lightly grasp lightweight dumbbells, one in each hand. Keep elbows in while flexing the elbow. Pause and return to original position. Avoid hyperextension at the elbow, but perform through a full range-of-motion.

Triceps Dip

Using a bench, perform a traditional triceps dip.

LOWER BODY EXERCISES

Strengthening the buttocks, quadriceps, and hamstrings improves balance, circulation, and stamina. Maintain neutral body alignment throughout each exercise. Be careful with clients who have lower extremity circulation problems.

Buttocks and hamstrings

The leg press effectively trains the buttocks and hamstrings and should be done with light resistance. If a leg press machine is unavailable, perform squats without resistance or with very light resistance since this exercise can drastically increase blood pressure. Have the client stand with feet shoulder width apart. Contract the abdominal muscles and bend the knees until the hips are parallel to the floor. Slowly return to an erect position without locking the knees. Exhale while lowering the hips; inhale when returning to the standing

---

Ischemia—an insufficient blood supply to an organ; usually due to artery blockage. An ischemic attack typically results in tissue death. Ischemia of the heart can cause a heart attack. Ischemia of the brain causes a stroke.

position. For added resistance, hold one dumbbell in each hand and squat. Lunges in a stationary position are also effective.

Quadriceps

The leg extension targets this muscle group. Position client as directed by the instruction panel. Maintain neutral body alignment. Extend at the knees until the legs are straight but not locked. Pause and return to original position.

NUTRITIONAL CONSIDERATIONS

Nutritional therapy helps manage blood glucose levels in people with either type 1 or type 2 diabetes. By obtaining the appropriate nutrients in the proper amounts, the diabetic minimizes the risk of hypoglycemia, long-term complications, excess weight gain, undesirable lipid levels, and overall quality of life. Obviously, specific nutritional advice differs for different individuals based on age, medication, lifestyle factors, and usual eating patterns; however, the ADA sets general suggestions that apply to most diabetics.[10,26,27]

ENERGY-YIELDING NUTRIENTS

Carbohydrates

Carbohydrates are important in a diabetic's diet and should supply most of the daily kilocalories consumed. In fact, the recommendations for diabetics are similar to the recommendations for the general population. To ensure normal blood glucose levels, diabetics must monitor the timing of carbohydrate intake; they should strive to consume a similar amount each day; and intake should be evenly spaced throughout the day. Interestingly, the *amount* of carbohydrates consumed in one sitting has a greater impact on blood glucose levels than the actual *source* of dietary carbohydrate, so intake during any one sitting should be moderate. Diabetics, however, should *still* select high-fiber, whole-grain products over highly processed simple sugars and starchy foods since high-fiber foods affect blood glucose less. They should also include various vegetables such as spinach, carrots, and broccoli to help meet their vitamin and mineral needs. Contrary to popular belief, diabetics do not have to completely avoid sugary foods; instead, they should typically select foods with little added sugar and be sure to count any sugary foods toward their daily carbohydrate allowance.

Type 1 diabetics must learn to carefully plan insulin injections to avoid hyperglycemia or hypoglycemia as discussed earlier in this chapter. This is particularly true for those who exercise.

Overall, diabetics should not restrict carbohydrate intake to less than 130 g per day. Their actual intake should vary based upon activity level and insulin therapy. Additionally, they should include approximately 14 g of fiber per 1,000 kcal consumed. All diabetics should closely monitor carbohydrate intake using Exchange Lists or Carbohydrate Counting to achieve glycemic control.

Protein

The body uses dietary protein to build, repair, and maintain tissues. Because protein has various functions, a deficiency can severely impair every organ system. To maintain normal activity, people need 0.8 g of protein per kilogram of body weight. That equals about 55 g of protein for a 150-lb person, an amount far below the average intake for Americans. Average intake is closer to 1.6 g/kg of body weight—twice as much as we need!

The ADA suggests that no more than 15% to 20% of a diabetic's total daily energy intake be in the form of proteins. This equals 75 to 100 g per day on a 2,000 kcal per day diet and assumes normal renal functioning. Unfortunately, many high-protein sources are also high in saturated fat and cholesterol, so the diabetic, like members of the general population, should choose proteins from lean sources. Chicken is a healthy choice, as long as the skin is removed. Pork loin and sirloin are also healthy options. In addition, legumes include fair amounts of protein. In fact, soy protein provides health benefits independent from those associated with its low fat content. Protein intake exceeding 20% of total daily kilocalories is discouraged in diabetics since the consequences are unknown.

Diabetics suffering from kidney disease would likely benefit from diets lower in protein since excess protein burdens the kidneys. Why? To answer that question, consider how the body processes proteins. Under normal conditions and with a healthy diet, a combination of carbohydrates, fat, and small amounts of protein provides energy for the body. To use protein for energy, the liver must remove the nitrogen-containing components from amino acids. It removes this nitrogen in the form of ammonia. Because ammonia is toxic, the liver almost immediately converts this ammonia into a less toxic compound called urea by combining two molecules of ammonia with carbon dioxide. Urea then enters the blood, travels to the kidneys, and is filtered by nephrons in the kidneys. Because the body normally only uses small amounts of protein for energy, the kidneys easily process the resulting urea as long as the body is hydrated. A diet high in protein (or low in carbohydrates), however, forces the liver to rely more on proteins for energy. This promotes urea production and places a greater demand on the kidneys. It also necessitates an increased water intake to ensure that the kidneys effectively filter urea. Obviously, someone with kidney disease needs to limit kidney stress, so limiting protein intake and maintaining adequate hydration are essential.

Limiting red meat in the diet might slow the progression of kidney disease in those with early stage nephropathy. According to a recent study published in the American Journal of Clinical Nutrition, replacing red meat with skinless chicken decreased the risk of complications in type 2 diabetics by decreasing blood cholesterol levels and minimizing albumin in the urine. In addition to reducing their red meat intake, subjects in this particular study also followed an overall low-protein, lacto-vegetarian diet for several weeks during the trial period. Although researchers could not discern whether the reduced red meat intake or the overall reduced protein intake contributed to the observed benefit, they encouraged limiting dietary intake of red meat and its associated saturated fat and cholesterol to improve heart health.[28]

Fat

Dietary fat adds flavor to food, provides essential fatty acids, and can be a part of a healthy diet. Recommendations for the general population suggest limiting daily fat intake to 20%

TABLE 9-10	ALCOHOL EQUIVALENTS
Drinks	**Equivalent**
1	12 oz beer
1	5 oz wine
1	1½ oz hard liquor (rum, vodka, whiskey)
1	10-oz wine cooler

to 35% of total kilocalories with less than 10% deriving from saturated and trans fats. The remaining portion of dietary fats should primarily come from unsaturated fats, particularly the monounsaturated fats (which are negatively correlated with cardiovascular disease). In addition, total dietary cholesterol for the average person should not exceed 300 mg per day.

Because diabetics are at an increased risk for cardiovascular disease, they must carefully control their intake of total fat, saturated fat, and cholesterol. Saturated fat should be limited to less than 7% of total daily intake and dietary cholesterol should be less than 200 mg per day. To obtain an adequate intake of omega-3 fatty acids, the diabetic should strive to consume two or more servings of fish per week.

Alcohol

Diabetics can safely include alcohol in their diets. Experts suggest that diabetic males consume no more than two alcoholic beverages per day, while diabetic females consume no more than one alcoholic beverage per day (see Table 9.10), amounts similar to the general population. Because insulin users have an increased risk for hypoglycemia, they should only consume alcohol in conjunction with food. All diabetics should be aware of the fact that many mixed drinks and wine coolers contain juices that are high in carbohydrates; therefore, these drinks can significantly increase blood glucose levels.

VITAMINS AND MINERALS

Diabetics have the same vitamin and mineral requirements as the general population. Vitamin and mineral supplements appear to provide no benefit for diabetics who do not have actual deficiencies. For those at increased risk for cardiovascular disease, limiting dietary sodium intake to less than 2,000 mg per day seems effective. Reducing sodium intake to less than 2,300 mg per day is advisable for all other diabetics, including those with hypertension.

WATER

QUICK REFERENCE

AI for total water intake:
Men: 3.7 L/day
Women: 2.7 L/day

All exercisers need adequate water to prevent dehydration and assist in thermoregulation. Since diabetics are at an increased risk for complications associated with inadequate hydration levels, they need to be especially careful about their fluid intake.

A water imbalance in a diabetic can cause a relative increase in blood glucose concentration, or hyperglycemia. As mentioned earlier, the symptoms of hyperglycemia include frequent urination, excessive thirst, and glucose in the urine. If diabetics suspect hyperglycemia, they should immediately treat it to avoid further complications. The steps to treat hyperglycemia vary for different individuals, but the first step is to measure blood glucose. If blood glucose is elevated but under 240 mg/dL, exercise helps. If over 240 mg/dL, however, the diabetic should check for ketones in the urine. If ketones are present, avoid exercise since exercising at this point can actually elevate blood glucose levels even more. If ignored, hyperglycemia can result in diabetic coma while the body incompletely breaks down fatty acids for fuel. Diabetic coma occurs along with ketoacidosis. As mentioned in an earlier section, the body produces substances called ketone bodies as it uses fatty acids for fuel. Certain cells in the body can actually use ketone bodies for energy, so low levels are perfectly acceptable and normal. As soon as production exceeds use, however, ketones begin to accumulate in the blood. Since many ketone bodies are also keto acids, excesses result in ketoacidosis—the condition in which blood pH drops. Ketoacidosis then interferes with normal metabolic functioning. Table 9.11 lists symptoms of ketoacidosis.

Dehydration also interferes with thermoregulation, or the ability of the body to maintain a normal internal temperature. The body cools itself through evaporation, radiation, convection, and conduction. The primary means are evaporative and radiative cooling. Evaporative cooling occurs as sweat evaporates from the skin surface. Water, which is the primary component of sweat, transports a huge amount of heat without its temperature being affected. When a person is dehydrated, this thermoregulatory mechanism falters.

Radiative cooling occurs as blood vessels in the dermis dilate, a condition that diverts a greater quantity of blood away from deeper vessels and closer to the skin's surface. As the blood passes near the surface of the skin, heat radiates from blood vessels into the surrounding environment; this cools the blood. Diabetics, who often suffer from circulation problems, lose some of this ability and often have difficulty cooling off during exercise. Hydration levels become particularly important to avoid heat illness.

Overall, the recommendations for water intake are similar for both the diabetic and the general population. In general, everyone should drink a minimum of 64 oz of water

TABLE 9-11 SYMPTOMS OF KETOACIDOSIS

Ketones in the urine

Shortness of breath

Dry mouth and excessive thirst

Fruity-smelling breath

Nausea

daily. In addition to this minimum amount, people should consume enough water to replace any water lost through excess sweating. A simple plan suggests that exercisers drink two to three 8-oz glasses of water 2 hours prior to exercise, another one to two cups 10 to 15 minutes before exercise, and then one to one-and-a-half cups every 15 minutes during exercise to avoid dehydration. After exercise, two to three cups per pound of body weight lost helps restore normal fluid levels.

> ### QUICK REFERENCE
>
> The goals of dietary intervention in the treatment of diabetes are to maintain normal blood glucose levels, to minimize incidences of hypoglycemia in insulin-dependent diabetics, to achieve and maintain weight-loss in type 2 diabetics, and to maintain healthy blood pressure and blood lipid profiles, all of which reduce the risk for diabetes-related complications.

SUMMARY

Exercise has inherent risks for any population; however, the benefits typically far outweigh these risks, even in the diabetic population. At the very least, exercise changes the way the body handles insulin, making it more sensitive and responsive to circulating levels. It can lower blood glucose levels and possibly even reduce the amount of medication needed. In addition, exercise encourages weight management, blood pressure control, and blood circulation. It lowers total cholesterol level, reduces LDL, and increases HDL—factors that promote a healthier heart. As long as they take certain precautions and as long as they have physician clearance, most diabetics can safely exercise for the long term. See Table 9.12 for additional tips for managing diabetes. Type 2 diabetics, who are typically resistant to the effects of insulin, usually benefit from moderate weight loss, increased physical activity, and lower kilocalorie diets. A loss of only 10 to 20 lb seems to improve blood lipid levels, blood pressure, and insulin resistance. The ADA recommends a 7% loss of weight and a minimum of 150 minutes of activity per week to achieve and sustain a healthy weight.

TABLE 9-12   TIPS FOR MANAGING DIABETES
Closely monitor blood glucose
Take medications as prescribed
Monitor blood pressure
Achieve and maintain a healthy weight
Eat foods that are low in fat and high in fiber
Exercise daily or almost every day
Drink plenty of water
Stop smoking
Check the condition of the feet daily

CASE STUDY

A 21-year-old client with type 1 diabetes comes in for a personal training appointment. She has been exercising routinely for 1 year, has achieved and maintained a healthy weight her entire life, and usually has good control of blood glucose. She says that she checked her blood glucose level 15 minutes earlier and had a reading of 65 mg/dL.

■ How do you proceed with this client?

■ Is this level safe for exercise?

■ Explain what you would do.

THINKING CRITICALLY

1. List and briefly explain three tests used by physicians to diagnose diabetes. Why is it so important to detect the presence of diabetes early?
2. Name and describe the organ responsible for maintaining blood glucose levels. What hormones does it release? Describe the functions of these hormones. What happens when this organ malfunctions?
3. Describe the general differences in type 1 and type 2 diabetes. What are some risk factors associated with each? How are these two conditions managed?
4. List several complications associated with diabetes. Choose three and elaborate on their causes.
5. Explain some functions of the liver. Why is this organ so important?
6. What is hyperglycemia and why is it so dangerous? How should a client handle hyperglycemia?
7. Explain why diabetics, particularly type 1 diabetics, are at an increased risk for hypoglycemia.
8. What are some of the specific benefits of exercise for diabetic clients?
9. Briefly describe a general one-day exercise plan for a diabetic client.
10. Describe the basic carbohydrate, protein, and fat needs of a diabetic client. Explain the importance of diet to the diabetic.

REFERENCES

1. DeCoste K, Scott L. Diabetes update: promoting effective disease management. Am Assoc Occup Health Nurs J 2004;52(8):344–355.
2. National Diabetes Information Clearinghouse. www.diabetes.niddk.nih.gov
3. Zanobetti A, Schwartz J. Are diabetics more susceptible to the health effects of airborne particles? Am J Respir Crit Care Med 2001;164:831–833.
4. Diabetes: Type I Annual Report. www.ebscohost.com. Health Source – Consumer Edition Database. Number 20498521. 2005. 1–15.
5. Harrison SA, Di Bisceglie AM. Advances in the understanding and treatment of nonalcoholic fatty liver disease. Drugs 2003;63:2379–2394.
6. Adami H, Cho W, Nyren O, et al. Excess risk of primary liver cancer in patients with diabetes mellitus. J Nat Cancer Inst 1996;88:1472–1477.

7. El-Seraq H, Richardson P, Everhart J. The role of diabetes in hepatocellular carcinoma. Am J Gastroenterol 2001;96:2462–2467.

8. La Vecchia C, Negri E, Decarli A, et al. Diabetes mellitus and the risk of primary liver cancer. Int J Cancer 1997;73:204–207.

9. Fong D, Aiello L, Gardner T, et al. Retinopathy in diabetes. Diab Care 2004;27:S84–S87.

10. American Diabetes Association Position Statement. Nephropathy in Diabetes. Diab Care 2004; 27:S79–S83.

11. Pigman H, Gan D, Krousel-Wood M. Role of exercise for type 2 diabetic patient management. South Med J 2002;95(1):72–77.

12. Kavookjian J, Elsvick B, Whetsel T. Interventions for being active among individuals with diabetes: a systemic review of the literature. Diab Educ 2007;33(6):962.

13. Roberts C. Type 2 diabetes and exercise. Prim Health Care 2003;13(4):27–31.

14. Watts S, Anselmo J. Nutrition for diabetes—all in a day's work. Nursing 2006;36(6):46–48.

15. American Diabetic Association. www.diabetes.org

16. Cox K, Burke V, Morton A, et al. Independent and additive effects of energy restriction and exercise on glucose and insulin concentrations in sedentary overweight men. Am J Clin Nutr 2004;80(2): 308–316.

17. Jeng C, Ku C, Huang W. Establishment of a predictive model of serum glucose changes under different exercise intensities and durations among patients with type 2 diabetes mellitus. J Nurs Res 2003;11(4):287–293.

18. Slentz C, Torgan C, Houmard J, et al. Long-term effects of exercise training and detraining on carbohydrate metabolism in overweight subjects. Clin Exerc Physiol 2002;4(1):22–29.

19. Virtanen SM, Laara E, Hypponen E, et al. Cow's milk consumption, HLA-DQB1 genotype, and type 1 diabetes: a nested case-control study of siblings of children with diabetes. Childhood diabetes in Finland study group. Diab 2000;49(6):912–917.

20. Hassmen P, Koivula N, Uutela A. Physical exercise and psychological well-being: a population study in Finland. Prev Med 2000;30(1):17–35.

21. Aldana S, Barlow M, Smith R, et al. A worksite diabetes prevention program: two-year impact on employee health. Am Assoc Occup Health Nurs J 2006;54(9):389–395.

22. American College of Sports Medicine. ACSM's Guidelines for Exercise Testing and Prescription. 8th Ed. Philadelphia: Lippincott Williams & Wilkins, 2010:232–237.

23. Cayley W. The role of exercise in patients with type 2 diabetes. Cochrane for clinicians. American Family Physician. 2007. Available at: www.aafp.org/afp/

24. Jiminez C, Corcoran M, Crawley J, et al. National Athletic Trainer's Association position statement: management of the athlete with type I diabetes mellitus. J Athl Train 2007;42(4):536–546.

25. Kraus W, Levine B. Exercise training for diabetes: the "strength" of the evidence. Ann Int Med 2007;147(6):423–425.

26. Joslin Diabetes Center. New nutrition guidelines for people with type 2 diabetes or pre-diabetes who are overweight or obese. Ascribe Newswire: Health. 4/6/05. p. 9–12.

27. Venables M, Shaw C, Jeukendrup A, et al. Effect of acute exercise on glucose tolerance following post exercise feeding. Eur J Appl Physiol 2007;100(6): 711–717.

28. de Mello V, Zelmanovitz T, Perassolo MS, Azevedo MJ, Gross JL. Withdrawal of red meat from the usual diet reduces albuminuria and improves serum fatty acid profile in type 2 diabetes patients with macroalbuminuria. Am J Clin Nutr 2006;83:1032–1038.

SUGGESTED READINGS

Skinner J. Exercise Testing and Exercise Prescription for Special Cases. 3rd Ed. Baltimore: Lippincott Williams and Wilkins, 2005.

Woolf-May K. Exercise Prescription: Physiological Foundations. UK: Churchill Livingstone Elsevier, 2006.

EXERCISE FOR PEOPLE RECOVERING FROM CANCER

10

According to the American Cancer Society (ACS), one half of all men and a little over one third of all women will develop some form of cancer during their lifetimes. In 2008, doctors diagnosed nearly 1,500,000 new cancer cases, a total that does not even include first-time skin cancer diagnoses. Add an additional one million cases of basal cell and squamous cell carcinomas to that total to get a true sense of cancer's prevalence. Sadly, more than 1,500 people per day die of cancer for a total of over 565,000 deaths each year; that means one out of every four people dies of cancer. This makes cancer the second most common cause of death in the United States, surpassed only by cardiovascular disease.[1,2]

> ### QUICK REFERENCE
> The following lists cancers in the United States with an annual incidence of ≥35,000 cases:
>
> - Urinary bladder cancer
> - Breast cancer
> - Colon and rectal cancer
> - Endometrial cancer
> - Kidney cancer
> - Leukemia
> - Lung cancer
> - Melanoma
> - Non-Hodgkin lymphoma
> - Pancreatic cancer
> - Nonmelanoma skin cancer
> - Thyroid cancer

A combination of risk factor identification, new early detection methods, and advances in therapy improves the prognosis for cancer victims. According to Dr. Julie Gerberding, Director of the Centers for Disease Control and Prevention, "the significant decline in cancer death rates demonstrates important progress in the fight against cancer that has been achieved through effective tobacco control, screening, early detection, and appropriate treatment." This means that a growing number of cancer victims can expect to live well into old age and would likely benefit from health promotion efforts and lifestyle changes.

This is important because cancer survivors remain at risk for recurrence of initial cancer, development of second cancers, and the emergence of additional chronic diseases.[3] In addition, cancer treatment protocols themselves tax the body and cause many negative side effects that often linger for years after treatment cessation.[4] Exercise and diet might alleviate some of these symptoms and therefore be viable adjuncts to traditional modes of therapy.

Studies demonstrate that people who are active from childhood through adulthood not only live longer lives, but they also have healthier lives than those who are sedentary[1,5-8] In addition, regular activity slows age-related functional decline, improves well-being, and promotes healthy weight management. Interestingly, research shows that benefits accrue even if individuals do not become active until late in life. That means that even previously sedentary cancer survivors can benefit by increasing activity level. But what are the guidelines for this population? What precautions are important for cancer survivors? This chapter addresses these issues.

ANATOMICAL AND PHYSIOLOGICAL CHANGES DURING THE DEVELOPMENT OF CANCER

NORMAL CELL GROWTH

Cells are the basic structural and functional units of the body that usually congregate together to form tissues. The body is composed of nearly 70 trillion cells, which vary in size, structure, and function. Although there are at least 250 different varieties, most cells are formed of a cell membrane, cytoplasm, and a single nucleus.

The cell membrane acts as the cell's outer boundary that separates the intracellular fluid from the extracellular fluid. The cell membrane, however, does more than simply separate the cell's contents from the outside; it also acts as a selective barrier that regulates movement into and out of the cell.

The cytoplasm includes both cytosol and organelles. Cytosol, the liquid yet viscous portion of cytoplasm, contains dissolved substances such as glucose, amino acids, fatty acids, and proteins. In addition, it is the site of many important chemical reactions necessary for cell functioning. The organelles are specialized structures in the cytoplasm that permit specific functions. Examples of organelles include mitochondria, ribosomes, endoplasmic reticulum, golgi bodies, the cytoskeleton, and lysosomes.

The nucleus is the third major component of the cell. It contains the genetic material necessary for cellular functioning. Genetic material, also known as DNA, exists in the form of chromatin in a nondividing cell and in the form of chromosomes in a cell preparing for cell division. DNA is a double-stranded molecule composed of billions of nucleotides (Fig. 10.1). Each nucleotide consists of a sugar, a phosphate, and a nitrogen-containing base. Along each strand of DNA, the sugar of one nucleotide bonds with the phosphate of another nucleotide, so each DNA strand essentially consists of a sugar–phosphate backbone with nitrogen-containing bases projecting toward and bonding with the nitrogen-containing bases of the second DNA strand.

In general, each set of three nitrogenous bases along each DNA strand specifies a particular amino acid. Therefore, DNA can essentially be thought of as a series of amino

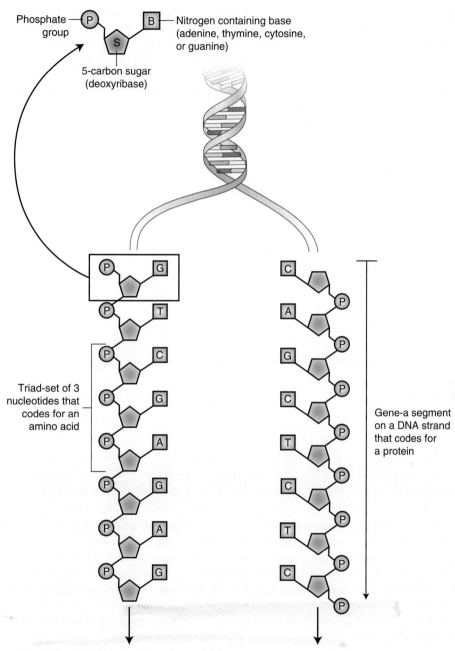

Phosphate group

Nitrogen containing base (adenine, thymine, cytosine, or guanine)

5-carbon sugar (deoxyribase)

Triad-set of 3 nucleotides that codes for an amino acid

Gene-a segment on a DNA strand that codes for a protein

FIGURE 10.1 ■ DNA molecule.

acids. (Note: some DNA segments are noncoding and do not specify amino acids.) Because amino acids are the building blocks of proteins, DNA molecules ultimately contain the blueprints for every protein made in the body. Each cell, therefore, has all of the information necessary to synthesize every protein it requires to function. This is why it is crucial for a cell to replicate genetic information prior to cell division; replication ensures that each new daughter cell receives this information so that it, too, can make all of the proteins required for normal functioning.

QUICK REFERENCE

The specific segment along DNA that codes for a given protein is called a gene. There are an estimated 20,000 to 30,000 genes in the human genome.[9]

The cell cycle encompasses a series of changes that a cell undergoes from initial formation until cell division. In general, the cell cycle of normal body cells consists of interphase and mitosis. During interphase, a cell grows in size, produces additional organelles, and participates in the activities for which it is specialized. If the cell is destined to divide, it must also replicate its DNA during this time. By the end of interphase, a cell has extra organelles and exact copies of its DNA to pass along to its daughter cells. At this point, mitosis occurs. The individual phases of mitosis are not important right now. What is important is to understand that mitosis results in two daughter cells. Each daughter cell has an exact copy of the DNA required to produce all proteins necessary for normal cellular functioning.

QUICK REFERENCE

The human body is made up of parts with increasing complexity. These "levels of body organization" include the chemical, cellular, tissue, organ, organ system, and organism levels. See figure 10.2. The overall organism, therefore, is based upon the chemical level which includes molecules such as DNA. Any problems at the chemical level can disrupt functioning at each subsequent level which can ultimately result in disease or death of the organism.

Healthy cells have a specific structure, function, and growth rate that enable them to perform their jobs.[10] The number of times a cell divides is strictly regulated and varies for different cells. Epidermal cells, for instance, constantly divide. In fact, it only takes 4 to 6 weeks for a brand new epidermal cell to move from its deepest location to the surface of the skin where it sloughs off. Epithelial cells lining the digestive tract are replaced even more frequently; new cells replace worn-out cells every 3 to 5 days.

There seems to be an internal "mitotic clock" that predetermines the number of times most human cells divide, but both internal and external factors influence this rate. For example, *hormones* and *growth factors* stimulate new cell proliferation and are used in medical procedures to hasten the healing process of damaged tissue. *Space availability* is another factor that can enhance or inhibit new cell growth. In most circumstances, healthy cells actually stop dividing once surrounded by other cells, a process called

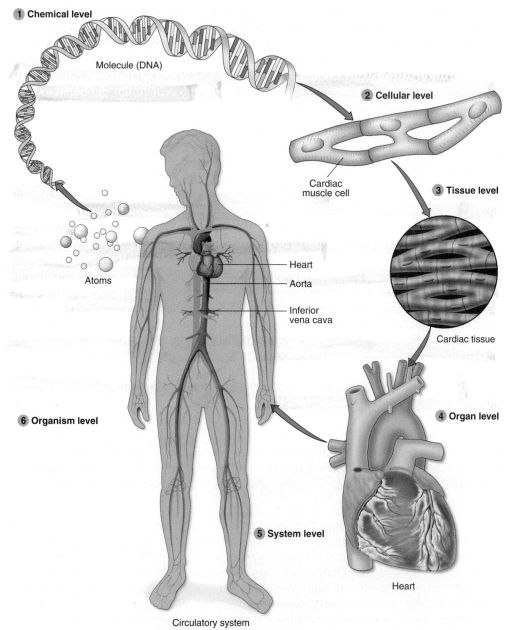

1 **Chemical level**

Molecule (DNA)

2 **Cellular level**

Cardiac
muscle cell

3 **Tissue level**

Atoms

Heart
Aorta
Inferior
vena cava

Cardiac tissue

6 **Organism level**

4 **Organ level**

5 **System level**

Heart

Circulatory system

FIGURE 10.2 ■ The entire organism is based on the chemical level of organization. Atoms combine to form molecules and macromolecules; macromolecules form cells; collections of cells form tissues; a combination of three or more tissues forms an organ; organs with common functions comprise organ systems; and organ systems ensure survival of the organism. (From Premkumar K. The Massage Connection: Anatomy and Physiology. Baltimore: Lippincott Williams & Wilkins 2004.)

contact inhibition. Lastly, old, worn-out cells undergo a natural process of cell death called **apoptosis** to make way for new cells. Overall, an appropriate rate of cell division is crucial for normal growth, development, and tissue repair. Without restraints, excessive cell division forms masses of tissue that can interfere with normal functioning. Fortunately, **tumor suppressor genes** normally code for proteins that inhibit cell division at times when cells divide too rapidly. In a sense, they prevent tumor development and often trigger apoptosis of tumor-producing cells.

WHAT IS CANCER?

Cancer is not a single disease. In fact, over 100 different types of cancer exist. They are distinguished based on their site of origin and the type of cell they affect. According to the National Cancer Institute, cancer cells can originate from just about any cell in the body; their main distinguishing characteristic is that they are **malignant**. The major categories of cancer are carcinomas, sarcomas, lymphomas, and leukemia. *Carcinomas,* such as lung, breast, prostate, stomach, and colon cancers, are the most common forms of cancer in the United States. They typically affect **epithelial cells** lining external or internal body surfaces. *Sarcomas* develop in soft tissues. Soft tissues include muscle and **connective tissues** such as bone, adipose, and cartilage. *Lymphomas* occur in lymphatic organs such as the lymph nodes and spleen, so they affect the immune system. They are further classified as Hodgkin's lymphoma (the most common form of lymphoma) or non-Hodgkin's lymphoma. *Leukemia* is a fourth class of cancer that affects immature blood cells as they form in the red bone marrow. Different types of leukemia exist, but they are all characterized by the rapid growth of white blood cells.

The word "cancer" refers to the rapid development and growth of abnormal cells that infiltrate and destroy normal body cells (Fig. 10.3). Cancer cells are sometimes isolated to

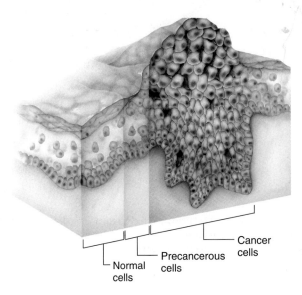

Normal cells   Precancerous cells   Cancer cells

FIGURE 10.3 ■ Cancer is a destructive (malignant) growth of cells, which invades nearby tissues and may metastasize to other areas of the body. Dividing rapidly, these cells tend to be very aggressive. (Asset provided by Anatomical Chart Co.)

a specific area, but they usually travel through the body and attack secondary tissues. Most importantly, and as mentioned earlier, cancer is not a single, specific disorder; instead, different forms affect various body tissues, have different modes of action, and require different management techniques. The only common characteristics among the different forms of cancer are that they all exhibit an unregulated, uncontrollable, and limitless capacity to reproduce, and they can easily migrate in the body. When cancers spread to secondary sites, they are still named for their organ of origin.

HOW DOES CANCER DEVELOP?

The human body normally balances cell division, cell growth, and cell death. Although the rate of cell division varies for different cells, it occurs at a pace that guarantees that viable, new cells are available to replace those undergoing apoptosis. This ensures that sufficient healthy tissue remains to sustain normal functioning.

Carcinogenesis, or the formation of cancer, can result from a multitude of factors (Table 10.1). It characteristically develops slowly and often goes undetected for years. The two most commonly studied contributing factors to cancer development are inherited genetic mutations and genetic mutations that result from chronic exposure to carcinogens.

Some people are born with an inherited genetic defect in their DNA that predisposes them to cancer. As a result, whenever their DNA replicates prior to cell division, that genetic mutation passes on to newly formed cells. If the mutation stimulates excessive cell proliferation or interferes with growth inhibition, affected cells can divide uncontrollably and eventually form masses. Interestingly, it is not uncommon for minor DNA mutations to develop during the process of replication. Fortunately, cells have built-in protective mechanisms that often detect and repair these mutations before replication completes. In cases where a cell cannot repair a mutation, the cell often self-destructs. In essence, it sacrifices itself to save the body.

Exposure to environmental carcinogens or tumor viruses can also alter genetic material. As mentioned earlier, cell proteins often identify mutated genes and either repair them or initiate apoptosis. Therefore, no matter what the source, the body has "protective"

Apoptosis—programmed cell death. A normal process that allows new cells to replace aging cells.

Tumor suppressor gene—codes for proteins that regulate mitosis and prevent uncontrolled cell division; also promotes apoptosis of overactive cells.

Malignant—the ability to spread to other parts of the body and invade and destroy tissues.

Epithelial cells—cells that line body and organ surfaces. Classified by cell shape and number of layers present.

Connective tissue—tissue found in between other tissues in the body. Forms a framework for the body and supports body organs and structures.

Carcinogenesis—a change or mutation in the DNA of a cell.

Carcinogen—a cancer-causing agent.

TABLE 10-1   FACTORS THAT CONTRIBUTE TO THE DEVELOPMENT OF CANCER

Factor	Description
Family history of cancer	Nearly 10% of all cancers have a heredity component
Age	Cancer risk begins increasing at age 40 and then increases dramatically at age 50. This is possibly because of the cumulative effects of exposure to environmental carcinogens.
Environment	Exposure to UV radiation from the sun, asbestos, benzene, or ionizing radiation from x-rays increase the risk for cancer
Tobacco use, excessive alcohol use, diet, and physical inactivity	Tobacco use increases the risk of lung, esophagus, pharynx, larynx, mouth, stomach, and liver cancers. Alcohol use increases the risk for breast and liver cancer—even at low intake levels. High-fat diets increase the risk for breast, colon, and prostate cancers. Physical inactivity increases the risk for breast and colon cancers.
Exposure to certain viruses	Human immunodeficiency virus (HIV), human papillomavirus (HPV), Hepatitis B or C, Human Herpes Virus 8, and Epstein-Barr virus are linked to liver, anal, and genital cancers as well as some lymphomas. These oncogenic viruses are thought to invade normal cells, alter their genetic material, and permit uncontrollable growths of tumors in susceptible individuals.
Exposure to certain bacteria	*Helicobacter pylori* and *Chlamydia trachomatis* are thought to slightly increase the risk of stomach cancer and cervical cancer, respectively
Chronic inflammation of the esophagus from acid reflux, chronic inflammation of the urinary bladder and pancreas from parasites, or chronic inflammation of the colon from inflammatory bowel disease	Long-term exposure to inflammatory mediators increases the risk for cell mutations, uncontrollable cell proliferation, and oncogene activation—all of which contribute to cancer development.

Source: American Cancer Society. Available at: www.cancer.org; National Cancer Institute. Available at: www.cancer.gov; Shacter E. Chronic inflammation and cancer. Oncology 2002;16(2):217–232.

or "regulatory"' proteins that takes care of mutated cells before they proliferate. If, however, damage occurs to the genes that code for these "protective" or "regulatory" proteins, they no longer function as intended. Consequently, mutated cells survive, proliferate, accumulate, and form **tumors**. Thus, cancer can arise when some sort of mutation alters the genes that produce the proteins that control cell division.

THE ROLE OF ONCOGENES AND TUMOR SUPPRESSOR CELLS IN CANCER DEVELOPMENT

Although nearly 30,000 genes exist in the human genome, only a few of these contribute to cancer development and progression. **Proto-oncogenes** are genes that code for proteins that promote normal cell division and typical cell growth. When functioning normally, proto-oncogenes ensure that new cells form at an appropriate rate to replace those lost through apoptosis. When mutated, however, proto-oncogenes form **oncogenes**, genes that produce proteins that permit uncontrolled cell growth.[11,12] Fortunately, a second type of gene controls the activity of oncogenes. This second type of gene was mentioned earlier. It is the tumor suppressor gene, which codes for proteins that inhibit cell division or stimulate apoptosis when the rate of cell division exceeds need. Problems develop when tumor suppressor genes mutate and lose their ability to inhibit tumor growth. In some cases, their mutations actually *stimulate* tumor cell proliferation. Once formed, tumors are self-sufficient; they release growth factors that stimulate **angiogenesis**, or the formation of their own blood vessel network. The newly formed blood vessels then enable the tumor cells to survive, thrive, and grow—often until they interfere with the functioning of nearby tissues. In fact, tumors actually divert blood, nutrients, and gases from healthy tissues to support themselves. In addition to supplying the tumor with necessary nutrients and oxygen, this vast blood vessel network provides the tumor cells with the means by which to travel to other areas of the body, a process known as **metastasis** (Fig. 10.4). Metastasis occurs even when only a few tumor cells break away from the primary tumor, spread to other parts of the body, and begin developing in new locations. This is how secondary tumors form from primary tumors. As angiogenesis within a developing tumor continues, lymphatic vessels also proliferate and provide an additional means of metastasis that takes advantage of the lymphatic system.[11,12]

As early as 1941, Rous and Kidd[13,14] described chemical carcinogenesis as a two-step process that involves initiation and promotion. Initiation occurs when a cell is exposed to a cancer-causing agent that permanently alters the cell's genetic make-up. Examples of initiators include errors in DNA replication, ineffective repair enzymes, or exposure to a carcinogen such as radiation. Damage from an initiator, however, is not sufficient to lead to cancer. Exposure to a promoter, however, can stimulate proliferation of the altered cell and subsequent tumor growth. Promoters include pollution, viruses, and other toxins. Some toxins, such as tobacco smoke, are considered complete carcinogens because they act as both an initiator and a promoter; therefore, they carry higher risk.[1,10,15]

QUICK REFERENCE

Research demonstrates that cancer risk is more strongly related to lifestyles factors and exposure to environmental carcinogens than to heredity.[16]

Tumor—a growth that results from excessive cell division; serves no functional purpose in the body.

Proto-oncogenes—genes that code for proteins that encourage cell growth.

Oncogenes—result from mutated proto-oncogenes; oncogenes are genes that allow uncontrolled cell division. They basically allow cells to continue to divide even when they should not, and thus promote the formation of cancerous growths.

Angiogenesis—development of new blood vessels.

Metastasis—movement, usually through the blood stream, of cancer cells from one location in the body to another. Tumors produced by metastasis are sometimes called secondary tumors. Metastasis is the cause of 90% of cancer-related deaths.

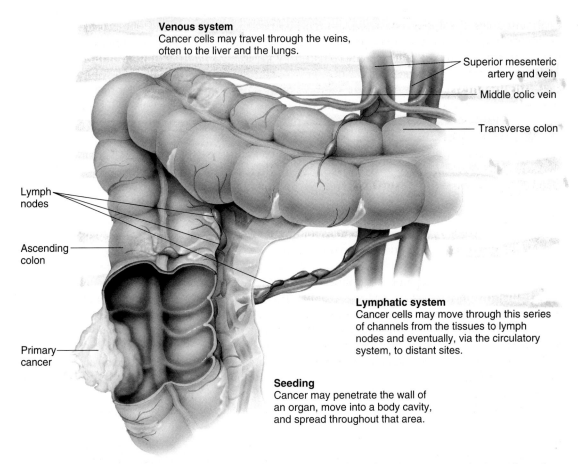

Venous system
Cancer cells may travel through the veins,
often to the liver and the lungs.

Superior mesenteric
artery and vein

Middle colic vein

Transverse colon

Lymph
nodes

Ascending
colon

Lymphatic system
Cancer cells may move through this series
of channels from the tissues to lymph
nodes and eventually, via the circulatory
system, to distant sites.

Primary
cancer

Seeding
Cancer may penetrate the wall of
an organ, move into a body cavity,
and spread throughout that area.

FIGURE 10.4 ■ How cancer spreads. Cancer cells may invade nearby tissues or metastasize (spread) to other organs. Cancer cells may move to other tissues by any or all of three routes: venous system, lymphatic system, or seeding. (Asset provided by Anatomical Chart Co.)

BENIGN VERSUS MALIGNANT TUMORS

Benign tumors, which are noncancerous growths composed of cells that resemble normal cells, result from excessive, local cell growth that typically does not spread. In fact, benign tumors are usually enclosed within a capsule, a structure that limits their ability to metastasize. In general, benign growths are nonthreatening and are often not detected for years. Once they reach a certain size, however, they can limit range of motion, compress nearby organs or blood vessels, or stimulate glands to produce excess hormones. In these cases, benign tumors usually need to be removed. Examples of benign tumors include lipomas, chondromas, and adenomas.

Lipomas are painless, moveable fat masses that are soft to the touch. They grow slowly and only rarely develop into cancer. Most people who have lipomas do not require treatment unless the lipoma becomes painful or limits range of motion around a joint. If necessary, surgeons can easily remove them. A relatively recent removal method involves using ultrasound waves to pulverize the cells.

Chondromas are benign tumors of cartilage cells—most frequently hyaline cartilage cells. They are the most common benign tumors of the chest wall, but they also occur at the ends of long bones. A capsule also surrounds this type of tumor, so it rarely metastasizes and is easily removed.

Adenomas usually arise from secretory cells such as those forming glands; consequently, any glandular tissue in the body can develop an adenoma. Adenomas are commonly associated with the adrenal, pituitary, and salivary glands. In many instances, adenomas cause glands to release excessive amounts of hormone. This can cause various symptoms depending upon which gland is affected. In most cases, the presence of an adenoma does not increase the likelihood of developing a carcinoma. An adenoma associated with the colon, rectum, or lungs, however, is a strong predictor of cancer. Physicians typically recommend surgical removal of adenomas, but medication is sometimes just as effective.

Benign tumors rarely develop into cancer and are often completely asymptomatic. If present, possible symptoms include pressure, pain, anemia, itching, restricted blood flow to organs, or various other symptoms if the affected organ is a gland. The only viable treatment is surgical removal since benign tumors rarely respond to radiation or chemotherapy.

Malignant tumors are composed of cells that invade healthy tissues, proliferate rapidly, develop extensive blood vessel networks, and then metastasize to other areas of the body. They differ structurally and functionally from normal body cells, are less organized than benign tumors, and often resist treatment. If not treated and eradicated, they cause death. Examples of malignant tumors include myeloma, angiosarcoma, lymphoma, sarcoma, leukemia, and neuroblastoma. Myeloma is a tumor of the bone marrow. Although rare, an angiosarcoma develops in the endothelial lining of blood vessels, particularly in those of the breast and skin. Lymphomas, one of the four major types of cancer, are usually malignant and spread rapidly through the lymphatic system. Sarcomas affect connective tissues, particularly bone cells and muscle cells. Leukemia, or cancer of the blood, is characterized by abnormal white blood cell production. Neuroblastoma, a rapidly spreading tumor, develops in nerve cells. See Table 10.2 for properties of malignant tumors.

TABLE 10-2   PROPERTIES OF MALIGNANT TUMORS

Property	Description
Aggressive	Proliferate and grow without limits
Invasive	Attack, enter, and destroy healthy tissue
Failure to mature	Rarely reach a stage where they stop dividing
Loss of contact inhibition	Continue to reproduce even when they contact one another and begin to pile up. Normal cells stop proliferating upon contact with other cells.
Metastasize	Spread to secondary locations in the body where they proliferate, attack, and destroy healthy tissue

COMMON CAUSES OF CANCER

Because there are so many types of cancer, it is unlikely that a single cause will ever be determined. Furthermore, there will likely never be a single cure either. Researchers, however, have been able to pinpoint several factors that promote cancer development (Table 10.2). Nearly 40% of all cancers seem to result from exposure to environmental carcinogens, particularly tobacco and excessive alcohol. Another 33% are related to dietary intake. The remaining cases are likely due to factors such as age, sex, and stress level.

Tobacco Use

The number one preventable risk factor for cancer is tobacco use. According to the National Cancer Institute, 87% of all lung cancer incidences and 30% of all deaths from cancer can be attributed to cigarette smoking. In fact, cigarettes kill more Americans than alcohol, car accidents, suicide, AIDS, homicide, and illegal drugs combined.[1] Sadly, tobacco use is not only a problem for adults; an estimated 22.1% of all high school students admit to smoking regularly. Shockingly, even 8.1% of all middle school students smoke.[1,7]

QUICK REFERENCE
The ACS estimates that 20.8% of all adults in the United States smoke and that one out of every five deaths in the United States is from cigarette smoking.

Tobacco use not only promotes lung cancer. It also increases the risk for cancers of the larynx, mouth, throat, esophagus, urinary bladder, pancreas, stomach, cervix, and kidneys. In addition, tobacco use in general also increases the risk for heart disease, stroke, chronic obstructive pulmonary disorders (like emphysema), aneurisms, gum disease, bone deterioration, and eye disease.[1]

Astonishingly, more than 4,000 chemicals are found in cigarettes. Sixty of these are known carcinogens. Some examples of cigarette components include carbon monoxide, tar, ammonia, arsenic, nicotine, acetone, benzene, cadmium, formaldehyde, hydrazine, and hydrogen cyanide (Fig. 10.5). Some of these components are used in rat poison, nail polish, paint removers, jet fuel, embalming fluids, household cleaners, rubber cement, and batteries.[7,17–19]

Heredity

Although not all cancers are hereditary, nearly 10% result from mutated genes passed along to offspring of cancer sufferers. Examples of inheritable cancers are breast, cervical, colon, stomach, prostate, and ovarian cancer. Of course, not everyone who has a family history of cancer develops cancer; however, the risk is greater, so precautions are necessary. Genetic testing for some forms of cancer is currently available.

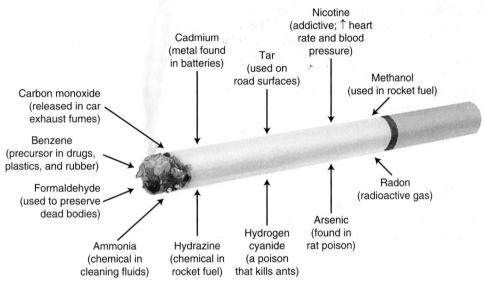

FIGURE 10.5 ■ Some of the ingredients found in a cigarette.

Age

Cancer affects all age groups, ethnicities, and income levels, but more than 75% of all cases occur in those over the age of 55. Some experts suggest that the increased age-related risk is because of the accumulated exposure to environmental toxins and pollutants that occurs over a lifetime. Breast, colorectal, and prostate cancer risk significantly increases with age.

Impaired Immune System Functioning

Certain states of immune deficiency, such as contracting HIV, are associated with a higher rate of malignant tumors. Perhaps a weakened immune system allows cancerous cells to continue to grow without interruption.

Exposure to Ultraviolet Radiation

Excessive exposure to ultraviolet (UV) radiation from the sun, especially if that exposure results in burned skin, increases the risk of developing skin cancer. Although everyone is at risk for skin cancer, certain groups are more susceptible. They include those with fair skin, freckles, and a family history of melanoma as well as those who spend a lot of time outdoors and neglect to wear sunscreen. To decrease risk, avoid exposure to the sun between 10 AM and 4 PM; wear sunscreen with a minimum SPF of 15; wear protective clothing such as hats and sunglasses; and stay in the shade during midday.

Exposure to Viruses

Approximately 15% of all cancers result from exposure to viruses such as the human papilloma virus (HPV), Hepatitis C, Hepatitis B, and Epstein-Barr virus. In some cases, the virus itself carries a gene that creates an oncogene once inside the host cell. In other cases, the virus stimulates a proto-oncogene in the invaded cell. In either case, rapid and uncontrolled viral replication ensues and cancerous cells develop.

Some types of HPV, which actually includes a group of more than 100 viruses, are commonly implicated in cervical cancer. Using a condom during sexual intercourse reduces the risk of contracting this virus and thereby reduces the risk of developing this particular cancer. In addition, a vaccine is now available that protects against this virus. According to the Centers for Disease Control, 11- and 12-year-old girls should receive a series of three injections over the course of 6 months. Girls and women between the ages of 13 and 26 who did not receive the injections previously are also encouraged to get vaccinated.

Diet and Lack of Physical Activity

According to the ACS, about one third of all cancer deaths are related to poor diet and a sedentary lifestyle in adulthood. Excessive alcohol intake, in particular, is associated with an increased risk of mouth and throat cancer. These, like many other risk factors for cancer, are modifiable and need to be addressed.

DIAGNOSIS

Developing tumors often elicit no signs or symptoms in their early stages. In fact, they often go unnoticed until they are fairly large and put pressure on surrounding organs or tissues. This can take years or even decades. Once a tumor is suspected, a physician usually orders medical tests such as blood tests, x-rays, computed tomography scans, or an endoscopy to confirm the presence of a growth. Common early detection methods include the Pap exam for cervical cancer, a colonoscopy for colon cancer, a mammogram to detect breast cancer, and a prostate-specific antigen blood test for prostate cancer. To determine malignancy, physicians remove and examine cells from the tumor by performing a procedure called a biopsy. There are different techniques for biopsies—a fine needle biopsy removes a small number of cells; a large needle biopsy removes a greater number of cells; an incisional biopsy removes a small piece of the tumor; and an excisional biopsy removes the entire tumor. After a biopsy, the cells are analyzed in a lab and the results help delineate treatment options.

If the biopsy comes back negative, the tumor is benign and can be left alone unless it is causing symptoms. An example of a benign tumor that requires surgical removal is a uterine tumor that exerts pressure on the urinary bladder or rectum or causes excessive bleeding during menstruation. If a tumor is malignant, however, removal is imperative. Before deciding upon a treatment option, physicians need to *stage* the cancer. This simply means that they need to describe the size of the tumor, determine if it has damaged nearby tissues, and ascertain if it has metastasized to other areas of the body. Once staging is complete, treatment begins. Of course, the earlier cancer is detected, the better the prognosis.

The Quick Reference below presents some possible warning signs and symptoms of cancer. Because the actual signs and symptoms vary based on cancer type, this list is broad and could indicate various less serious conditions. If any of these are present, however, visit a physician for a thorough examination.

QUICK REFERENCE

Early warning signs or symptoms of cancer include the following:

- Unexplained fatigue
- Muscle weakness
- Unusual weight loss despite no changes in diet or activity
- Persistent headache
- Pain that will not go away
- Changes in bowel movements or urinary habits
- Persistent cough or hoarseness
- Feelings of depression
- Sores or wounds that do not heal
- Unusual bleeding (blood found in saliva, stools, vaginal discharge, urine)
- Indigestion or difficulty swallowing
- Persistent fever

TREATMENT OPTIONS FOR MALIGNANT TUMORS

Treatment options depend upon the cancer's location, type, and developmental stage. They also depend upon a person's age and health status prior to diagnosis. In any case, treatment can include surgery, radiation, chemotherapy, or immunotherapy (also known as biologic therapy). Ideally, the goal of treatment is to remove all cancerous cells with minimal damage to healthy tissue; however, in some advanced stages of cancer, the goal is to limit the spread of an incurable cancer or to minimize its symptoms. If a malignancy is detected before metastasis, surgery can often "cure" the cancer. A lumpectomy, for example, can successfully remove cancerous tissue from the breast. In more advanced stages of breast cancer, however, the entire breast might need to be removed. Unfortunately, because malignant tumors can spread even before the primary tumor is located, surgery often needs to be followed by radiation or chemotherapy to ensure complete elimination of cancerous cells.

Radiation therapy offers hope in cases of localized cancer. During radiation treatment, a radiologist administers ionizing radiation that is intended to shrink tumors and kill cancerous cells by damaging their DNA. Although radiation also harms nearby noncancerous cells, these healthy cells can usually recover in between bouts of radiation treatment. Radiation seems to be effective against cancers of the breast, brain, prostate, pancreas, and uterus. Even if radiation does not completely destroy a cancerous mass, it often shrinks it enough so that a minimally invasive surgical procedure can remove any remaining abnormal tissue. Side effects of radiation therapy include skin rashes, nausea, vomiting, and diarrhea, but newer techniques minimize these.[1,7,20]

Chemotherapy involves the cyclic administration of drug cocktails. Drug cocktails, which are combinations of two or more cancer-fighting drugs, prove to be more effective than a single drug alone. The drugs may be taken orally, or they may be injected. After an initial injection, the cancer patient waits for a period of 3 to 4 weeks, called the recovery period, before receiving a second injection. The average cycle is 6 months; however, if one cycle does not eliminate the cancer, it is often followed by a second cycle.

Chemotherapy is usually used in cases where cancer has spread into the blood stream or lymphatic system. The drugs are designed to attack, kill, and inhibit reproduction of any rapidly dividing cell. Consequently, chemotherapeutic drugs often damage rapidly dividing healthy cells. Fortunately, most healthy cells repair themselves in between treatments—something cancerous cells cannot do. Chemotherapeutic drugs have progressed significantly over the past few decades. Once thought to elicit symptoms much worse than the cancer itself, chemotherapy drugs are now often well tolerated by cancer victims. Of course, some individuals experience mild side effects, but only a few cannot tolerate chemotherapy at all.[1,7]

QUICK REFERENCE

Common side effects of chemotherapy include the following:

■ Nausea
■ Vomiting
■ Temporary hair loss
■ Decreased immune functioning
■ Fatigue

Immunotherapy is a relatively new treatment method that attempts to prompt a person's own immune system to fight off cancerous cells. Because it is so new, research on its effectiveness is not yet available. The exact method used depends upon cancer type, so a complete discussion of immunotherapy is beyond the scope of this book. One type of immunotherapy involves administering interferons, cytokines, and antibodies, substances also naturally produced by a healthy immune system, to destroy foreign cells. Vaccines and stem cell implantation are additional methods that hold promise for certain forms of cancer.[1,20,21] Overall, the goal of immunotherapy is to inhibit cancer cell growth, repair normal but damaged body cells, and enhance immune response so that the body can destroy cancer cells more effectively on its own.

Angiogenesis inhibitors interfere with the blood vessel formation that typically accompanies tumor development. Their effectiveness depends upon the type of tumor present and the route of delivery. Unfortunately, tumors often develop vast blood vessel networks despite the action of angiogenesis inhibitors since these inhibitors have limited action. Avastin is an example of an angiogenesis inhibitor used in conjunction with other chemotherapy drugs to treat colon and rectal cancer that have metastasized. Although Avastin has not been shown to cure these cancers, it appears to increase the survival rate of users.[7,22]

Overall, cancer cell behavior is totally unpredictable. Thus, each type of cancer requires specialized treatment. In other words, what works for one type of cancer does not necessarily work for another type. This is why discovering a cure is so difficult.

PRECAUTIONS DURING EXERCISE

With advances in technology, a diagnosis of cancer is no longer an absolute death sentence. In fact, many cancer survivors undergo treatment, have positive prognoses, and enjoy a quality of life equivalent to those who have never before had cancer. According to 2008 statistics from the ACS, the overall 5-year survival rate for cancer is up to 65%, so a significant number of people are in remission. Unfortunately, cancer and the side effects associated with cancer treatment often leave survivors with limited functional ability, severe fatigue, debilitating pain, nausea, vomiting, diarrhea, severe weight loss (often in the form of lean tissue), emotional challenges, and an increased risk of infection and dehydration. Therefore, physicians have traditionally discouraged exertion and encouraged rest. The past few decades, however, mark the first time in history that cancer patients are reentering the world of exercise to try to slow deterioration and minimize side effects. Current focus in cancer care is on patient rehabilitation that improves quality of life by increasing functional abilities through activity.[23] With that in mind, this section explores the various factors that might impede a cancer victim's exercise ability.

FATIGUE

The number one side effect of cancer and cancer treatments such as radiation and chemotherapy is a debilitating fatigue that seems to exist no matter how much rest or sleep a cancer survivor gets. It is a tiredness that interferes with normal functioning and leaves the sufferer feeling irritable, impatient, and unmotivated.[24] Fatigue is also the most difficult problem to address because it consists of both physiological and psychological exhaustion that together interfere with the ability to concentrate, remember, and think clearly.[4,25] Fitness professionals must ascertain the degree of this type of fatigue to determine when they should encourage clients to work through the fatigue and when they should suggest clients avoid exercise for the day. Sometimes the fatigue subsides within the first 5 to 10 minutes of activity. If not, offer the client frequent breaks during a workout to encourage continued participation. The most important tactic, however, is to explain to clients that fatigue is a natural part of the recovery process and to offer options for addressing it.

QUICK REFERENCE

Tips to help manage cancer-related fatigue[1]:

■ Get adequate, but not too much, sleep and rest
■ Increase daily activity
■ Add exercise to the daily routine
■ Eat nutritional foods including lots of fruits and vegetables
■ Drink adequate water

LOSS OF FUNCTIONAL CAPACITY BECAUSE OF CHRONIC PAIN, NAUSEA, AND VOMITING

Cancer and cancer therapy can cause pain and multiple impairments depending upon the specific location of the cancer.[23] Some people report high levels of pain, while others are relatively unaffected; however, chronic pain after surgery is common. Sometimes pain develops when large amounts of healthy tissue are removed along with the cancerous tissue. In most instances, physicians prescribe medications that control and often eliminate all discomfort. Even if they elicit no pain, surgeries can damage nerves and limit range of motion around nearby joints. Damaged nerves then impair the actions of the organs they innervate, so fitness professionals must be cautious when designing exercise programs. Certain exercises should be avoided until the affected area heals. The intensity, duration, type, and frequency of exercise typically need readjusting until wounds have healed; however, the rate of progression depends solely on an individual's rate of recovery.

Nausea, vomiting, and diarrhea are also common side effects of radiation and chemotherapy, so an exercise schedule must be flexible enough to accommodate bouts of discomfort. In some cases, initiating exercise actually reduces feelings of nausea within the first few minutes; in other cases, it exacerbates nausea. If it seems to worsen their nausea, clients should avoid exercise for at least 24 hours. Cancer patients who have experienced excessive vomiting or diarrhea might experience electrolyte imbalances and dehydration, so they must be certain to consume both liquids and foods prior to exertion. Health and fitness professionals should be prepared no matter what the scenario is.

If a client's treatment protocol affects the lungs or heart, be careful with all forms of cardiovascular training. Watch for bleeding injuries in those on blood thinners. What would be an inconsequential cut for a typical client can become a life-threatening event in a cancer patient.

CACHEXIA

Cachexia, the physical wasting syndrome accompanied by loss of muscle mass, fat mass, overall weight, and appetite, occurs in up to 75% of cancer patients—particularly in those who are in the advanced stages of cancer. It tends to be more common in those who have cancers of the pancreas, esophagus, and stomach, and it can result in electrolyte imbalances, reduced strength, severe weakness, and fatigue. Since cancer survival is related to the total amount and rate of weight loss, the outlook for patients experiencing cachexia is bleak. In cases of cachexia, treatment with nutrient supplementation rarely reestablishes a healthy weight. In fact, so little is known about cachexia that it is associated with 20% of the total deaths from cancer. A few treatment options have shown promise in extreme cases, but none has been effective in the long term.[26]

Researchers know that cachexia is a complex metabolic disturbance, and they are desperately looking for methods to combat it. Most cancer patients suffering from cachexia lack the energy and ability to exercise, so little is known about the impact of exercise on this condition. Perhaps future research can investigate the effect of resistance training on the preservation of lean muscle mass and alleviation of severe fatigue. The average fitness professional, however, will likely not encounter those with cachexia.

EMOTIONAL ISSUES (ANXIETY, DEPRESSION, LOW SELF-ESTEEM)

Cancer survivors often go through a multitude of emotions ranging from anger at initial diagnosis, depression upon acceptance of the diagnosis, anxiety as they explore treatment options, and elation when they first realize their cancer is in remission. All of this emotional upheaval can stress interpersonal relationships and result in social isolation. This can significantly impair a cancer survivor's desire to participate in an exercise program.

INCREASED RISK FOR INFECTION

Chemotherapy, radiation therapy, and immunotherapy are all designed to kill cancer cells. Unfortunately, they often kill healthy body cells as well. In fact, these treatments have a substantial impact on white blood cells, the cells in the body that help fight and protect against foreign invaders. Consequently, immune function often weakens during cancer treatment. Frequent hand washing helps reduce the risk of contracting viral or bacterial infections, but a chemotherapy or radiation patient should be extra cautious when working out in a fitness center where germ count is usually high. Cancer patients should avoid exercise altogether when blood counts are low since they have an increased risk for anemia and infection.

RISK FOR DEHYDRATION

Dehydration often occurs during chemotherapy since large quantities of water are necessary to help the kidneys filter the cancer-fighting drugs. Inadequate hydration promotes fatigue and dizziness, so cancer patients, especially those who exercise, should ensure adequate fluid intake.

> *QUICK REFERENCE*
>
> Cancer survivors should avoid exercise for 24 hours after periods of vomiting and diarrhea; if body temperature exceeds 101°F; if acute nausea persists upon initiation of exercise; or if breathing difficulty, chest pain, or unusual muscular weakness develop during the initial stages of activity.[27]

ADDITIONAL PRECAUTIONS

- Cancer patients undergoing radiation therapy should avoid chlorinated water.
- Survivors who have had a bone marrow transplant should avoid public places such as fitness centers for at least 1 year after treatment. Those with low white blood cell counts should avoid public areas until white blood cell count is within normal limits (as indicated by a physician).

- Cancer patients with indwelling catheters should avoid swimming pools and any training that could dislodge the catheter.
- Cancer patients with significant peripheral neuropathies (pain, tingling, or loss of sensation in a limb) should avoid activities that require extreme balance since they have limited feelings in the affected extremity.

BENEFITS OF EXERCISE

Because so many people are now surviving and thriving after cancer diagnosis, focus is now on improving the quality of life. In fact, exercise both during and after cancer treatment might be one of the most beneficial adjuncts to cancer therapy because it gives cancer survivors some control over their own lives. Most existing research has investigated the effects of exercise on breast, prostate, and colon cancer survivors, but these results likely apply to those who have other forms of cancer as well. Granted, cancer survivors experience challenges and obstacles uncommon to other populations. For example, certain treatments impair muscular, cardiovascular, pulmonary, and neurological functioning; however, the fact remains that several of these difficulties can be addressed with relatively minor adjustments and modifications to typical exercises. In addition, many cancer survivors can experience the same benefits from exercise that are experienced by the general population. Furthermore, exercise helps survivors handle and overcome many of the side effects of cancer and cancer treatments.

Overall, most research shows that exercise reduces fatigue, limits chemo-induced nausea, increases functional capacity by increasing lean mass, and improves psychological functioning in cancer patients.[27–30] Moreover, some studies suggest that exercise reduces the likelihood of cancer recurrence and minimizes overall risk for additional chronic diseases.

QUICK REFERENCE

Benefits of exercise during cancer treatment include the following:

- Less fatigue
- Improved functional capacity
- Maintenance of or increased muscle mass
- Reduced risk of bone loss
- Reduced risk of cardiovascular disease
- Improved mood and self-esteem
- Decreased nausea, vomiting, and diarrhea
- Improved appetite
- Improved quality of life

REDUCED FATIGUE

As mentioned, the number one complaint from cancer treatment patients is a debilitating fatigue that does not subside with increased sleep or improved nutrition.[31] It affects an estimated 70% to 100% of cancer patients receiving radiation therapy, chemotherapy, or immunotherapy. The exact cause is unknown, but it might be related to the anemia common among cancer patients. In the past, medical personnel advised patients to avoid physical activity since higher activity levels tended to promote fatigue.[24,32,33] Several of the latest studies, however, suggest that regular cardiovascular exercise following cancer treatment *decreases* the incidence of fatigue and actually *improves* energy levels.[24,31–35] In fact, many recent studies demonstrate that regular aerobic exercise over a period of 6 months significantly increased cardiovascular conditioning which likely improves endurance.[4] Exercise has also been shown to decrease fatigue in patients with Hodgkin Disease and prostate cancer.[24]

REDUCED INCIDENCE OF NAUSEA, VOMITING, AND DIARRHEA

Additional adverse effects of chemotherapy and radiation treatment include nausea, vomiting, and diarrhea.[31] In numerous studies, breast cancer patients undergoing chemotherapy reported that nausea subsided within a few minutes of initiating aerobic exercise.[1,36,37] When nausea does not subside within the first few minutes of exercise, clients should postpone exercise for at least 24 hours.[27] Overall, exercise promotes healthier digestive tract functioning and reduces the incidence of gastrointestinal distress in the long term.

IMPROVED FUNCTIONAL CAPACITY

Cancer patients who do not remain active during chemotherapy tend to decondition rapidly.[27] Inactive muscles atrophy, which means they lose size, strength, endurance, and flexibility. Continued muscle stimulation, however, minimizes the loss of muscle mass and stimulates muscle growth and strength, factors that improve overall functional capacity.[35] Both cardiovascular and resistance exercise preserve lean mass. Resistance training in particular also enhances communication between the nervous and muscular systems.

Cardiovascular training helps maintain normal cardiorespiratory functioning, VO_{2max}, and oxygen delivery to cells by improving heart and lung functioning. This promotes a healthy blood pressure, blood volume, red blood cell count, and gas exchange—factors that make activities of daily living easier and more enjoyable.

IMPROVED PSYCHOLOGICAL FUNCTIONING AND SELF-ESTEEM

In addition to decreasing fatigue and improving physical functioning, exercise enhances emotional well-being, improves self-esteem, and decreases incidences of anxiety and depression.[35,38] This is true even when cancer treatment has failed. Why? This might be because exercise restores energy levels by improving cardiorespiratory functioning, a factor that directly affects feelings of self-confidence and hope.[2,39] Additionally, exercise improves gastrointestinal functioning, reduces chronic inflammation, enhances immune function, and reduces the incidence of obesity, all factors that improve self-image and outlook on life.[39] This should not be surprising given that exercise has been associated with decreased anxiety and improved mood in the general population.

DECREASED RISK OF RECURRENCE FOR SOME CANCERS

Studies consistently show that participation in cardiovascular exercise decreases the recurrence of breast cancer in women.[4] In one study, moderate aerobic exercise for 25 to 45 minutes per day significantly improved survival of breast cancer patients.[2] Perhaps this is because it lowers the amount of circulating insulin and various growth factors that stimulate rapid cell growth. Exercise is also associated with decreased estrogen levels, a factor that could directly benefit breast cancer survivors since risk increases proportionately with increases in blood estrogen levels.

Authorities agree that exercise coupled with proper energy intake helps achieve and maintain a healthy weight. Since being overweight or obese is clearly related to the development of breast, colon, endometrial, esophageal, and kidney cancers, maintaining a healthy weight through exercise and diet likely decreases risk. In a recent report, the American Cancer Institute suggested that maintaining a body mass index of 20 to 25 is one of the most important factors in preventing cancer. It seems that avoiding overweight and obesity would also reduce the risk of recurrence.

In a study of 65-year-old men with early stage prostate cancer, researchers found that moderate aerobic exercise (for a total of 3 hours per week) decreased the risk of prostate cancer progression.[40] If regular exercise lowers the recurrence rate of breast and prostate cancers, perhaps it can also lower the recurrence of other types of cancer through its effects on the immune system, hormones, and weight.[41] Since cancers vary in how they develop, progress, and respond to treatment, though, exercise might not be the answer for every type. Whether exercise exerts a direct effect on cancer recurrence or not, the impact it has on energy levels and self-confidence might be enough to improve overall survival rate.

DECREASED RISK FOR OTHER CHRONIC DISEASES

Cancer survivors are at an increased risk for chronic diseases such as cardiovascular disease, stroke, diabetes, obesity, and osteoporosis. Most existing research indicates that an active lifestyle in the cancer-free population decreases risk for these chronic diseases. Although studies related to the effects of exercise on the incidence of cardiovascular disease and diabetes in cancer survivors are lacking, it seems that increased physical activity could provide cancer survivors with the same protection experienced by those without cancer.

Osteoporosis is another common concern for patients undergoing cancer treatment. In fact, breast cancer survivors have a five times greater risk of experiencing an osteoporosis-related vertebral fracture 1 year following treatment than their healthy counterparts. This is likely because many chemotherapeutic agents also contain bone-demineralizing agents that weaken bones. This can be particularly dangerous because chemotherapy patients often lose significant muscle mass making them prone to imbalance and falls.[42] According to a study that investigated the side effects of prostate cancer treatment, researchers noted that men undergoing therapy experienced an average loss of 3% to 5% of bone mass each year during treatment. To prevent this loss, cancer patients should participate in regular weight-bearing exercise (though precise recommendations on frequency and duration were not addressed).[43] Overall, weight-bearing exercise not only preserves muscle mass and bone tissue; it also improves endurance, balance, and functional abilities.

RECOMMENDATIONS FOR EXERCISE

As mentioned, exercise is a fairly new "treatment option" for many types of cancers, so research and precise recommendations are currently lacking. The American College of Sports Medicine (ACSM) and the ACS, however, offer some basic guidelines. The ACS convened a group of experts to evaluate existing research on the impact of nutrition and physical activity on cancer survival and treatment tolerance. This group of experts recognizes a continuum of cancer survival, a range that includes a treatment phase, a recovery phase, an after-recovery phase, and a living-with-advanced-cancer phase. Different phases demand different exercise and nutrition protocols, so exercise testing and prescription must be individualized.[44] ACSM has also evaluated existing research and has made general recommendations for this special population.

EXERCISE TESTING

According to Carole Schneider's article in ACSM's Fit Society,[45] ACSM suggests that cancer patients and their trainers work closely with physicians in designing exercise routines since each patient experiences different limitations and varying tolerance levels. The first step is for cancer patients to seek medical clearance from their physicians prior to any exercise testing or other physical activity. Once a medical clearance is provided, fitness professionals should collect complete medical histories and perform comprehensive fitness evaluations including tests for cardiopulmonary functioning, muscular strength and endurance, and flexibility. Adaptations for certain exercise tests are necessary since many cancer patients have limited mobility or impaired functioning because of the type of cancer present and/or the type of treatment protocol they have undergone. Furthermore, cancer and cancer therapy interfere with cardiovascular fitness, muscular strength and endurance, body composition, flexibility, and gait and balance, so results can be misleading.[46] ACSM specifically recommends a graded treadmill or bicycle ergometer test to assess cardiovascular functioning, a spirometer test for pulmonary functioning, dumbbells or resistance machines for muscle strength and endurance tests, and the modified sit-and-reach for flexibility.[45]

QUICK REFERENCE
ACSM recommends medical supervision of symptom-limited or maximal exercise testing for this population.[46]

In addition to careful exercise testing, ACSM suggests that fitness professionals working with cancer patients obtain additional specialized training that prepares them for the unique challenges imposed by working with this diverse group.[45,46] Thoroughly screen clients for comorbidities and obtain as much information from physicians as possible to include complete blood counts, lipid profiles, and pulmonary function test results if available.[46] See Table 10.1 in *ACSM's Guidelines for Exercise Testing and Prescription*, 8th Ed for details on contraindications and precautions in this group.

EXERCISE PRESCRIPTION

Based on the results of exercise testing, fitness professionals should design an individualized exercise program that should be evaluated every 6 months until cancer treatment is stopped. Unlike the general population, progression for cancer survivors is often less predictable. As a result, trainers need to reassess often and be prepared to readjust prior to each workout. The overall goal of exercise for this population is to minimize the general deconditioning that often results from cancer treatment so that the side effects of therapy are better tolerated.[47] General guidelines based on ACS and ACSM recommendations include the following[1,25,27,44,46,47]:

- Make sure clients have a complete medical examination prior to exercise initiation and obtain a written medical clearance for any vigorous activity. If there is any question whatsoever regarding the safety of a given exercise for a particular client, seek physician approval before incorporating that exercise into the workout.
- Plan to monitor blood pressure and heart rate, before, during, and after exercise. Stop all activity if dizziness, nausea, or chest pain occurs.
- Begin each workout with a 5- to 10-minute warm-up that stimulates blood flow to working muscles. Include limbering movements and mild stretching. Some authorities suggest taking a resting heart rate prior to warming up. If heart rate exceeds 100 bpm, check with a physician before continuing. If heart rate is well below 100 bpm, check it again at the end of the warm-up. At this point, heart rate should be up by 10 to 20 bpm and should be accompanied with mild sweating. To return the body to a resting state, follow each workout with a 5- to 10-minute cooldown that includes stretching.
- Start each workout slowly and build up even more gradually than for traditional patients. Progression in the longer term should consist of increases in frequency and duration rather than in intensity. Postpone increases in intensity until treatment is completed.
- Most research has investigated the impact of *cardiovascular* training on cancer survivors. Stationary bicycles, treadmills, and outdoor walking programs have been the focus of most studies, and these activities seem to offer positive results. Interval training in particular elicits the greatest effect on physical and psychological functioning in breast cancer survivors.[25] Plan for frequent short breaks during the aerobic session to accommodate therapy-related fatigue.

- Actual intensity depends upon an individual's functional status and history of exercise prior to cancer diagnosis and treatment.[47] Previously active cancer patients can typically continue their usual routines but likely need to decrease intensity during treatment. In general, intensity should be low-to-moderate (60% to 80% of maximum heart rate) to prevent taxing the immune system. Avoid continuing any activity that in previous workouts has been followed by stiffness, delayed soreness, severe muscle fatigue, pain, or bleeding. The presence of any of these signs usually implies that intensity during the previous workout was too high. Often, intensity may be increased once treatment is completed.

- To monitor exercise intensity, heart rate may be taken. Since some cancer patients are on blood pressure medications or other drugs that affect heart rate, this might not be the best choice for monitoring intensity. Teach clients to use the Borg Scale of exertion and encourage a light-to-moderate intensity (RPE of 11 to 14) based on this scale. See Appendix A for the Borg Rating of Perceived Exertion Scale.

- ACSM recommends aerobic training on 3 to 5 days per week at an intensity of 40% to 60% VO_{2R}. Clients should work up to 20 to 60 minutes of activity to minimize nausea, decrease fatigue, and improve quality of life. For those with severe fatigue, encourage, multiple 10 to 20 minute segments throughout the day. ACS concurs and suggests a minimum of 30 minutes of moderate-to-vigorous activity on at least 5 days per week.

- Resistance exercise is beneficial and feasible for many cancer patients. Free weights, weight machines, and resistance bands are acceptable choices. The type and extent of resistance work are highly variable and depend upon many factors such as range of motion around joints, location of tissue removal, wound healing, and overall balance. In general, ACSM suggests resistance training 2 to 3 days per week with at least 48 hours of rest in between each session. They recommend an intensity of 40% to 60% of 1 RM for one to three sets of 8 to 12 repetitions each. As the client progresses, additional sets may be safely added. If clients prefer to avoid traditional weight lifting, yoga, Pilates, and other core training techniques substantially improve strength, endurance, and flexibility. They also help manage stress, stabilize blood pressure, and improve immune system functioning. The ACS encourages some sort of strength training to help preserve bone and muscle mass, which are often diminished during treatment.[1,28–30,46]

- Static stretching and range of motion exercises improve flexibility and should be done on 2 to 7 days per week. Perform four repetitions per exercise and hold stretches for at least 10 to 30 seconds to improve flexibility around joints. Include stretches for all major muscles. In addition to improving range of motion, stretching offers a time to relax the mind and focus on how good the workout felt.[28–30]

- Plan a whole body workout that targets all major muscle groups on 1 day rather than doing a split routine that requires working half the body on 1 day and the other half on another day. Whole body exercise performed every other day is best for this group because it gives them a complete 24-hour period during which to recover. It is also an easier schedule with which to comply.

- Clients who have a body temperature that exceeds 101°F should avoid exercise for at least 24 hours or until body temperature returns to normal.[27]
- Clients should wait at least 24 hours following chemotherapy treatments or blood withdrawals to ensure that the drugs are in the system long enough to exert their effect and to ensure appropriate blood volume. This reduces incidences of nausea, dizziness, and fatigue.[27]
- As with all exercisers, clients should drink plenty of water before, during, and after exercise to ensure proper hydration and thermoregulation.
- Because exercise during cancer treatment is just as important for psychological well-being as it is for physiological well-being, personal trainers should encourage enjoyable activities that build confidence and facilitate independence.[28–30]
- Clients with diminished bone mass should avoid high-impact activities and contact sports to minimize risk for fracture. Swimming, walking, and bicycling are safer options.
- Patients with terminal cancer often experience cachexia or muscle wasting, which limits ability.
- Clients with low white blood cell counts or those who have undergone a bone marrow transplant need to avoid exercise in public places since their immune systems are compromised. Those with indwelling catheters or feeding tubes—along with those undergoing radiation therapy—should avoid swimming.
- Short-term benefits of exercise include better functioning, lower resting heart rate, decreased subcutaneous fat, stabilized body weight, and increased muscular strength and endurance, which make daily activities more tolerable and enjoyable.[25]

QUICK REFERENCE

To encourage clients to continue exercise,

- Set realistic short-term goals and explain how to measure progress
- Set realistic long-term goals to encourage commitment to exercise
- Make the workout fun
- Offer words of encouragement to build confidence
- Add variety to the workout to keep the client interested
- Encourage activity with family and friends
- Use exercise logs to document progress
- Allow the client to have input into their routine

ADDITIONAL CONCERNS

As cancer survivors complete therapy and move into remission, they can typically follow ACSM's general exercise guidelines. Again, certain permanent limitations might exist because of surgeries, but overall recommendations for frequency, duration, and intensity resemble those for the general population. As always, fitness professionals need to adjust the actual exercise prescription to meet the individual client's needs.[28–30]

QUICK REFERENCE

Contraindications to vigorous exercise in cancer patients include the following[25,47]:

- Acute onset of nausea following exercise initiation
- Chest pain
- Decreased heart rate and blood pressure with increased workload
- Irregular pulse during exertion
- Disorientation and confusion
- Dizziness or blurred vision
- Intravenous chemotherapy within the last 24 hours
- Leg pain or cramping
- Bone weakness from long-term use of Prednisone
- Numbness in legs or hands
- Pallor or cyanosis
- Difficult or shallow breathing, especially in cases of pulmonary tumors
- Unusual muscle weakness
- Vomiting within the last 24 to 36 hours

SAMPLE EXERCISES

Cardiovascular exercise benefits cardiorespiratory and musculoskeletal functioning and should be done for a minimum of 3 to 5 days per week as tolerated. Low-impact activities such as walking or stationary cycling are best during the initial training period. Begin with short segments of activity and gradually increase duration as the patient adapts. Since cancer patients experience more frequent relapses in exercise conditioning than the average client, be prepared for setbacks. During episodes of minor fatigue, encourage clients to continue training if possible. If they cannot continue, recommend rest so that the next exercise session will be better tolerated.

Resistance exercises should target the muscles of the chest, back, arms, abdomen, and legs and include the lat pull down, seated row, chest press, incline press, biceps curl, triceps extension, leg extension, leg curl, and leg press. Perform one to three sets of each exercise using a weight that can be lifted for 8 to 12 repetitions, with an upper limit of 15 repetitions for deconditioned or frail clients. Remember that bones often become more fragile during and immediately after cancer therapy, so undue stress from heavy weights might cause fracture. In addition, balance problems sometimes persist temporarily during and following therapy. Therefore, weight machines or resistance bands might be preferable in the early stages of training before strength, balance, and capacity develop. In addition, be aware of surgery locations. The specific exercises that are contraindicated depend upon the location of tumor removal and the actual amount of tissue removed. Overall, cancer survivors can typically perform the same exercises recommended to the general population.

NUTRITIONAL CONSIDERATIONS[48,49]

EATING TO PREVENT CANCER DEVELOPMENT: THE ROLE OF INITIATORS, PROMOTERS, AND ANTIPROMOTERS

The results of years of research suggest that consuming certain foods increases the risk of developing cancer, while consuming others actually reduces the risk. In fact, certain foods are considered cancer **initiators**, some are considered cancer **promoters**, and still others are actually **antipromotors**.[49]

As an example of an initiator, consider grilled or smoked meat, poultry, or fish (Table 10.3). Grilling or broiling red meat, poultry, or fish produces a charred appearance on the food, and this char contains carcinogens called heterocyclic amines (HCAs). HCAs increase the risk for cancers of the breast, colon, stomach, and prostate in humans. In addition, the vapors that form as fat drips from foods grilled on an open flame are also carcinogenic. These vapors contain the carcinogen polycyclic aromatic hydrocarbons, or PAH. They rise from the fire and tend to adhere to the food as it continues to cook. Once consumed, the food and its associated carcinogens can then damage the digestive tract lining as they pass through each section. Fortunately, the liver typically detoxifies any remaining toxins once they are absorbed.[50,51]

Another potential carcinogen is acrylamide, a substance produced when certain carbohydrate-rich foods such as potatoes are fried or baked at high temperatures. The FDA is currently investigating the effects of the small amounts found in the human food supply. The general consensus is that even though acrylamide increases the risk of cancer in animals, it unlikely harms humans because it is consumed in such low amounts.[49]

Nitrites are food additives that preserve color, enhance flavor, and prolong shelf life by preventing rancidity and microbial growth. They are common in cured meats, especially

TABLE 10-3   SUGGESTIONS FOR GRILLING FOODS

Suggestion	Reason
Grill vegetables instead of meats	Still get that grilled taste
Marinate meat before grilling	Significantly reduces the amount of HCAs
Trim excess fat from meats and choose lean cuts	Less fat drips during cooking
Precook meats in the oven or microwave	Helps ensure meat is thoroughly cooked and still gives a grilled taste
Cook kebobs	Small cuts of meat spend less time on the grill and produce fewer carcinogens than larger cuts that must cook longer
Place foil on the grill and puncture it, then cook the meat on top of the foil	Allows fat to drip from the meat into the grill but blocks the vapors from contacting the food
Lower the temperature, flip the meat more frequently, and plan to cook for a longer period of time	Reduces carcinogen formation
Remove any charred or burnt portions from the food before eating	

Information available from the American Institute for Cancer Research at www.aicr.org.

bacon. The problem with nitrites is that the body converts them into nitrosamines, substances that cause cancer in animals. The cancer-causing effect on humans, however, is nonexistent because the amounts used in food preparation are so minimal. In fact, cigarette smokers inhale nitrosamines in an amount 100 times than consumed by regular bacon eaters. Even the amount of nitrosamines in the "new car smell" of a brand new automobile—and the amount found in some cosmetics—is much higher than the amount consumed in the average diet.[48,49]

All of the preceding are examples of cancer initiators. Cancer promoters do not actually cause a cell to mutate into a cancerous cell. Instead, promoters accelerate cancer cell proliferation once cancer has been initiated. In human studies, high kilocalorie diets seem to promote cancer development. Animal studies also show a specific and consistent link between high fat intake and cancer promotion, but the precise relationship in human trials is not as clear. Enough evidence exists, however, to suggest that diets high in saturated fat and trans fat promote cancer development.[48,49]

Antipromoters include foods and food components that protect against cancer. Examples of antipromoters include fruits, vegetables, and fatty fish. Fruits and vegetables contain fiber and **phytochemicals** in addition to various vitamins and minerals, which act as **antioxidants**. The phytochemicals in cabbage, cauliflower, and broccoli seem especially effective against the development of colon cancer. Fiber appears to inhibit cancer cell growth by binding to cancer-causing agents in the digestive tract and preventing their absorption. In addition, a high fiber diet is associated with healthy weight maintenance, another factor that reduces cancer risk.

Overall, a healthy diet that inhibits cancer development encourages plenty of fruits, vegetables, and whole grains; limits red meats, fat, salt, sugar, and alcohol; and encourages appropriate energy intake.

Initiators—factors, in this case foods or food preparation techniques, that give rise to cancer; they are carcinogenic.

Promoters—factors, in this case foods or food preparation techniques, that do not form cancer cells but encourage growth of cancerous cells once these cells exist.

Antipromoters—factors, in this case foods and food components, that reduce the risk of developing cancer.

Phytochemicals—nonnutritive substances found in plant sources thought to have protective biological effects in the body. Examples include isoflavones in soy products, lycopene in tomatoes, flavenoids in fruit, and lutein in dark green vegetables. Different phytochemicals have different modes of action. Some act as antioxidants; some have hormone effects; some effect enzyme action; some inhibit cancer cell replication; and some physically block pathogens from binding to body cells.

Antioxidants—molecules that protect the body from free radical damage. Free radicals form as a result of normal metabolism but increase in number when a person is exposed to pollution, UV radiation, and cigarette smoke. Free radicals act by mutating DNA, damaging cell proteins, and destroying cell membranes. Antioxidants, such as vitamin C, vitamin E, beta carotene, and selenium, deactivate free radicals and protect the body's cells.

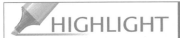

HIGHLIGHT   Foods That Protect Against Cancer

The American Institute on Cancer Research (AICR) has an excellent Web site that provides practical information on dietary manipulations that might reduce the risk of cancer development. According to results from studies conducted by the AICR, numerous foods offer protection from cancer. The AICR Web site lists the following as possible antipromoters of cancer: legumes, berries, cruciferous vegetables, leafy green vegetables, flaxseed, and garlic. Legumes, also commonly known as beans, contain various phytochemicals including saponins, protease inhibitors, and phytic acid. Saponins, abundant in soybeans, seem to slow tumor cell growth and inhibit cancer cell division. In addition, they decrease total blood cholesterol levels, which lowers the risk for heart disease. Protease inhibitors slow cancer cell division as well, but they also protect body cells indirectly by inhibiting the release of damaging chemicals from tumor cells. Phytic acid, found abundantly in cereals and legumes, appears to significantly inhibit the growth rate of existing tumors.[50]

Berries, like many other fruits, are high in fiber and vitamin C. Studies indicate that fiber decreases the risk of colorectal cancer, while vitamin C reduces the risk of esophageal cancer. Some berries are also rich in ellagic acid, a phytochemical that has antioxidant properties and interferes with cancer cell proliferation. Raspberries and strawberries are excellent sources of ellagic acid.[50]

Broccoli, cauliflower, and cabbage—also known as cruciferous vegetables—seem to protect against cancers of the mouth, pharynx, esophagus, and stomach. They contain large quantities of glucosinolates, crambene, and isothyiocyanates that seem to completely stop cancer cell growth.[50]

Dark green leafy vegetables such as spinach, romaine lettuce, and collard greens contain large quantities of carotenoids, saponins, and folate. The carotenoids act as powerful antioxidants that protect against free radical damage, particularly in the breasts, lungs, stomach, and skin. The saponins, as mentioned earlier, inhibit cancer cell growth and reproduction in general. Folate seems to protect against pancreatic cancer, a very serious and often deadly form of cancer.[50]

Flaxseeds and flaxseed oil are also protective. Flaxseeds themselves contain large amounts of the phytochemical lignin, a plant chemical that mimics the effects of estrogen in the body. Lignin seems to lower the risk of several cancers. Although flaxseed oil lacks lignin, it is a good source of the healthy omega-3 fatty acids thought to reduce the risk for heart disease and some cancers. In general, those who include flaxseed in their diets tend to have lower rates of colon, breast, skin, and lung tumors. Supplements are still not recommended, though, because high intakes of flaxseed and flaxseed oil reduce blood clotting and interfere with medications such as blood thinners.[50]

For more information, visit the AICR Web site at www.aicr.org.

EATING WELL AFTER CANCER DIAGNOSIS

Although research has identified dietary factors that reduce the risk of *developing* cancer, information regarding the best diet to reduce the risk of cancer *recurrence* is limited. There is no doubt, however, that diet is an important component of cancer treatment.

Energy Needs

During cancer treatment, the body is not only fighting off the disease; it is also rebuilding tissues. Therefore, it usually requires additional energy to meet this increased demand. That means more carbohydrates for energy and more protein for tissue repair, enzyme formation, and hormonal balance. Ideally, those diagnosed with cancer are already eating healthy diets and are at healthy weights prior to beginning treatment. In many cases, well-nourished individuals tolerate chemotherapy and radiation better than those who are malnourished. The healthiest diet during treatment includes various plant-based foods, at least five servings per day of fruits and vegetables, limited intake of high-fat foods, reduced amounts of cured, smoked, or pickled foods, alcohol in moderation (if at all), and increased lentils and soy products with reduced meat intake—a diet similar to the one suggested for cancer prevention. Healthy snacks such as cereal, cheese, whole grain crackers, fruits, ice cream, milk, nuts, vegetables, and yogurt help meet the increased energy requirements.

Unfortunately, however, several factors interfere with the ability to consume a healthy and adequate diet during cancer treatment. Loss of appetite accompanied with nausea and vomiting result in inadequate intake and subsequent weight loss. Patients can counter this by consuming smaller meals and frequent snacks high in protein and healthy carbohydrates. Soreness in the mouth or throat along with problems with the teeth and gums make eating painful. If this is the case, avoid dry, coarse food so that eating is less uncomfortable and more pleasurable. Temporary loss of taste and smell sensations also interferes with appetite and is quite difficult to handle. Convince a patient with these symptoms to eat by emphasizing the importance of energy for tissue repair and immune system functioning. Additional problems include diarrhea and/or constipation, both of which affect nutrient absorption, so patients should avoid foods that exacerbate either condition. Raw fruits and vegetables, for example, can worsen diarrhea, while inadequate water and fiber intake worsen constipation. Lastly, the treatment itself can interfere with the body's handling of nutrients. In these cases, a cancer survivor's diet might be healthy and packed with all necessary nutrients, but the body might not be able to absorb the nutrients from the digestive tract. And even if the nutrients are absorbed, they might not be handled properly, or they might even be disposed of before they are used. These cases need special attention from the team of experts working with the cancer survivor.

Ironically, the overall best method for countering many treatment side effects is to avoid nutritional deficiencies by continuing to ingest food and beverages on a regular basis. The first goal for cancer patients is to try to consume an adequate amount of energy to prevent lean tissue loss and to maintain normal nutrient levels. If lack of appetite is a problem, encourage patients to consume small amounts of high-energy, high nutrient foods at meal times and add in-between-meal snacks. Sometimes the only means of obtaining additional kilocalories is for these patients to consume liquid meal replacements *in addition to*, not in lieu of, food. In serious cases of malnutrition, tube feeding or total parenteral nutrition might be required.

Carbohydrates

Carbohydrates are the preferred source of energy for most body cells. In addition, an adequate intake of carbohydrates is necessary for body cells to adequately burn stored body fat for energy. A diet filled with fruits, vegetables, and whole grains ensures adequate vitamins, minerals, and phytochemicals. Include various vibrantly colored sources to receive the greatest amount of micronutrients. Limit the intake of simple carbohydrates since they typically add little more than empty kilocalories to the diet. Instead, include complex carbohydrates, which also contain fiber, a component associated with lower risks of cancer.

Proteins

Proteins are needed to rebuild tissue, form antibodies and hormones, transport oxygen through the blood, and ensure that chemical reactions are occurring at an appropriate rate. Without an adequate intake of protein, recovery time and risk for infection increase dramatically. Many foods are high in protein and relatively low in fat. Dairy products such as cheese, low-or-no-fat milk, yogurt, and powdered milk (added to other foods) are great sources. Hard-boiled eggs included in salads offer a complete source of protein. Lean red meats, poultry, and fish are also high in protein, iron, and zinc and are healthy when baked. Legumes, nuts, and seeds are additional healthy sources of protein.

Fat

Fat serves several purposes in both the body and the diet. In the body, fats, or triglycerides, provide insulation, cushion organs, and serve as a reservoir of concentrated energy. In foods, triglycerides enhance flavors, provide energy, allow for absorption of fat-soluble vitamins, and supply essential fatty acids. Consequently, a healthy diet supplies just enough fat to meet its needs.

All dietary fats, however, are not created equally. Saturated fats, which are usually solid at room temperature, are found primarily in animal-based foods such as red meats, poultry, whole milk, butter, and lard. Most people know that limiting dietary saturated fat reduces the risk for cardiovascular disease. However, the evidence linking saturated fats with cancer is less conclusive. Some preliminary findings suggest that high-fat diets promote cancer development once cancer exists, but this might be because high-fat diets are also high in kilocalories.[52,53] Since certain studies show a positive correlation between high kilocalorie intake and cancers of the breast and prostate, perhaps the high energy content of high-fat diets is the culprit.

Omega-3 fatty acids, found primarily in fish, are associated with a reduced risk of some cancers, including breast, prostate, colon, and pancreatic cancers. These fatty acids seem to prevent severe lean tissue wasting and enhance the effects of certain cancer treatments such as chemotherapy.[54] According to the University of Maryland Medical Center (UMMC), low blood levels of omega-3 fatty acids are associated with an increased risk of colon cancer, but animal studies showed that supplemental omega-3 actually stimulated cancer growth in cases of metastasized colon cancer. These UMMC researchers, therefore, do not recommend supplements until further research clarifies the relationship between omega-3 fatty acids and colon cancer promotion. The researchers also speculate that adequate omega-3 fatty acids improve treatment for those with breast cancer, though the exact mechanism is unclear. Additional laboratory studies suggest that omega-3 fatty acids actually inhibit prostate cancer progression. Still, further research is necessary before supplements can be recommended. Good food sources include fatty fish (salmon, halibut, mackerel, and tuna), flaxseed, flaxseed oil, canola oil, soybean products, pumpkin seeds, and walnuts.[55–58]

Trans fats are fats that rarely occur naturally in foods. The large amounts found in the general food supply result when manufacturers transform unsaturated fats into fats that resemble saturated fats through a process called hydrogenation. Why do manufacturers hydrogenate fats and thus produce trans fats? First, hydrogenated fats have a longer shelf life than unsaturated fats, so manufacturers can prolong the life of their products. Secondly, hydrogenated fats are firmer than unsaturated fats, so manufacturers can turn liquid vegetable oils into spreadable margarines. The problem with trans fats is that the body treats them just as if they were saturated fats since they look just like saturated fats. That means that trans fats are just as unhealthy as saturated fats and should be limited in the diet. Common sources of trans fats include margarines, pastries, and other snack foods. Check nutrition labels for trans fat content.

QUICK REFERENCE

Cancer survivors who lose their appetites because of treatment-related nausea, temporary loss of taste, or overall fatigue should try to consume smaller meals more frequently throughout the day. They should consume foods separately from liquids since liquids quickly fill the stomach and reduce stomach capacity. In addition, those with diminished appetites should consume most of their meal within a 20-minute time period. It takes about 20 minutes for the brain to register satiety, so a person with a small appetite can, within reason, ingest a greater quantity if they eat relatively rapidly. Cancer patients who are unable to consume enough food to meet their daily energy needs might need to invest in healthy nutritional meal replacements for additional kilocalories.

Alcohol

According to the American Institute for Cancer Research, excessive alcohol intake increases the risk for cancers of the mouth, pharynx, larynx, esophagus, and liver. Alcohol is a lipid solvent, which means it dissolves the lipids out of cell membranes. Once damaged, the cell membrane is no longer an effective barrier to potential toxins. If the cell does not die from exposure to the alcohol itself, it becomes vulnerable to carcinogens, which easily enter and damage DNA. In addition to promoting damage to the DNA, excessive alcohol intake interferes with the functioning of the B vitamin folate. Folate is necessary for DNA repair and replication, so with insufficient folate availability, DNA is more susceptible to permanent, irreversible damage.[50]

QUICK REFERENCE

To provide the greatest protection against cancer, the AICR suggests avoiding alcohol intake altogether; however, a moderate intake, defined as no more than two drinks per day for men and no more than one drink per day for women, seems relatively safe. One drink is the equivalent of a 12 oz can of beer, 5 oz of wine, or 1.5 oz of 80-proof hard liquor.

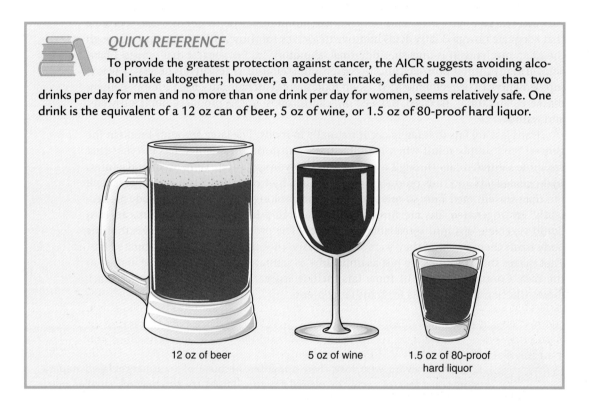

12 oz of beer   5 oz of wine   1.5 oz of 80-proof
                                             hard liquor

Vitamins and Minerals

Although they do not supply energy, vitamins and minerals are required for many body processes. Vitamins in particular are necessary to access the energy found in carbohydrates, proteins, and fats; help maintain healthy body tissues; and act as regulators in various processes. Minerals are necessary components of several body structures, are crucial for muscle contraction and nerve impulse propagation, and are required for hormone functioning. A diet that includes various carbohydrates and protein usually supplies sufficient vitamins and minerals.

Approximately 64% to 81% of cancer survivors report using vitamin and/or mineral supplements despite the fact that the biological effects of supplements in this particular population are not well established. In fact, ingesting megadoses of supplements is likely not beneficial to cancer survivors at all.[59] Advocates of vitamin and mineral supplementation believe that if recommended amounts are good, then larger amounts must be better. Cancer survivors, and everyone else for that matter, should be wary of this type of thinking. Excesses of certain vitamins and minerals directly cause harm. In other cases, excesses of one might interfere with the action of another. Additionally, certain mega-doses actually minimize the effectiveness of chemotherapy and radiation therapy. Granted, these treatments often diminish appetite, which obviously interferes with nutritional status, but cancer patients should discuss supplement options with a physi-cian prior to taking any.[60] Studies are currently investigating the effects of supplemental beta carotene (associated with a lower mortality from all cancers), vitamin E (thought to inhibit cancer formation by attacking free radicals), and vitamin C (which is associated with lower risks of mouth, larynx, esophagus, and stomach cancers); however, there is not enough existing evidence to suggest that cancer patients take supplements of any of these. Instead, they should consume various fruits, vegetables, and whole grains for an adequate intake.

Water

Proper hydration is necessary for every process in the body. In addition, it ensures an adequate body temperature. In general, the average person should consume at least 64 oz of water per day plus additional amounts to replace losses through sweat. Since diarrhea and vomiting are common side effects of cancer treatment, cancer survivors need to be especially careful about ingesting adequate fluids.

HEALTHY EATING AFTER TREATMENT ENDS

According to the ACS, research has not shown a direct relationship between diet and cancer recurrence; however, eating a healthy diet full of fresh vegetables, fruits, and whole grains is encouraged. A dietitian can help establish the best eating plan and ensure an appropriate energy intake that maintains a healthy weight and adequate vitamin and minerals. General suggestions include the following:

- Obtain information regarding dietary restrictions from a doctor and dietician.
- Choose various foods from all food groups.
- Include at least 5 to 7 servings per day of fruits and vegetables.
- Eat whole grains and other high fiber foods.
- Decrease total dietary fat intake with an emphasis on limiting saturated and trans fats.
- Avoid salt-cured, smoked, and pickled foods.
- Avoid alcohol if possible, or at the very least, limit intake.
- If overweight, consider losing weight by reducing total energy intake and increas-ing activity level.

SPECIAL CONCERNS FOR THOSE WITH ADVANCED CANCER

Advanced cancer is defined as cancer that can no longer be cured, so the goal is to relieve pain, ease fear, and preserve independence for as long as possible. During this stage of cancer, patients usually have a poor appetite, persistent nausea and vomiting, bloating, difficulty swallowing, and constipation. They are encouraged to eat anything that is appealing and tolerable to them, but they should still try to consume nutritious foods that help maintain strength, energy, weight, and the ability to resist infection. In the advanced stages of cancer, hospice care is common and the physician is crucial in determining appropriate care.

QUICK REFERENCE

Factors that reduce the risk for cancer include:

- Achieving and maintaining a healthy weight
- Eating various fruits and vegetables, at least five servings per day
- Consuming 100% whole grain products to increase fiber intake
- Limiting intake of red meats and processed meat products
- Choosing fish, poultry, and legumes as alternatives to red meat
- Limiting alcohol consumption (no more than two drinks per day for men; no more than one drink per day for women)
- Participating in at least 20 to 60 minutes of cardiovascular activity 3 to 5 days per week

SUMMARY

An ounce of prevention is worth a pound of cure. How true this old adage is with regard to cancer. Because so many lifestyle habits contribute to the chances of developing this life-threatening disease, people should establish habits early in life that reduce overall risk. Unfortunately, in today's society, millions of people either have or have had cancer, so it is truly a pervasive disease. Obviously, the sooner a physician diagnoses cancer, the sooner treatment begins, and the better the outlook.

Years ago, medical professionals were reluctant to recommend exercise as a component of the treatment plan for cancer patients. Perhaps the medical team thought those suffering from cancer could not handle the additional stress of exercise. Or perhaps they believed that exercise for this group was too risky. No matter what the reason, increased physical activity was rarely suggested to those with cancer. More recent research, however, has demonstrated that remaining active during and after cancer treatment empowers cancer survivors and gives them a sense of independence and control. No matter what a person's initial fitness level, physical activity improves strength, decreases fatigue, improves mood, and increases the desire to live. Yes, activities must be modified, but educated fitness professionals can develop programs that meet the needs and capabilities of just about anyone.

A healthy diet is also vital for cancer survivors. Cancer and cancer treatment can strip the body of lean tissue, so to prevent this wasting and to ensure better tolerance of therapy, the cancer patient needs an adequate intake of kilocalories and nutrients. Those who eat healthy diets tolerate treatment better and tend to have positive attitudes—factors that improve quality of life and potential for recovery.

CASE STUDY

A cancer survivor underwent surgery 3 months ago to remove his prostate gland. He is currently at the end of his first cycle of chemotherapy and only has two more treatments to go. After performing a complete physical examination that found no preexisting heart or pulmonary conditions, his doctor referred this patient to you. Currently, the patient's blood pressure, blood glucose level, and weight are all within normal limits. He complains of frequent diarrhea and experiences nausea for about 5 days after chemotherapy, but other than that, he feels fine.

■ Discuss the type of exercise testing and exercise prescription you would suggest for this patient. Include recommendations on frequency, time, type, and duration of activity. Also give specific examples of exercises you would have him perform.

THINKING CRITICALLY

1. Discuss the differences between normal cell and cancer cell development and growth.
2. What are proto-oncogenes and tumor suppressor cells? How do they contribute to cancer development?
3. List four different treatment methods for cancer and discuss the advantages and disadvantages of each.
4. What is a malignancy? How does it differ from a benign growth?
5. List at least three common causes of cancer and discuss each thoroughly. How might risk for cancer be reduced?
6. What are some special precautions for cancer survivors who decide to exercise?
7. How does exercise improve functional capacity in cancer survivors?
8. Discuss some of the major dietary concerns for cancer patients undergoing treatment.
9. Why is alcohol intake not advised for this special population?
10. What factors reduce the risk for cancer recurrence in cancer survivors?

REFERENCES

1. American Cancer Society. Available at: www.cancer.org
2. Supplements vs. exercise for heart disease and cancer: the "vitamins" in your legs. Harv Mens Health Watch 2007;12(4):2–4.
3. James A, Campbell M, DeVellis B, et al. Health behavior correlates among colon cancer survivors: NC STRIDES baseline results. Am J Health Behav 2006;30(6):720–730.
4. Damush T, Perkins A, Miller K. The implementation of an oncologist referred, exercise self-management program for older breast cancer survivors. Psychooncology 2005;15:884–890.
5. Fenster C, Weinsier R, Darley-Usmar V, et al. Obesity, aerobic exercise, and vascular disease: the role of oxidant stress. Obes Res 2002;10:964–968.
6. McTiernan A. Moderate physical activity is critical for reducing the risk for chronic disease in older

women. Sci Daily. 2003. Available at: www.sci-encedaily.com

7. National Cancer Institute. Available at: www. cancer. gov

8. Winett J, Carpinelli R, Hu F, et al. Exercise intensity and risk of chronic disease. JAMA 2000; 284:1784–1785.

9. United States Department of Energy. Office of Science. Human Genome Project. Available at: www.genomics.energy.gov

10. Drouin J, Pfalzer L. Cancer and Exercise. National Center on Physical Activity and Disability. 2008. Available at: www.ncpad.org

11. Croce C. Oncogenes and cancer. N Engl J Med 2008;358(5):502–511.

12. Emory University. Available at: www.cancerquest. com

13. Rous P, Kidd J. The activating, transforming, and carcinogenic effects of the rabbit papilloma virus (SHOPE) upon implanted tar tumors. J Exp Med 1941;71:787–812.

14. Rous P, Kidd J. Conditional neoplasma and sub-threshold neoplastic states: as study of tar tumors in rabbits. J Exp Med 1941;73:365–389.

15. Eker P, Sanner T. Assay fro initiators and promoters of carcinogenesis based on attachment-independent survival of cells in aggregates. Cancer Res 1983;43:320–323.

16. Chlebowski R. Reducing the risk of breast cancer. N Engl J Med 2000;343(3):191–198.

17. Campaign for tobacco free kids. Available at: www. tobaccofreekids.org

18. National Institute on Drug Abuse. Available at: www.nida.nih.gov

19. Tobacco News and Information. Available at: www.tobacco.org

20. Shangling L, Wang H, Zhonghui Y, et al. Enhancement of cancer radiation therapy by use of adenovirus-mediated secretable glucose-regulated protein 94/gp96 expression. Cancer Res 2005;65: 9126–9131.

21. Parks J, Benz C. Immunotherapy Cancer Treatment. Support Cancer Care. 2007. Available at: www.cancersupportivecare.com

22. United States Food and Drug Administration. Available at: www.fda.org

23. Fialka-Moser V, Crevenna R, Korpan M, et al. Cancer rehabilitation, particularly with aspects on physical impairment. J Rehabil 2003;35:153–162.

24. Watson T, Mock V. Exercise as an intervention for cancer-related fatigue. Phys Ther 2004;84(8): 736–743.

25. Kirshbaum M. Promoting physical exercise in breast cancer care. Nurs Stand 2005;19(40):41–48.

26. Martignoni M, Kunze P, Friess H. Cancer cachexia. Mol Cancer 2003;2:36.

27. Young-McCaughan, S. Exercise in the rehabilitation from cancer. Medsurg Nurs 2006;15(6):384–388.

28. Courneya K. Exercise interventions during cancer treatment: biopsychosocial outcomes. Exerc Sport Sci Rev 2001;29(2):60–64.

29. Courneya K. Exercise for breast cancer survivors: research evidence and clinical guidelines. Phys Sportsmed 2002;30(8):33–42.

30. Courneya K. Exercise in cancer survivors: an overview of research. Med Sci Sports Exerc 2003;35(11): 1846–1852.

31. Smith G, Toonen T. Primary care of the patient with cancer. Am Fam Phys 2007;75(8):1207–1214.

32. Mock V, Pickett M, Ropka M, et al. Fatigue in patients with cancer: an exercise intervention—report on the FIRE® project. Program and abstracts of the 26th Congress of the Oncology Nursing Society; May 17–20, 2001; San Diego, California. Discussion Session. National Cancer Institute. Available at: www.cancer.gov

33. Mock V, Pickett M, Ropka M, et al. Fatigue and quality of life outcomes of exercise during cancer treatment. Cancer Pract 2001;9:119–127.

34. Holmes M, Chen W, Feskanich D, et al. Physical activity and survival after breast cancer diagnosis. J Am Med Assoc 2005;293(2):2479–2486.

35. Knobf M, Musanti R, Dorward J. Exercise and quality of life outcomes in patients with cancer. Semin Oncol Nurs 2007;23(4):285–296.

36. McNeely M, Campbell K, Rowe B, et al. Effects of exercise on breast cancer patients and survivors: a systemic review and meta-analysis. Can Med Assoc J 2006;175(1):34–41.

37. Winningham M, MacVicar M. The effect of aerobic exercise on patient reports of nausea. Oncol Nurs Forum 1988;15(4):447–450.

38. Pinto B, Trunzo J. Body esteem and mood among sedentary and active breast cancer survivors. Mayo Clin Proc 2004;79:181–186.

39. Harriss D, Cable T, George K, et al. Physical activity before and after diagnosis of colorectal cancer. Sports Med 2007;37(11):947–960.

40. Giovannucci E, Yan L, Leitzmann M, et al. A prospective study of physical activity and incident and fatal prostate cancer. Arch Intern Med 2005; 165:1005–1010.

41. Torti D, Matheson G. Exercise and prostate cancer. Sports Med 2004;34(6):363–369.
42. Schwartz A, Winters-Stone K, Gallucci B. Exercise effects on bone mineral density in women with breast cancer receiving adjuvant chemotherapy. Oncol Nurs Forum 2007;34(3):627–633.
43. Daniel H, Dunn S, Ferguson D, et al. Progressive osteoporosis during androgen deprivation therapy for prostate cancer. J Urol 2000;163:181–186.
44. Doyle C, Kushi L, Byers T, et al. Nutrition and physical activity during and after cancer treatment: an American Cancer Society guide for informed choices. Cancer J Clin 2006;56:323–353.
45. Schneider C, Carter S. The role of exercise in recovery from cancer treatment. Rocky Mountain Cancer Rehabilitation Institute. ACSM Fit Society Page. Winter 2003;6:9.
46. American College of Sports Medicine. ACSM's Guidelines for Exercise Testing and Prescription, 8th Ed. Philadelphia: Lippincott Williams & Wilkins, 2010:228–232.
47. Rosenbaum E, Manual F, Rosenbaum R, et al. Exercises for cancer supportive care. Available at: www.cancersupportivecare.com/exercises
48. Balch P. Prescription for dietary wellness. New York: Avery Publishing, 2003. ISBN 1583331476.
49. Whitney E, Rolfes S. Understanding Nutrition. 11th Ed. USA: Wadsworth Publishing, 2008.
50. American Institute of Cancer Research. Available at: www.aicr.org
51. Petersen, T. SrFit—The Personal Trainer's Resource for Senior Fitness. Tonganoxie, Kansas: The American Academy of Health and Fitness, 2004.
52. Khor G. Dietary fat quality: a nutritional epidemiologist vis. Asia Pac J Clin Nutr 2004; 13:S22.
53. Stoeckli R, Keller U. Nutritional fats and the risk of type 2 diabetes and cancer. Physiol Behav 2004; 83(4):611–615.
54. Barclay L. New Nutrition and exercise guidelines for cancer survivors. Available at: www.medscape.com
55. Aronson W, Glaspy J, Reddy S, et al. Modulation of omega-3/omega-6 polyunsaturated ratios with dietary fish oils in men with prostate cancer. Urology 2001;58(2):283–288.
56. de Deckere E. Possible beneficial effect of fish and fish n-3 polyunsaturated fatty acids in breast and colorectal cancer. J Urol 2000;163:181–186.
57. Freeman V, Meydani M, Yong S, et al. Prostatic levels of fatty acids and the histopathology of localized prostate cancer. J Urol 2000;164(6):2168–2172.
58. Griffini P, Fehres O, Klieverik L, et al. Dietary omega-3 polyunsaturated fatty acids promote colon carcinoma metastasis in rat liver. Cancer Res 1998;58(15):3312–3319.
59. Velicer C, Ulrich, C. Vitamin and mineral supplement use among U.S. adults after cancer diagnosis: a systemic review. J Oncol 2008;26(4):665–673.
60. Fairfield K, Stampfer M. Vitamin and mineral supplements for cancer prevention: issues and evidence. Am J Clin Nutr 2007;85(1):289S–292S.

11 EXERCISE FOR PEOPLE WITH ASTHMA

Asthma is characterized by chronic **inflammation** of the airways and **hyperactive bronchi** that temporarily narrow the respiratory passageways. Ultimately, these conditions result in the classic signs of an asthma attack—shortness of breath, tightness in the chest, coughing, and wheezing. In fact, the word "asthma" literally means to pant or gasp for air. Actual symptoms—and the severity of symptoms—vary from person to person; furthermore, they differ from day to day in any given individual. Additionally, symptoms can be mild, moderate, or severe enough to cause death.

The number of asthma sufferers is increasing. Currently, nearly 23 million people in the United States—or 1 out of every 14 Americans—has asthma. This includes 7 million children who are younger than age 18.[1] Asthma is slightly more common in African Americans than in Caucasians and in females than in males.[2] Asthma was responsible for about 4,000 deaths during 2005, but loss of lives is not the only cost associated with this condition.[1] An estimated one quarter of all emergency room visits (the equivalent of 2 million in the year 2001) result from asthma attacks and contribute to the annual $10 billion in asthma-related health care costs. Add an additional $8 billion from lost productivity to this total, and the annual monetary cost of asthma exceeds $18 billion! To top that off, an additional $5 billion is spent annually on prescription medications and treatments for acute asthma attacks and chronic inflammation.[3]

According to the Asthma and Allergy Foundation of America, "40,000 people miss school or work, 30,000 people experience an asthma attack, 5,000 people visit the emergency room, 1,000 people are admitted into the hospital, and 11 people die" as a result of asthma on a daily basis.[2] Because of asthma's pervasiveness, every American should be aware of its consequences, and fitness professionals, in particular, should be ready to work with asthmatic clients.

QUICK REFERENCE
People between the ages of 11 and 18 are affected the most by asthma.[4]

ANATOMICAL AND PHYSIOLOGICAL CHANGES IN THOSE WITH ASTHMA

NORMAL RESPIRATORY SYSTEM FUNCTIONING

Understanding asthma requires a basic knowledge about respiratory system functioning. The respiratory system includes the nasal cavity, pharynx, trachea, lungs, bronchi, and bronchioles (Fig. 11.1). The trachea, or windpipe, divides into left and right primary bronchi, each of which travels to its corresponding lung. The right primary bronchus forms three secondary bronchi that penetrate lung tissue on the right side, while the left primary bronchus forms two secondary bronchi that enter the left lung. These secondary bronchi continue to divide repeatedly until they ultimately form several **terminal bronchioles** deep within each lung. This pattern of branching actually resembles an inverted tree in which the trachea is the trunk and the primary bronchi and its many divisions form the branches of the tree. Inhaled air, therefore, passes through a series of smaller and smaller branches until it reaches the terminal bronchioles. The terminal bronchioles end at **alveoli**, small air sacs that make up lung tissue (Fig. 11.2). Overall, there are at least 300 million alveoli in each lung, and these alveoli provide a huge surface area through which oxygen may diffuse. Because inhaled oxygen must enter the blood to reach body cells, the lungs are richly supplied with blood vessels. In fact, numerous pulmonary capillaries surround each alveolus and facilitate gas exchange between these two structures. They allow oxygen to move into blood vessels, while carbon dioxide moves into alveoli.

Inflammation—indicated by redness, swelling, heat, and pain. A major indicator of asthma is abnormal and excessive inflammation in the respiratory passageways that interferes with airflow to the lungs.

Hyperactive bronchi—when smooth muscle lining the airways responds to certain stimuli by contracting. A prolonged contraction narrows the airways and restricts airflow to the lungs. Inflammation and hyperactive bronchi, when combined, promote asthma attacks.

Terminal bronchioles—the branches of the respiratory passageways that terminate with alveoli. The trachea branches into right and left primary bronchi; each primary bronchus branches into secondary bronchi, which, in turn, branch into tertiary bronchi, and so on. As the walls of the respiratory passageways thin, bronchioles form.

Alveoli—microscopic air sacs with thin walls located in the lungs. The sites of gas exchange in the lungs. Each lung contains millions of alveoli.

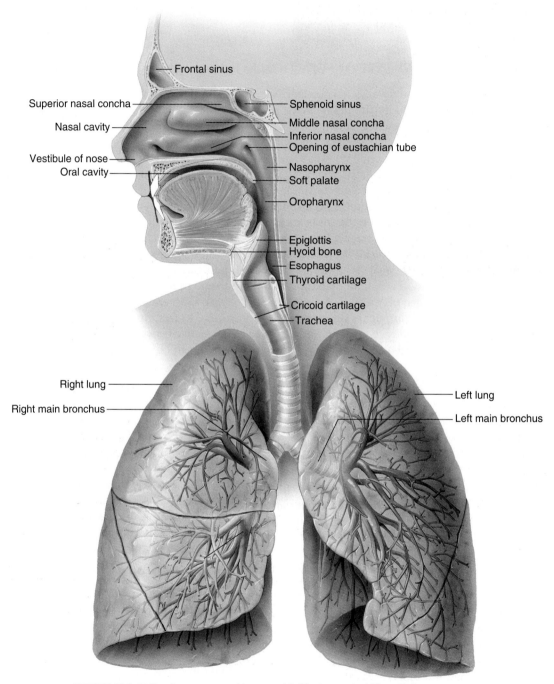

FIGURE 11.1 ■ Respiratory system. (Asset provided by Anatomical Chart Co.)

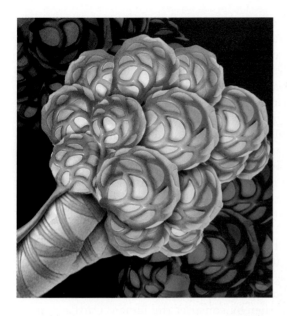

FIGURE 11.2 ■ Alveoli and surrounding pulmonary capillaries. (Asset provided by Anatomical Chart Co.)

The respiratory passageways are hollow structures enclosed by walls composed of several layers of different tissue types. Overall, their role is to filter, moisten, and warm inhaled air to avoid damaging the delicate lung tissue and to facilitate gas exchange. Air passes through the **lumen** of the respiratory tract. If the lumen dilates, more air passes through; if it constricts, less air passes through. *Filtration* prevents coarse particles found in inhaled air from entering deep lung tissue since these particles can easily damage lung tissue. *Warming* and *moistening* inhaled air enhance oxygen diffusion from alveoli into the pulmonary blood vessels. Nose hairs act as initial filters; they prevent large particles from entering the pharynx. The mucous membrane lining found along the respiratory passageways acts as a second filtration system. Cells scattered throughout this lining (which is composed of pseudostratified ciliated columnar epithelium) release mucus to trap most of the foreign particles that elude the nose hairs. Other cells within this lining have **cilia** on their surfaces that beat in unison to move trapped and potentially hazardous particles away from the lungs and into the mouth where they may be swallowed or spit out. Together, mucus and cilia inhibit the entry of foreign particles into the lungs and thus protect lung tissue from physical trauma.

Lumen—an opening. In the case of the respiratory passageways, it is the opening through which inhaled and exhaled air passes. Constricting the lumen restricts air movement. Dilating the lumen promotes air movement.

Cilia—fine, hairlike extensions that actively beat in unison to move substances, including mucus and trapped particles. Abundant in the respiratory passageways, they prevent the entry of harmful substances into the lungs.

Heat radiating from blood vessels deep inside the lining warms air, while water evaporating from mucus moistens air. Warming inspired air is important because cold air can actually "shock" the respiratory system and constrict small bronchioles in the lungs. If the bronchioles constrict, less air enters and less oxygen is available for gas exchange. Moistening inspired air is important because if the alveoli lining dries out, alveoli simply collapse and are incapable of gas exchange. The moisture in warm, humid air and the water that vaporizes from mucus help prevent alveoli collapse. Thus, inhaling warm, moist air eases oxygen diffusion into pulmonary capillaries and prevents the drying and cooling of the airways.

In addition to the mucous membrane lining, the respiratory passageways contain additional tissue layers. Most importantly, the trachea contains a cartilage layer that ensures an open passageway. Cartilage, unlike the epithelial tissue that contacts the lumen, is somewhat rigid, so it prevents collapse of the trachea during breathing. To understand the significance of this, think of sucking air through a flimsy straw. Strong suction would cause the straw to collapse. If the inside lining of the straw is sticky, the lining might stick to itself after strong suction. If this were to happen, air would not flow through the straw again. Now apply the same conditions to the trachea. If the trachea were to collapse inward during breathing, the entire mucous lining would likely stick to itself, and thereby constrict the lumen. Cartilage, however, prevents collapse and ensures an open airway. The cartilage layer does not completely encircle the trachea's lumen. Instead, it is a C-shaped ring with a thin layer of smooth muscle that connects the two posterior ends together. This arrangement is important because the esophagus abuts the trachea on its posterior side. If the cartilage ring completely encircled the trachea, a relatively large **bolus** of food might not pass through the esophagus very easily. The pliable smooth muscle, however, permits easy passage.

The structure of the cartilage layer changes somewhat as the trachea branches into the primary bronchi. The individual C-shaped cartilage rings lengthen and ultimately completely encircle the tubes. As smaller and smaller bronchioles form, however, the rings eventually thin and actually disappear entirely, while the smooth muscle layer develops and eventually entirely encircles the smaller bronchioles. As tube diameter shrinks, the inner lining changes as well. The pseudostratified ciliated columnar epithelium begins producing less mucus and contains fewer cilia as the branches approach the alveoli. Alveoli are lined by an exceedingly thin layer of tissue designed to facilitate gas diffusion.

Respiration refers to the overall exchange of oxygen for carbon dioxide. But why are oxygen and carbon dioxide levels so important? In general, oxygen is required by cells so that they can make ATP, the energy necessary for cellular functioning. While creating ATP aerobically, cells release carbon dioxide as a by-product. If left to accumulate in the blood, carbon dioxide can dangerously lower pH, which would greatly interfere with metabolic processes. Thus, intrinsic mechanisms work to maintain oxygen and carbon dioxide levels at **homeostasis**.

Respiration itself consists of ventilation, external respiration, internal respiration, and cellular respiration. *Cellular respiration* occurs at the cellular level and involves mitochondria—organelles known as the powerhouses of cells since they produce large quantities of ATP. To ensure an adequate supply of ATP, oxygen must be available to act as the final electron acceptor at the end of the electron transport chain. Carbon dioxide, which is simply a waste product that results from cellular respiration, must be removed before it accumulates in the blood. Both carbon dioxide and oxygen are transported in the blood. Oxygen, most of which is bound to hemoglobin in red blood cells, moves easily into cells, while carbon dioxide, which accumulates inside metabolically active cells, moves easily out of cells into the blood. This process is called *internal respiration*. Blood vessels then transport carbon dioxide to the lungs where carbon dioxide diffuses from pulmonary blood vessels into alveoli, while oxygen from alveoli diffuses into blood. This process is called *external respiration*. *Ventilation* is simply the movement of air into and out of the lungs, a process that ensures oxygen availability. It includes both inhalation and exhalation.

During normal breathing, air enters the respiratory pathway via the nose and mouth. When air enters the nose, it circulates throughout the nasal cavity and the **paranasal sinuses**, hollow spaces lined with pseudostratified ciliated columnar epithelial tissue. As mentioned earlier, this epithelial tissue warms, moistens, and filters air before permitting it to enter deeper passageways. Air entering through the mouth, however, is not exposed to the nasal cavity or the paranasal sinuses; therefore, it is usually insufficiently warmed, moistened, and filtered as it passes through the respiratory tree. In fact, air inhaled through the mouth actually removes more moisture from the mucous lining than air inhaled through the nose.

RESPIRATORY CHANGES WITH ASTHMA

An asthma attack occurs when inflammation in the lining of the respiratory passageways interferes with air movement through the tubes and when its smooth muscle layer constricts and narrows the lumen (Fig. 11.3). During inflammation, the airways become red and swollen and produce copious amounts of mucus. The larger airways have cells with abundant cilia, so they manage to move excess mucus out of their lumens; however, the smaller bronchioles have fewer ciliated cells. Consequently, the secretions accumulate and obstruct these smaller passageways. If inflammation is not treated and reduced, the smooth muscle lining begins to twitch and involuntarily constrict the airway. Ultimately, a combination of inflammation and **bronchoconstriction** complicates breathing and ultimately reduces airflow into alveoli, which subsequently deprives body cells of oxygen.

Bolus—a semisolid mass of food swallowed at one time.

Homeostasis—the ability of the body to maintain relatively constant internal conditions despite ever-changing external conditions.

Paranasal sinuses—cavities within different bones of the skull that are lined with a specialized type of tissue that helps warm, moisten, and filter air.

Bronchoconstriction—narrowing of the respiratory passageways. It decreases airflow and thus promotes breathlessness, wheezing, and coughing.

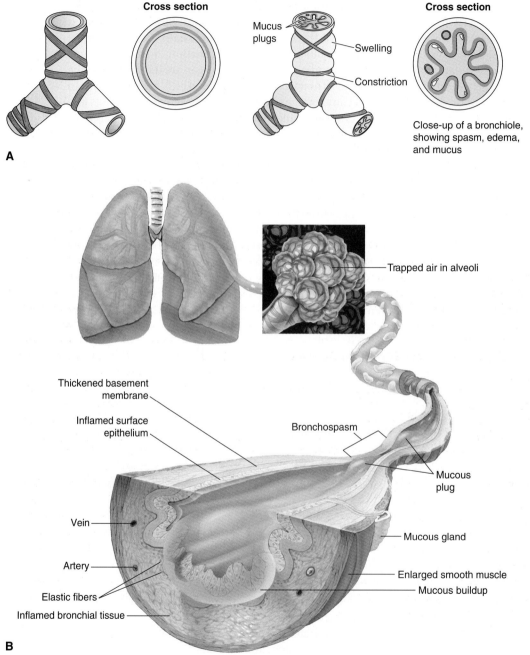

Cross section

Mucus plugs

Swelling

Constriction

Cross section

Close-up of a bronchiole, showing spasm, edema, and mucus

A

Trapped air in alveoli

Thickened basement membrane

Inflamed surface epithelium

Bronchospasm

Mucous plug

Vein

Artery

Elastic fibers

Inflamed bronchial tissue

Mucous gland

Enlarged smooth muscle

Mucous buildup

B

FIGURE 11.3 ■ Normal versus asthmatic bronchiole. **A.** Normal bronchioles (*left*) and bronchioles in asthma (*right*) (From Willis MC. Medical Terminology: A Programmed Learning Approach to the Language of Health Care. Baltimore: Lippincott Williams & Wilkins, 2002). **B.** Asthmatic bronchus (Provided by Anatomical Chart Co.).

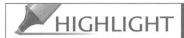

HIGHLIGHT   Diffusion of Gases

Diffusion is a passive process that occurs because of concentration gradients. The word "passive" means that energy is not required to move a substance because the substance is moving from an area of higher concentration to an area of lower concentration, or down its concentration gradient.

Consider the following example. A young man sprays a large amount of cologne onto his wrists prior to entering a lecture hall. After he enters, he sits at the very back of the classroom for the duration of the lecture. Although students in the front row do not initially smell the cologne, the molecules of cologne eventually move from the area of higher concentration (on the young man's wrists) to an area of lower concentration (the front of the classroom). Why does this happen? The molecules of cologne are in constant motion; therefore, they are likely to collide with one another frequently in the area where they are in greatest concentration (just as students are more likely to physically bump into one another in a crowded room). As these particles of cologne collide in the area of high concentration, they "bounce" farther and farther away from each other until they are evenly distributed throughout the classroom and equilibrium is reached (just as the group of students would spread out if more room became available). At equilibrium, the particles continue to move; they are just less likely to collide with other particles than when they were concentrated.

Apply this concept to the diffusion of oxygen and carbon dioxide across the permeable membranes of alveoli and blood vessels. To understand this discussion, remember that the pulmonary arteries transport blood low in oxygen from the heart to the lungs, while the pulmonary veins transport blood high in oxygen back to the heart.

The oxygen content in the alveoli is always higher than the oxygen content in the pulmonary arteries—a factor that facilitates the movement of oxygen out of the alveoli. This is because the lungs are filled with freshly oxygenated blood following each inhalation. As blood low in oxygen passes near the alveoli, oxygen moves from the alveoli into the blood vessels. This oxygenated blood then travels by way of the pulmonary veins back to the heart so that the heart can deliver it to the rest of the body. Now consider the carbon dioxide content within the pulmonary arteries and alveoli. The pulmonary arteries carry blood high in carbon dioxide from the heart to the lungs to eliminate excesses. The alveoli, which continuously release carbon dioxide during each exhalation, maintain a low concentration of carbon dioxide. Thus, carbon dioxide continues to move from the pulmonary arteries (an area of high carbon dioxide concentration) into the alveoli (which are always low in carbon dioxide). Overall, therefore, oxygen always moves from the alveoli into the blood vessels from an area of higher oxygen content to an area of lower oxygen content, and carbon dioxide always moves from the blood vessels into the alveoli.

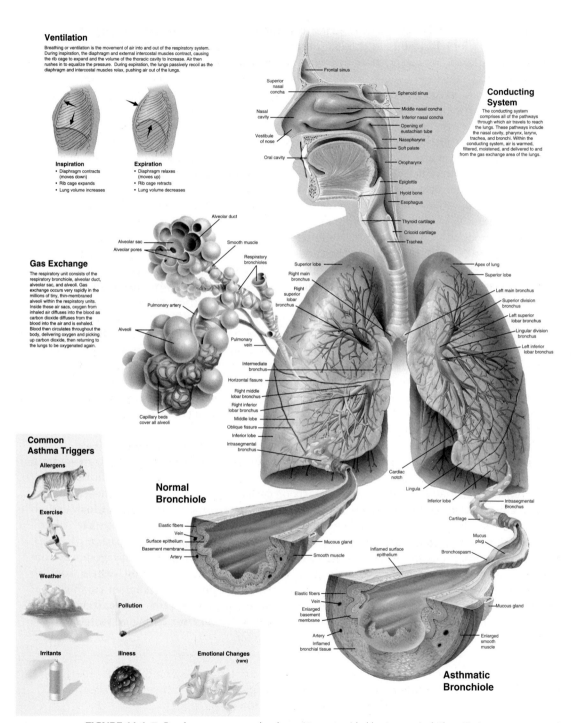

Ventilation

Breathing or ventilation is the movement of air into and out of the respiratory system. During inspiration, the diaphragm and external intercostal muscles contract, causing the rib cage to expand and the volume of the thoracic cavity to increase. Air then rushes in to equalize the pressure. During expiration, the lungs passively recoil as the diaphragm and intercostal muscles relax, pushing air out of the lungs.

Inspiration
• Diaphragm contracts (moves down)
• Rib cage expands
• Lung volume increases

Expiration
• Diaphragm relaxes (moves up)
• Rib cage retracts
• Lung volume decreases

Conducting System

The conducting system comprises all of the pathways through which air travels to reach the lungs. These pathways include the nasal cavity, pharynx, larynx, trachea, and bronchi. Within the conducting system, air is warmed, filtered, moistened, and delivered to and from the gas exchange area of the lungs.

Gas Exchange

The respiratory unit consists of the respiratory bronchiole, alveolar duct, alveolar sac, and alveoli. Gas exchange occurs very rapidly in the millions of tiny, thin-membraned alveoli within the respiratory units. Inside these air sacs, oxygen from inhaled air diffuses into the blood as carbon dioxide diffuses from the blood into the air and is exhaled. Blood then circulates throughout the body, delivering oxygen and picking up carbon dioxide, then returning to the lungs to be oxygenated again.

Frontal sinus
Superior nasal concha
Sphenoid sinus
Middle nasal concha
Nasal cavity
Inferior nasal concha
Opening of eustachian tube
Vestibule of nose
Nasopharynx
Soft palate
Oral cavity
Oropharynx
Epiglottis
Hyoid bone
Esophagus
Thyroid cartilage
Cricoid cartilage
Trachea

Alveolar duct
Alveolar sac
Alveolar pores
Smooth muscle
Respiratory bronchioles
Superior lobe
Apex of lung
Superior lobe
Right main bronchus
Left main bronchus
Right superior lobar bronchus
Superior division bronchus
Pulmonary artery
Left superior lobar bronchus
Lingular division bronchus
Alveoli
Left inferior lobar bronchus
Pulmonary vein
Intermediate bronchus
Horizontal fissure
Right middle lobar bronchus
Right inferior lobar bronchus
Middle lobe
Cardiac notch
Oblique fissure
Lingula
Inferior lobe
Intrasegmental bronchus
Capillary beds cover all alveoli
Inferior lobe
Intrasegmental Bronchus
Cartilage

Common Asthma Triggers

Allergens

Exercise

Weather

Pollution

Irritants

Illness

Emotional Changes (rare)

Normal Bronchiole

Elastic fibers
Vein
Surface epithelium
Basement membrane
Artery
Mucous gland
Smooth muscle

Inflamed surface epithelium
Bronchospasm
Mucus plug

Asthmatic Bronchiole

Elastic fibers
Vein
Enlarged basement membrane
Mucous gland
Artery
Inflamed bronchial tissue
Enlarged smooth muscle

FIGURE 11.4 ■ Respiratory system and asthma. (Asset provided by Anatomical Chart Co.)

In general, both inflammation and airway constriction occur in response to exposure to **allergens** or other irritants in the environment. In fact, the airways of individuals without asthma initially constrict when such irritants first enter; however, healthy passageways quickly dilate to permit easier air movement as breaths become deeper. This response helps rid the airways of irritants and ensures an adequate oxygen supply.

People with asthma, on the other hand, experience sustained airway constriction—even when they take in deeper breaths. This prolongs narrowing of the respiratory passageway and promotes breathing difficulties. Why does this happen? Some experts believe that asthma sufferers lack a specific chemical necessary for airway dilation; thus, their airways cannot relax like healthy airways. An additional culprit is the inflammatory response, a normal component of the immune system that overreacts under certain circumstances. One factor that stimulates the inflammation of the respiratory passageways is exposure to allergens and other irritants. Allergen invasion of the airways triggers several processes in the body. First, blood flow increases to transport macrophages and neutrophils (two types of white blood cells) to the area of invasion where they can engulf the allergens. Additionally, capillaries become leakier as chemicals such as histamine are released by damaged cells. Blood from deeper tissues travels to the area of invasion, which results in localized heat and redness. Capillary dilation allows for fluid accumulation, or swelling, and pain occurs in response to the presence of chemicals often produced by the allergens themselves. These factors account for the redness, heat, swelling, and pain characteristic of inflammation. Unfortunately, asthmatics often experience an extreme inflammatory response that causes excess fluid accumulation and mucus production that significantly interfere with proper breathing. Furthermore, continual bouts of inflammation can permanently damage airways, a factor that promotes further inflammation and continued airway constriction.[5] Figure 11.4 provides a summary of the effects of asthma on the respiratory system.

The precise causes for asthma are unknown; however, a genetic component appears to exist. If one parent has asthma, each child has a 33% chance of developing asthma. If both parents have asthma, the risk increases to 70%.[2]

Environmental factors also affect the likelihood of developing asthma. Some studies suggest a positive correlation between diets high in processed and fast foods (and subsequently low in fiber, fruits, and vegetables) and the development of childhood asthma. Other experts believe that children are overexposed to indoor allergens and dust mites because they stay inside so much (to watch television, use the computer, or play video games). Furthermore, low–birth-weight babies, who have an increased risk for asthma and numerous other conditions, have a higher survival rate than in the past; therefore, the pool of susceptible individuals is increasing. Additionally, fewer infants are breastfed, so a greater number do not receive the natural anti-inflammatories and antibodies

---

Allergen—a substance that elicits an immune response in susceptible individuals. Allergens, though not necessarily harmful to all people, are perceived as pathogenic (potentially damaging) by the immune systems of sensitive individuals.

present in breast milk that protect against asthma. Lastly, there is a movement in developed nations, particularly in the United States, toward cleaner and more sanitized environments for children. These efforts are admirable, but they also limit a child's exposure to (and subsequent immunity from) a vast array of allergens and other pathogens. Although no conclusive evidence exists, many experts believe that the prevalence of asthma is increasing partly because children are not adequately exposed to pathogens; therefore, their immune systems are not sufficiently challenged.[5]

MANAGING ASTHMA

Avoid Triggers

Currently, no cure for asthma exists; however, sufferers can manage their condition with a few lifestyle adjustments (Table 11.1). Most importantly, asthma sufferers must avoid triggers since triggers promote asthma attacks. Triggers include anything that causes acute inflammation and/or the constriction of the respiratory passages. They vary among different individuals, but the most common inflammatory triggers (also known as allergic triggers) include air pollutants, mold, pollen, animal dander, cockroaches, respiratory system infections, and dust mites. Nonallergic triggers, which cause only a minor constriction of the airways, include intense exercise, emotional stress, and inhaling cold or dry air, cigarette smoke, paint fumes, or fireplace smoke.[5,6]

> ### QUICK REFERENCE
>
> The risk for an asthma attack often increases at night. Although the precise reason is uncertain, experts believe that the body releases certain night-time chemicals that detrimentally affect lung functioning. Additionally, body temperature tends to decrease at night; this in turn cools the airways, which promotes constriction.

TABLE 11-1 MANAGING ASTHMA

Tips for decreasing frequency of asthma attacks	Explanation
Avoid triggers.	Triggers include mold, pollen, animal dander, dust mites, and air pollutants.
Learn to breathe properly.	Breathe through the nose; avoid hyperventilating.
Avoid respiratory infections.	Colds, flu, sore, throats, and sinus infections are the major contributors to asthma attacks in children.
Avoid medications that make asthma symptoms worse.	Certain high blood pressure, glaucoma, migraine, and diabetes medications worsen asthma symptoms in some people.
Exercise appropriately.	Use the suggestions described throughout this chapter.
Maintain a healthy weight.	Excess weight stresses the cardiorespiratory system and makes breathing difficult.
Eat a healthy diet.	Although it is unknown whether or not diet can prevent or cure asthma, a healthy diet might decrease the severity of symptoms.

QUICK REFERENCE

Common triggers for asthma attacks include

- Irritants in the air
- Nasal allergies
- Animal dander
- Cold or very dry air
- Strenuous exercise
- Emotional stress
- Respiratory infections (cold, sore throat, bronchitis)
- Strong smells
- Smoke
- Intensified asthma symptoms in some women prior to the monthly cycle

Take Prescribed Medications as Directed by a Physician

Medications can also control asthma symptoms and reduce asthma attack frequency. The two major asthma medications currently available are **bronchodilators** and anti-inflammatory drugs. Bronchodilators are used immediately prior to or during an asthma attack to instantly relax the bronchial tubes and prevent (or alleviate) constriction. Anti-inflammatories, on the other hand, are used for the long-term control of asthma. As their name suggests, they limit inflammation and swelling in the bronchial tubes and must be taken regularly. Ultimately, they protect airway linings by preventing irritation. This, in turn, decreases the number and severity of asthma attacks.[5,6]

Overall, those with *mild* asthma sometimes do not need anti-inflammatories. Instead, they can rely on bronchodilators during acute asthma attacks or prior to exercise. Those with *moderate* to *severe* asthma, however, usually require both anti-inflammatories and bronchodilators to appropriately manage symptoms and prevent acute attacks. Although some medications are available over the counter, asthma sufferers are safer if they consult with a physician and follow strict guidelines.[4] They should also be wary of herbal medications.

Monitor Airflow

To measure the amount of air exhaled from the lungs, asthma sufferers use a portable measuring device called a peak flow meter. The device is simple to use. Users blow into the tube and then check their scores on the needle. After completing three attempts, they take the highest score and compare it to a standard score that represents the amount of air a healthy person of the same age, gender, and height can exhale. A score below the standard suggests a constricted airway and a possible upcoming asthma attack.[5,6]

Bronchodilators—medications that ease air flow into the lungs by increasing airway diameter.

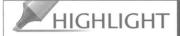 **HIGHLIGHT**   A Closer Look at Asthma Medications

Most asthmatics can successfully prevent or lessen the severity of acute asthma attacks if they take prescribed medications as indicated by a physician. In general, bronchodilators, corticosteroids, and anti-inflammatories are used to treat asthma.

Short-acting beta-2 agonist sprays (albuterol, pirbuterol, and terbutaline) should be used about 15 minutes prior to exercise; however, they are also beneficial after an episode of exercise-induced asthma (EIA). These bronchodilators are inhaled through the nostrils and usually begin working immediately. Their effects last up to 6 hours.

Long-acting bronchodilators (salmeterol, metaproterenol, and theophylline) are also available. They help control symptoms in special circumstances such as during the night or during a particularly high pollen season.

Corticosteroids help manage short-term airway inflammation by reducing existing inflammation (rather than by preventing inflammation). In effect, they ultimately decrease the risk of spontaneous muscle spasm in the smooth muscle lining—a factor that maintains an open airway and prevents acute asthma attacks. Some are taken orally (prednisone, methylprednisolone, and prednisolone), while others are inhaled (fluticasone, budesonide, and flunisolid).

Other anti-inflammatories work over the long term to prevent (rather than simply reduce) redness and swelling in the airways. Zafirlukast and zileuton belong to a class of anti-inflammatories known as leukotriene inhibitors that interfere with factors that promote inflammation. Advair is an inhaled drug that combines fluticasone (a corticosteroid) with salmeterol (a long-acting bronchodilator); thus, it reduces both airway inflammation and constriction.

Learn to Breathe Properly

Inhalation and exhalation are components of ventilation. Inhalation is an active process that requires the contraction of the diaphragm and external intercostal muscles. Before considering the roles of these muscles in inhalation, review the basic structure of the pleural membrane, the double-layered protective membrane surrounding each lung. The inner layer of the pleural membrane firmly attaches to the lung surface, while the outer layer firmly attaches to surrounding structures such as the diaphragm, sternum, ribs, and intercostal muscles. In between these two layers is a fluid that firmly holds the inner layer to the outer layer. It is this arrangement that facilitates breathing.

When relaxed, the diaphragm is a dome-shaped muscle that separates the thoracic cavity from the abdominal cavity. If the diaphragm remains relaxed, pressure inside the lungs equalizes to atmospheric pressure, so there is no net movement of air into or out of the lungs. When the diaphragm contracts, however, it flattens (Fig. 11.5). Since the outer layer of the pleural membrane attaches to the diaphragm, any movement of the diaphragm pulls on this outer layer, which then pulls on the inner layer, which ultimately pulls on the lungs and causes them to expand. Lung tissue expansion decreases the pressure within the lungs and creates a pressure gradient. Air from outside the body now moves from an area of

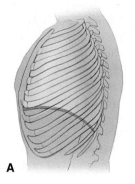 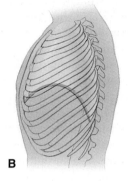

FIGURE 11.5 ■ Diaphragm: contracted **(A)** and relaxed **(B)**. (Asset provided by Anatomical Chart Co.)

A   **B**

higher pressure (in the atmosphere) to an area of lower pressure (within the lungs) through the process called inhalation. Since inhalation requires muscle contraction, and since muscle contraction requires energy, inhalation is an active process. At times of rest, diaphragm contraction is enough to maintain appropriate pressure gradients to ensure proper breathing. During exertion, however, additional muscles contract to help expand the lungs further. The external intercostals, for instance, contract and elevate both the sternum and the ribs. These structures also firmly attach to the outer layer of the lungs, so contraction of the external intercostals expands the upper portion of the lungs and creates a pressure gradient that facilitates additional air movement into the lungs. At the same time, accessory muscles in the neck, chest, and shoulders contract and thereby assist as demand increases.

Normal exhalation is a passive process. As long as lung tissue remains elastic and muscle tissue maintains contractile properties, exhalation occurs as the diaphragm—and the external intercostals—relax and as the elastic lung tissue recoils. These events increase pressure within the lungs, which forces air to move from the lung space (an area that now has higher pressure) to the external environment (an area of relatively low pressure) through a process called exhalation. The contraction of the abdominal muscles also assists in forcing air out of the lungs during intense exertion.

Because asthma sufferers often have difficulty breathing, they must use their intercostals and accessory muscles more than normal. This often results in overdeveloped muscles and a barrel-shaped chest, particularly when asthma attacks occur frequently.[7]

Asthmatics often practice poor breathing techniques, even when they are not experiencing an asthma attack. In fact, they frequently hyperventilate, which can drastically worsen asthma symptoms both in the short term and in the long term. Hyperventilation usually relies on the intercostals and accessory muscles more than the diaphragm; thus, breathing tends to occur in the upper rather than lower torso. Why does hyperventilation worsen asthma? During **hyperventilation**, breathing occurs through the mouth rather than through the nose. Air entering through the mouth is cool and dry, so it irritates the

> **Hyperventilation**—a pattern of breathing that results in rapid, shallow breaths. It occurs from overuse of the accessory breathing muscles and underuse of the diaphragm.

lining of the airways. Since the airways of asthmatics are already inflamed, additional irritation usually causes constriction. Thus, people with asthma must retrain themselves to breathe through the nose in between asthma attacks to reduce their severity and frequency. In fact, physicians often recommend breathing exercises to encourage diaphragmatic and nasal breathing.[7,8] Some studies show that long-term practice of these techniques once or twice daily decreases medication use by as much as 50%.[8]

Hyperventilation indirectly contributes to asthma because it tends to lower blood carbon dioxide (CO_2) levels. Low CO_2 levels usually encourage system-wide smooth muscle contraction—which also affects the smooth muscle lining of the airways. Furthermore, low CO_2 levels stimulate **mast cells** to release histamine, a chemical that initiates inflammation and subsequently narrows the airways.[7] The resulting inflammation and muscle spasms in the respiratory passageways increase the likelihood of an asthma attack.

> ### QUICK REFERENCE
>
> The Buteyko method, developed by Konstantin Buteyko, is a simple method that helps train asthmatics to breathe properly. For details on this method, see the article by Jonathan Brostoff and Linda Gamlin in the reference section of this chapter.

PRECAUTIONS DURING EXERCISE

During exercise, oxygen demand and carbon dioxide removal increase. Thus, the respiratory system and associated muscles must move a greater-than-usual quantity of air into and out of the lungs. Those suffering from asthma are at a disadvantage because their lungs normally function less than optimally, even at rest. Add the challenge of increased activity and this can promote an "exercise-induced" asthma attack, the primary concern for asthmatics who exercise.

Anyone who has asthma symptoms at rest can also experience exercise-induced asthma (EIA) when their activity level increases. However, EIA can also occur in those who do not typically experience asthma symptoms at low intensities. In either case, exercise acts as the trigger for an acute asthma attack that results in coughing, wheezing, and shortness of breath.[9,10] Symptoms do not arise immediately; instead, they tend to develop about 5 to 10 minutes after the start of exercise and then gradually resolve for the duration of activity. Within several minutes following exercise completion, however, the airways begin to tighten and symptoms develop once again. They become most severe about 5 to 15 minutes post exercise and subside after about 15 minutes. They usually completely resolve within 45 to 60 minutes following exercise.[9,11]

The basic theory behind EIA is as follows. As exercise intensity and oxygen demand increase, respiratory rate accelerates. Since the nostrils can take in only a limited quantity of air, exercisers typically begin to rely more on mouth breathing. Eventually, the amount of air breathed in through the mouth exceeds that breathed in through the nose, so much of the air is insufficiently filtered, warmed, and moistened as it passes into deeper respiratory passageways.[10] In fact, air is moistened only 60% to 70% relative to humidity during mouth breathing, whereas it is moistened up to 80% to 90% relative to humidity during nose breathing. Thus, as air breathed in through the mouth travels toward the lungs, moisture and heat are drawn out of the mucous lining. This dries and cools the lining and promotes further irritation, inflammation, and constriction.[10]

QUICK REFERENCE

Interestingly, those who experience EIA usually have a refractory period following an initial bout of exercise. This means that if, after an initial exercise session, they exercise again within 30 to 90 minutes of the first activity, airway tightening is significantly less likely and symptoms diminish.

In some cases, asthma sufferers claim to have an asthma attack 3 to 6 hours following exercise; however, research has not yet confirmed whether or not this attack is actually related to the exercise itself.[9]

Fortunately, EIA can be managed and its symptoms minimized with careful planning. Asthma sufferers should avoid exercising in dry, cool environments. They should participate in activities that involve short bursts of energy rather than those that require a constant pace for a long duration. Exercise in an indoor pool is beneficial for two major reasons. First, the air in this environment tends to be warm and moist, so it is less likely to dry the airways. Second, swimming places the body in a horizontal position, which facilitates mucus removal. One word of caution: if pool water contains excessive amounts of chlorine, the fumes can trigger an attack in some individuals—especially when the pool is confined indoors.

QUICK REFERENCE

Tips to reduce the risk of EIA[5,9]:

- Warm up prior to exercise and cool down following exercise.
- Participate in activities that require short bursts of energy (like baseball, tennis, or volleyball) and avoid those that require long-duration running (such as soccer, long-distance running, or bicycling).
- Breathe through the nose as much as possible; place a scarf over the mouth and nose to help warm air during mouth breathing, especially when outside in cold, dry air.
- Use bronchodilators as needed and prescribed.

Mast cells—cells that release various substances, including histamine and heparin. They are associated with allergic responses and contribute to asthma. They cause inflammation and muscle spasms in the airways, factors that promote asthma attacks.

EIA occurs in about 12% to 15% of the U.S. general population. Episodes are much more likely to occur in chronic asthma sufferers; in fact, 70% to 90% of those with chronic asthma experience EIA. Surprisingly, nearly 11% of Olympic athletes in the 1984 summer Olympics met the criteria for EIA.[12]

BENEFITS OF EXERCISE

Although increased physical activity is not a cure for asthma, asthma sufferers experience many of the same exercise-related health improvements as those without asthma. Therefore, they should include physical activity in their daily routines. This section explores some of the benefits associated with an active lifestyle.

IMPROVED OVERALL PHYSICAL CONDITIONING AND FUNCTIONAL CAPACITY

Exercise increases muscular strength and endurance, improves cardiovascular functioning, and enhances joint mobility, factors that enhance quality of life and functional capacity in everyone. Research shows that a well-conditioned asthmatic experiences a lower heart rate, greater heart rate reserve, reduced ventilation at peak levels, decreased episodes of **dyspnea**, improved maximal oxygen uptake, and lower blood lactate levels following long-term regimented exercise.[13–17] These improvements in turn ease daily activities and permit greater involvement in life. Additionally, though no conclusive evidence exists, some experts believe that asthmatics who routinely exercise might minimize episodes of EIA.[17]

Researchers are still investigating the role of exercise in asthma prevention. So far, studies on children do not show a relationship between regular activity and the incidence of asthma; however, increased physical activity does not adversely influence the frequency or severity of asthma attacks either, so doctors now encourage exercise because of all of the other benefits it provides.[17–19]

DECREASED HOSPITALIZATIONS

Because overall conditioning improves, asthmatic exercisers seem to have fewer physician consultations and decreased hospitalization rates. One study that investigated the impact of a long-term swimming program on asthmatic children found a 46% drop in physician consultations and a 64% decrease in hospitalizations after 2 years of compliance. Additionally, parents of two thirds of these same subjects reported that their children were taking lower medication doses than they were prior to initiating exercise.[17,19]

IMPROVED PSYCHOLOGICAL MOOD

As occurs in other populations, exercise seems to improve the mood of those with asthma, a factor that affects overall mental health.[5,9] Improved mental health in turn enables individuals to better deal with stress. Furthermore, since excess stress can act as a trigger for asthma attacks, exercise might indirectly control the severity of such attacks.[5] Exercise also reduces asthma-associated symptoms and gives exercisers a sense of control over their lives, which boosts their confidence.[9,13,17] Additionally, it eases activities of daily living, promotes interaction with other people, and encourages goal setting and achievement, factors that improve self-efficacy.[20]

DECREASED RISK FOR CHRONIC CONDITIONS

The primary long-term benefits of exercise are the same for asthmatics as they are for the general population.[15] Essentially, exercise reduces the risk for developing chronic conditions such as heart disease, stroke, diabetes, and obesity. Long-term training accomplishes this by improving heart rate, blood pressure, body composition, and vascularity. These in turn reduce the risk of high blood pressure, atherosclerosis, blood clots, and excess weight, factors that predispose individuals to heart attack.[21]

A large percentage of asthma sufferers are overweight or obese, so they should consider exercise as a means of achieving a healthier weight. It is important to note that research has not conclusively correlated weight loss with less severe asthma symptoms or fewer acute attacks.[22] Furthermore, some health professionals believe that many obese individuals are incorrectly diagnosed as being asthmatic "… when in fact they are simply short of breath, possibly because of the increased effort required for breathing."[5] Still, weight loss provides benefits for the obese whether they have asthma or not. And since some experts believe that excess weight triggers bronchoconstriction in asthmatics by putting excess pressure on the lungs, asthma sufferers who carry extra weight should try to lose it.

RECOMMENDATIONS FOR EXERCISE

Unfortunately, those with asthma tend to be less active and less fit than those without asthma.[22,23] Most research suggests that the lower fitness levels result from self-imposed inactivity rather than airway obstruction,[21] a fact that suggests that a major barrier is the fear of EIA episodes.

Although physicians once considered exercise unsafe for this population, most now recommend physical activity to asthma sufferers provided their condition is under control.[9,21] Furthermore, with proper education, training, and medication use, asthmatics can actually safely participate in nearly any form of activity. In fact, several individuals with asthma—including Jackie Joyner-Kersee, Greg Louganis, Tom Dolan, and Jim Ryan—have become elite athletes.[9]

EXERCISE TESTING

The American College of Sports Medicine offers exercise-testing guidelines for those with pulmonary diseases that predispose them to shortness of breath during exertion (see

Dyspnea—difficulty in breathing or shortness of breath.

ACSM's Guidelines for Exercise Testing and Prescription, 8th Ed, for more specific details on the suggestions presented in this section). These conditions include chronic bronchitis, emphysema, and asthma. To paraphrase general guidelines, ACSM suggests exercise testing to determine cardiopulmonary capacity, pulmonary function, and arterial blood gases and arterial oxygen saturation. They suggest that tests be given in shorter increments with slower progression rates since activity often results in dyspnea in this population. They also suggest test termination in cases of arterial oxygen desaturation. The preferred mode for exercise testing is walking, but stationary cycling without arm ergometry is also acceptable. This is because excessive arm movements often cause shortness of breath, which can interfere with exercise duration. For those with severe pulmonary disease, the 6-minute walk test is safe for assessing functional exercise capacity.

QUICK REFERENCE

People with pulmonary disease often have ventilatory limitations to exercise, so it might not be appropriate to predict peak VO_2 based on age-predicted maximal heart rate.[24]

EXERCISE PRESCRIPTION

In general, exercise guidelines for those with pulmonary disease are separated into two categories. The first applies to those who have well-controlled asthma or mild chronic obstructive pulmonary disorder (COPD). The second applies to moderate to severe COPD.[24] Overall, recommendations for the well-controlled group are similar to those of the general population with a few exceptions.[3,24–27]

QUICK REFERENCE

People with asthma must have their asthma under control prior to participating in exercise testing or prescription.

Obtain a medical clearance prior to allowing clients with pulmonary disorder to participate in any form of activity. Physicians can ensure that clients are taking appropriate medications at appropriate dosages and times.

ACSM's Aerobic Training Guidelines for Those With Controlled Asthma or Mild COPD

- Perform cardiovascular exercise 3 to 5 days per week for 20 to 60 minutes of continuous or intermittent activity.
- Experts have not yet determined optimal training intensity, so they suggest that those with COPD follow intensity guidelines for senior adults (see Chapter 5)

and that young people with asthma or cystic fibrosis follow guidelines for children and adolescents (see Chapter 4).

■ Walking or stationary cycling is generally safe and beneficial.

ACSM's Cardiovascular Guidelines for Individuals With Moderate to Severe COPD

■ Participate in cardiovascular exercise 3 to 5 days per week. Initial duration might only be a few minutes. Slowly increase duration as client's health improves, but base duration on tolerance level.

■ Intensity should be 60% to 80% of peak work rate, or base intensity on dyspnea ratings.

■ Walking or stationary cycling is the best mode.

Individuals belonging to either of these two groups also benefit from resistance and flexibility training. For flexibility training, follow the same guidelines used for the general population. Those with controlled asthma or mild COPD may follow resistance training guidelines for the general population. Those with moderate to severe COPD should follow recommendations for senior adults. See Chapters 2 and 5 for more details. Those with pulmonary disorders typically have weak inspiratory muscles, which interferes with exercise tolerance and causes dyspnea in sufferers. ACSM suggests training inspiratory muscles on 4 to 5 days per week at 30% maximal inspiratory pressure measured at functional residual capacity for a duration of 30 minutes (or two 15-minute segments). This can decrease dyspnea, increase exercise tolerance, and improve lung functioning.

Special Concerns for Asthma Sufferers

■ Before cardiovascular training, include a longer warm-up with a more gradual progression. This helps reduce the chest tightness that sometimes occurs after exertion and prevents or lessens the severity of EIA. A longer cool-down that includes stretching is also beneficial to prevent air within the lungs from drastically changing temperature, a factor that promotes EIA.[3]

■ The mode of cardiovascular exercise is important for asthmatics. EIA is most likely to occur with outdoor running; however, it might also occur with indoor running, outdoor bicycling, soccer, aerobic dance classes that involve excessive arm movements, or any activity performed outdoors in a cold, dry climate. In fact, any prolonged activity is potentially dangerous to the person with asthma. Intermittent activities, such as football, baseball, volleyball, gymnastics, wrestling, and tennis, are better choices. Walking and swimming are least likely to evoke episodes of EIA. Stationary cycling without arm movements is also safe.

■ Exercise at intensities that do not evoke symptoms. High-intensity activities at or above 80% to 90% of maximum heart rate cause more episodes of EIA than lower-intensity activities. Intermittent activities that include frequent rest periods are usually well tolerated.

■ Resistance training is important since many people suffering from asthma have been sedentary for most of their lives. Training muscles throughout the body helps develop functional capacity, while working the muscles of inspiration might improve breathing mechanics. Emphasize shoulder and arm work since many sufferers experience shortness of breath when participating in everyday activities that require elevation of the arms. Also include exercises that can be done with the arms below the heart.

■ Some authorities suggest yoga and meditation to teach better breathing. This type of training encourages deep, slow breaths and eases stress and anxiety. Proponents say that this relaxes blood vessels and reduces blood pressure, factors that might reduce the occurrence of acute attacks.

■ Most asthmatics can successfully prevent or lessen the severity of acute **bronchospasm** if they use prescribed bronchodilators prior to exercise as indicated by their physician. As mentioned earlier, 2 to 4 puffs of short-acting beta-2 agonist sprays should be used about 15 minutes prior to exercise. Ensure that asthmatic clients have their bronchodilators on hand before permitting them to begin exercise.

■ Asthma sufferers should avoid, or severely limit, activity when they have a viral infection or when their body temperature is low.

■ Pay attention to the air quality outside or in the gym, wherever you are exercising. If air quality is poor, move to a different location or postpone activity until air quality improves.

■ If symptoms develop, stop the exercise and have clients use inhalers. If the symptoms completely subside, clients can usually continue exercising without concern. If the symptoms return, have them stop the exercise again, use prescribed inhalers, and contact their physicians for further instructions.

SAMPLE EXERCISES

A diagnosis of asthma alone does not preclude anyone from strength training; however, asthmatics might have other preexisting conditions that make them vulnerable when performing certain exercises. As with other populations, screen clients with asthma for coexisting limitations. In general, asthma sufferers sometimes become breathless during daily activities that require them to lift their arms above their heads. Therefore, strength training should focus on improving both strength and endurance of muscles involved with these types of movements. Improved conditioning in asthmatic clients usually increases tolerance for normal activities of daily living without exacerbating asthma symptoms. Definitely include shoulder presses, lateral shoulder raises, biceps curls, and triceps extensions. Additionally, add in exercises that train the torso muscles—such as the chest press, chest flies, lat pull downs, and seated rows. Squats, leg presses, leg extensions, and leg curls effectively train the lower body. Include abdominal crunches to complete the full body workout. *No specific modifications are necessary; simply follow general guidelines as presented throughout this book and avoid increasing intensity too much.*

NUTRITIONAL CONSIDERATIONS

Overall, a healthy diet for the asthmatic population resembles a healthy diet for the general population. It includes a balance of carbohydrates, fats, and proteins and emphasizes fresh fruits and vegetables, whole grains, lean meats, fish, and monounsaturated and omega-3 fatty acids. See Appendix B for the specific dietary recommendations for different age groups.

Because diet promotes or prevents the development of many other diseases, researchers are currently investigating its effect on asthma. Although they have not yet conclusively discovered any miracle nutrients that prevent or cure asthma, they hypothesize that a few might influence symptom severity.

QUICK REFERENCE

Foods and nutrients that might affect asthma symptoms include

- Antioxidants
- Folic acid
- Magnesium
- Omega-3 fatty acids
- Water
- Calcium
- Salt
- Caffeine

ANTIOXIDANTS

Antioxidants are nutrients that fight free radicals and inhibit their ability to cause damage. In general, free radicals are highly reactive molecules found in varying quantities in the body at all times. In fact, they are natural by-products of normal metabolic processes, but their levels increase in response to exposure to UV radiation, cigarette smoke, air pollutants, or toxic chemicals. Under normal conditions, the body adequately handles free radicals and limits their devastating effects. Sometimes, however, the number of free radicals exceeds the body's ability to contain them, so they are free to destroy cell membranes, damage DNA, and cause inflammation. Keep in mind that asthma is partly classified as an inflammatory disease.

The body has several lines of defense that protect against free radicals. One of the most important defense systems includes the antioxidant vitamins and minerals that

Bronchospasm—an abnormal contraction of the smooth muscle lining of the respiratory passageways that constricts the airways. It is a common condition in chronic asthma and EIA and is usually indicated by coughing and wheezing.

essentially disable free radicals and prevent their activity. By neutralizing free radicals, these antioxidants might help reduce inflammation thereby preventing asthma symptoms and attacks.

Antioxidants include vitamin C, vitamin E, beta carotene, and selenium, nutrients abundantly found in fresh fruits and vegetables. Good sources of vitamin C include citrus fruits, Brussels sprouts, cauliflower, green peppers, broccoli, cantaloupe, strawberries, and lettuce. Vitamin E is found in margarine, salad dressings, shortening, leafy green vegetables, wheat germ, egg yolks, liver, nuts, seeds, whole grains, and fatty meats. Consume plenty of cantaloupe, sweet potatoes, carrots, spinach, and squash for an adequate supply of β carotene, and include seafood, meat, whole grains, fruits, and vegetables to meet the body's needs for selenium. Phytochemicals are additional substances thought to have antioxidant properties. They are found predominantly in fruits and vegetables such as tomatoes, broccoli, carrots, berries, soybeans, whole grains, and various teas and wine.

The best alternative is to increase dietary intake of these nutrients. Most supplements have not provided the same protective effects as foods.

FOLIC ACID AND MAGNESIUM

People suffering from asthma consistently show deficiencies in both folate and magnesium, so perhaps these nutrients play a role in asthma development. Folate is abundant in fortified and whole grains, liver, spinach, legumes, and seeds. Magnesium, which helps relax smooth muscle, is found in nuts, legumes, whole grains, dark green vegetables, seafood, and chocolate. Researchers are still investigating the relationship between asthma and deficiencies of these nutrients, but it is still prudent for those with asthma to obtain recommended intakes.

OMEGA-3 FATTY ACIDS

Omega-3 fatty acids act as natural anti-inflammatories, so asthmatics might benefit from an increased intake[28]; however, specific recommendations for asthma sufferers are currently not available since evidence showing a direct correlation is lacking.[29] Because omega-3 fatty acids provide several additional benefits (such as protection against heart disease), increasing their intake is certainly beneficial. Again, dietary sources are better choices than supplements. Simply consuming fatty fish (such as mackerel, salmon, herring, or tuna) two times per week significantly increases omega-3 fatty acid levels. Those who do not like fish can obtain an adequate intake by including walnuts, flaxseeds, flaxseed oil, canola oil, and soybeans in their diets.

CAFFEINE

Caffeine has effects similar to theophylline, a long-acting bronchodilator used to treat asthma. Consequently, researchers are investigating caffeine's potential use as a treatment for asthma symptoms. Some studies on asthmatic subjects show that low doses of caffeine relax the smooth muscle lining of the bronchioles for up to 4 hours, but its effectiveness on the long-term management of symptoms is still not clear.[30] Other studies show that *high* doses of caffeine seem to reduce the severity of EIA, while *low* doses have no apparent effect. In these studies, participants either consumed a placebo, a low dose of caffeine (3.5 to 5 mg/kg), or a high dose of caffeine (7 to 10 mg/kg) prior to an event. Overall, the high doses (the equivalent to three to five cups of very strong coffee) consumed 90 to 120 minutes prior to exercise reduced the severity of EIA in the subjects. Subjects taking the placebo or a lower dose of caffeine experienced no improvements at all.[31,32] Obviously, the amount of caffeine necessary for improvements is extremely high, and a high intake can cause frequent urination and dehydration since caffeine acts as a diuretic. Not only does dehydration negatively affect performance, but it can also be deadly. The threats associated with dehydration are even more pronounced in the asthmatic for reasons discussed in the next section. Additionally, the "effective dose" of caffeine is in excess of that permitted by the Olympic committee and other international competitions, so it is not recommended for asthmatics competing in elite athletic competitions.[29]

Overall, caffeine seems to be somewhat effective in managing EIA. Asthma sufferers, however, need to consider the potential problems that result from excess caffeine intake. Most importantly, they should not use caffeine to replace prescribed medications.

WATER

All exercisers need to remain hydrated, so water intake must match daily water loss. One of the most important functions of water is to enable the body to thermoregulate. This function becomes crucial during physical activity when contracting muscles produce large quantities of heat that must be dissipated. For an asthmatic, water intake is even more critical because water ensures a moist airway, and a moist airway prevents excessive mucus production and inflammation that, if present, eventually narrow the passageway and trigger bronchoconstriction. Adequate water also keeps lung tissue moist, which controls mucus production and facilitates gas exchange.

CALCIUM

The long-term use of oral steroids, and possibly inhaled steroids, reduces bone density.[5] Thus, asthmatics, particularly children and adolescents, who use steroids to manage their symptoms should be conscientious about their calcium intake. Adequate calcium and vitamin D intake is essential for bone health. See Appendix B for recommended intake levels of calcium and vitamin D.

SALT

As early as 1938, researchers noted that asthma symptoms were alleviated in those on a low-salt diet, so scientists have been investigating the relationship ever since.[33] The fact that asthma is becoming more common in industrialized nations where sodium chloride consumption continues to increase seems to support the hypothesis that salt might trigger asthma symptoms.[34-37] Recent research suggests that asthmatics reduce salt intake to decrease the intensity and frequency of asthma attacks.[38,39] Current dietary guidelines, which suggest no more than 2,400 mg of sodium per day, seem appropriate for the asthmatic.[29,38-40] Reducing sodium intake to this amount would be a great improvement considering that the average American consumes three to four times this amount!

SUMMARY

Although many people suffering from asthma avoid and often fear exercise, they should learn more about the benefits of increased physical activity and identify how they can manage episodes of EIA. Although exercise cannot cure asthma, it improves overall functional capacity, which, in turn, minimizes the stress of challenging activities. This ultimately eases actual and perceived exertion and hopefully reduces episodes of breathlessness, coughing, wheezing, and acute asthma attacks. As long as they practice certain precautions, continue to take their prescribed medications, and regularly consult with their physicians, most asthmatics can safely participate, and may even excel, in just about any form of physical activity.

CASE STUDY

A 30-year-old man with controlled asthma was referred to you by his physician. He is 5'9" tall and weighs 210 lb. Although he has never actually participated in a regular exercise program, he has always been relatively active. He walks a lot for his job and can be found doing work around the house and yard during his free time. He is taking a daily anti-inflammatory and has a bronchodilator.

■ What type of exercise program would you recommend to this client?

■ Describe the mode, frequency, duration, and intensity of exercise appropriate for him. Keep in mind that his ultimate goal is to lose 25 lb to reduce his risk for heart disease since his father is currently recovering from a heart attack.

THINKING CRITICALLY

1. Name and describe two conditions that characterize asthma. Explain how they cause the classic signs of asthma.
2. Explain the general structure and function of the respiratory system. How does asthma interfere with normal functioning?
3. Why must air be filtered, warmed, and moistened prior to entering the lungs?
4. What structures are involved with gas exchange in the lungs? Describe how gas exchange occurs. Be sure to name the major gases involved.
5. Explain thoroughly how a person can manage and live with asthma.

6. What muscles are involved with normal passive breathing? Explain how they function, both at rest and during exertion.
7. What is EIA? Describe how it develops.
8. Explain several benefits of exercise for the asthmatic client.
9. What are some special dietary considerations for a person suffering from asthma?
10. Why is proper hydration so important for those with asthma?

REFERENCES

1. Centers for Disease Control. www.cdc.gov
2. Asthma and Allergy Foundation of America. www.aafa.org
3. American Academy of Allergy, Asthma, and Immunology. www.aaaai.org
4. Peacock J. Perspectives in Disease and Illness (Chapter 1). USA: Capstone Press, 2000:5–12.
5. A.D.A.M. Well-Connected In-depth Health Information. www.well-connected.com
6. Peacock J. Perspectives in Disease and Illness (Chapter 4). USA: Capstone Press, 2000:27–33.
7. Brostoff J, Gamlin L, Brostoff M. Breathing exercises and the Buteyko Method. In: Asthma: The Complete Guide to Integrative Therapies. Rochester, VT: Healing Arts Press, 1999.
8. Anonymous. New breathing exercises help manage asthma. Immunotherapy Weekly, 2008;332.
9. Nieman D, ed. Asthma. In: The Exercise-Health Connection. Champaigne, IL: Human Kinetics, 1998.
10. Preboth M. Causes and treatment of exercise-induced asthma. Am Fam Physician 2000;61(7):2266.
11. Helenius I, Lumme A, Haahtela T. Asthma, airway inflammation and treatment in elite athletes. Sports Med 2005;35(7):566–574.
12. Hermansen C, Kirchner J. Identifying exercise-induced bronchospasm: treatment on distinguishing it from chronic asthma. Postgrad Med 2004;115(6):15, 16, 21, 22, 24, 25.
13. Basaran S, Guler-Uysal F, Ergen N, et al. Effects of physical exercise on quality of life, exercise capacity, and pulmonary function in children with asthma. J Rehabil Med 2006;38:140–135.
14. Counil F, Varray A, Matecki S, et al. Training of aerobic and anaerobic fitness in children with asthma. J Pediatri 2003;142:179–184.
15. Hallstrand T, Bates P, Schoene R. Aerobic conditioning in mild asthma decreases the hyperpnea of exercise and improves exercise and ventilatory capacity. Chest 2000;118(5):1460–1469.
16. Storms W. Can a regular exercise program improve your patient's asthma? J Respir Dis 2001;22(6):340.
17. Welsh L, Kemp J, Roberts R. Effects of physical conditioning on children and adolescents with asthma. Sports Med 2005;35(2):127–141.
18. Matsumoto I, Araki H, Tsuda K, et al. Effects of swimming training on aerobic capacity and exercise induced bronchoconstriction in children with bronchial asthma. Thorax 1999;54:196–201.
19. Wardell C, Isbister C. A swimming program of children with asthma: does it improve their quality of life? Med J Austr 2000;173:647–648.
20. Emtner M, Hedin A. Adherence to and effects of physical activity on health in adults with asthma. Adv Physiother 2005;7:123–134.
21. Worsnop C. Asthma and physical activity. Chest 2003;124(2):421–422.
22. Ford E, Heath G, Mannino D, et al. Leisure-time physical activity patterns among US adults with asthma. Chest 2003;124:432–437.
23. Pianosi P, Davis H. Determinants of physical fitness in children with asthma. Pediatrics 113(3):e225–e229.
24. American College of Sports Medicine. ACSM's Guidelines for Exercise Testing and Prescription. 8th Ed. Philadelphia: Lippincott Williams & Wilkins, 2010:260–264.
25. American Association of Cardiovascular and Pulmonary Rehabilitation. www.aacvpr.org
26. National Heart, Blood, and Lung Institute. Available at: www.nhlbi.nih.gov
27. Satta A. Exercise training in asthma. J Sports Med Phys Fitness 2000;40(4):277–283.
28. Stephensen C. Fish oil and inflammatory disease: is asthma the next target for n-3 fatty acid supplements? Nutr Rev 2004;62(12):486–489.
29. Mickleborough T, Gotshall R. Dietary components with demonstrated effectiveness in decreasing the severity of exercise-induced asthma. Sports Med 2003;33(9):671–681.

30. Bara A, Barley E. Caffeine for asthma. Cochrane Database of Systematic Reviews 2001, Issue 2. Art. No.: CD001112. DOI: 10.1002/14651858. CD001112.
31. Duffy P, Phillips Y. Caffeine consumption decreases the response to bronchoprovocation challenge with dry gas hyperventilation. Chest 1991;99(6): 1373–1377.
32. Kivity S, Aharon Y, Man A, et al. The effect of caffeine on exercise-induced bronchoconstriction. Chest 1990;97(5):1083–1085.
33. Stoesser A, Cook M. Possible relation between electrolyte balance and bronchial asthma. Am J Dis Child 1940;60(6):1252–1268.
34. Burney P. A diet rich in sodium may potentiate asthma: Epidemiologic evidence for a new hypothesis. Chest 1987;91:143S–148S.
35. Burney P, Britton J, Chinn S, et al. Response to inhaled histamine and 24 hour sodium excretion. Br Med J 1986;292:1483–1486.
36. Javaid A, Cushley M, Bone M. Effect of dietary salt on bronchial reactivity to histamine in asthma. Br Med J 1988;297:454.
37. Medici T, Schmid A, Hacki M, et al. Are asthmatics salt-sensitive? A preliminary controlled study. Chest 1993;104:1138–1134.
38. Gotshall R, Fedorczak L, Rasmussen J, et al. One week versus two weeks of a low salt diet and severity of exercise-induced bronchoconstriction. Med Sci Sports Exerc 2003;35(5):S10.
39. Mickleborough T, Gotshall R. Dietary salt intake as a potential modifier of airway responsiveness in bronchial asthma. J Altern Complement Med 2004;10(4):633–642.
40. Gotshall R, Mickleborough T, Cordain L. Dietary salt restriction improves pulmonary function in exercise-induced asthma. Med Sci Sports Exerc 2000;32:1815–1819.

SUGGESTED READINGS

Adams FV. The Asthma Sourcebook. CA: NTC/Contemporary Publishing Group, 1998.

Skinner J. Exercise Testing and Exercise Prescription for Special Cases. 3rd Ed. Baltimore: Lippincott Williams & Wilkins, 2005.

EXERCISE FOR PEOPLE WITH MULTIPLE SCLEROSIS

12

According to the National Multiple Sclerosis Society, 400,000 Americans and 2.5 million people worldwide have been diagnosed with multiple sclerosis (MS). Because the symptoms of this disease sometimes go unnoticed, especially early in its progression, many people who have MS have not been formally diagnosed.[1] Thus, the number of actual sufferers might be much higher. Diagnosis usually occurs between the ages of 20 and 50, and although MS is not normally fatal, it can dramatically interfere with quality of life.[2,3] MS tends to affect twice as many women as men and twice as many whites as other ethnicities.[1,2] Although it is not an inherited disease, the rate of occurrence among families is estimated at 20% (Table 12.1).[4]

The incidence of MS is increasing with nearly 200 new diagnoses each week.[1] Initial symptoms are blurred or double vision or red-green color distortion. Additional difficulties include lack of balance, incoordination, fatigue, general muscle weakness, speech disturbances, memory problems, and urinary incontinence (Table 12.2). In severe cases, partial paralysis results.[2,3,5] A diagnosis of MS, however, does not necessarily relegate sufferers to wheelchairs. On the contrary, two thirds of MS sufferers remain relatively mobile and are able to perform activities of daily living.[1]

MS is a progressive disorder that can cost sufferers considerably. The financial costs result from medical care and hospitalizations, but even more devastating are the personal

TABLE 12-1	RISK FACTORS FOR DEVELOPING MS
Risk Factor	**Description**
Sex	MS affects two to three times more women than men
Race	Whites are two times more likely to develop MS than blacks
Age	MS typically occurs in those between the ages of 20 and 50; it rarely occurs in those younger than 15 or older than 60
Geographical location	MS is more prevalent in temperate regions than in tropical regions
Genetics	Experts believe that some people are genetically predisposed to react to environmental triggers in a way that promotes MS development
Diet	Countries that consume large quantities of saturated fat tend to have higher incidences of MS than those that consume small quantities
Viral infection	Some viruses trigger demyelination and inflammation in genetically predisposed individuals; this is a major focus of current research

Source: Hamler B. Exercise for multiple sclerosis. A safe and effective program to fight fatigue, build strength, and improve balance. Hatherleigh Press, 2006; National Multiple Sclerosis Society. www.nationalmssociety.org.

TABLE 12-2   SYMPTOMS OF MS

The symptoms of MS vary greatly and often resemble those of other disorders.

- Physical and mental fatigue
- Visual disturbances (blurred or double vision; loss of color vision; abnormal pupil response)
- Muscle spasticity, with or without pain
- Loss of balance and coordination
- Urinary incontinence
- Depression or mood swings; unexplained anxiety

costs associated with a diminished quality of life.[2] MS not only affects people afflicted with it, but it also affects everyone around them.

ANATOMICAL AND PHYSIOLOGICAL CHANGES WITH MS

Experts do not yet know the precise cause of MS, but they classify it as an **autoimmune disorder** that affects the central nervous system (CNS). As mentioned in Chapter 2, the CNS includes nervous tissue found in the brain and spinal cord. Neurons are the major cells involved with nervous system functioning; they initiate and propagate nerve impulses and ultimately influence **effectors** (e.g., other neurons, muscles, or glands). To function, these effectors require stimulation from neurons. Problems result if a neuron is damaged since its effectors will subsequently be unable to fulfill their roles.

In MS, the immune system attacks and destroys a structure called the **myelin sheath**; hence, MS is often referred to as a **demyelinating disease**. The myelin sheath surrounds various segments of the neuron axon and speeds up impulse propagation along it (see Chapter 2 for further information on neuron structure). Without adequate myelin sheath, the rate of propagation slows and communication with effectors is impaired. Demyelination, which occurs during periods of relapse, is often followed by **remyelination**. Remyelination attempts to repair damaged myelin to restore axon function; however, it is a slow and often incomplete process that is usually accompanied by inflammation. After repeated bouts of demyelination, remyelination, and inflammation, sclerotic plaques rather than functional myelin sheath form.[4] Over time, this vicious cycle can damage actual axons. Since axons in the CNS are unable to repair themselves, impulse propagation along a damaged axon eventually ceases altogether. Subsequently, its effectors no longer receive stimulation and cannot function. Because it is impossible to determine which neurons will be destroyed during MS development, it is also impossible to predict which effectors will suffer. Thus, symptoms vary widely from person to person, but common complaints are overall fatigue, loss of balance, paralysis, blindness, and the inability to concentrate.[1,4]

Researchers do not understand why remyelination occurs in some MS sufferers but not in others. They know, however, that demyelinated axons often die, and they believe that the progressive nature of MS likely results from the cumulative loss of axons.

Researchers continue to investigate methods to stimulate remyelination in an attempt to slow disease progression and preserve axon function.[6,7]

> ### QUICK REFERENCE
> The axons of affected neurons are not always destroyed. When not destroyed, axons develop additional sodium channels in an effort to preserve functioning. This might explain why MS symptoms often oscillate.[1,4,6]

FACTORS THAT CONTRIBUTE TO THE DEVELOPMENT OF MS

Some experts believe MS is caused by an unknown environmental trigger, perhaps a virus.[3] Although conclusive evidence does not currently exist, ongoing studies are investigating the relationship between MS and over a dozen viruses and bacteria since many pathogens trigger demyelination and systemic inflammation in genetically predisposed individuals. Examples of viruses that might play a role in the development of MS include Epstein-Barr, measles, and human herpes virus-6.[1]

Because MS is more common in temperate areas rather than in tropical areas, researchers are investigating a possible link here as well. The inhabitants of sunny regions are continually exposed to ultraviolet (UV) radiation and therefore make larger amounts of vitamin D than those in less-sunny regions. Some experts believe that this higher vitamin D level provides protection against MS development and progression. This topic is addressed again in the nutrition section.

Some experts believe that MS might develop more readily in people born with a "… genetic predisposition to react to some environmental agent that, upon exposure, triggers

---

Autoimmune disorder—a condition in which a person's immune system attacks normal body cells. The specific signs and symptoms vary depending upon which cells or organs are attacked, but all involve overactive T cells (see Chapter 2 for further information on the immune system and T cells).

Effectors—cells that respond to impulses propagated by neurons. Effectors include muscles, glands, or other neurons.

Myelin sheath—a fatty covering that lines segments of neuron axons in both the CNS and peripheral nervous system (PNS). In the CNS, myelin sheath is formed by oligodendrocytes. In the PNS, it is formed by Schwann cells. Myelin sheath speeds up the rate of impulse propagation along a neuron allowing for more rapid communication with effectors. MS affects the myelin sheath of the CNS.

Demyelinating disease—any condition that damages myelin sheath and, therefore, interferes with neuron functioning.

Remyelination—the process by which myelin sheath is repaired. Occurs spontaneously but very slowly in some patients with MS.

an autoimmune response."[1,4] Experts have not been able to pinpoint any specific gene involved with MS. Most likely, a combination of genes acting together predisposes individuals to MS.[8] Technological advances will hopefully help discover the role genes play in MS development.[1]

CATEGORIES OF MS

In 1996, scientists from around the world established four categories of MS. *Relapsing-Remitting MS* is the most common form upon initial diagnosis. Sufferers exhibit periods of acute flare-ups during which neurological functioning deteriorates as the body's immune cells destroy existing myelin. This causes inflammation and lesions. A relapse can last from a few days to a few months and is followed by a period of remission during which symptoms might completely disappear as inflammation subsides and remyelination occurs. Remission can be almost instantaneous, or it can be slow and gradual.[1,9,10]

Primary progressive MS is a relatively rare form that often develops in those in their late 30s or early 40s. Sufferers experience a steady decline with no relapses or remissions, but the actual rate of deterioration varies. Improvements are infrequent and minor.[1,9,10]

Secondary progressive MS traditionally occurs in 50% of those diagnosed with relapsing-remitting MS. Its onset is usually within 10 years of initial diagnosis. After several years of relapses and remissions, sufferers begin to experience a slow but steady worsening of symptoms with or without flare-ups. In other words, the disease progresses in between relapses until relapses essentially merge into a continual progression of disease with no remissions.[1,9,10]

Progressive-relapsing MS is the rarest form. It is essentially primary-progressive MS with periods of relapse and remission in between. Unlike the relapsing-remitting form, this form is marked by progressive deterioration.[1,9,10]

There is currently no cure for MS; however, medications can slow progression once diagnosis has been made. Diagnosing MS, however, is not an easy task for many reasons. First, the symptoms of MS vary and resemble those of other conditions[1] such as spinal cord tumors, stroke, lyme disease, neurosyphilis, systemic lupus erythematosus, complicated migraine, diabetes, myasthenia gravis, and herpes simplex.[8] Thus, physicians have to "rule out" these other conditions before settling on a diagnosis of MS. Further complicating diagnosis is the fact that symptoms often come and go which makes it difficult to pinpoint triggers. Additionally, since there is no one diagnostic test for MS, diagnosis relies on a battery of tests that includes a full medical history, a neurological exam, magnetic resonance imaging (MRI), visual evoked potential (VEP) tests, lumbar puncture (spinal tap), and blood tests. The medical history and neurological examination help discover the presence of symptoms—and the triggers—that might indicate MS. MRI scans can locate plaques or lesions in the CNS. VEP tests can stimulate visual sensory pathways, record time of response, and determine electrical activity within the brain. A spinal tap withdraws and analyzes cerebrospinal fluid, the fluid that circulates throughout the brain and spinal cord. Blood tests help rule out other causes of symptoms.[1]

TREATMENT FOR MS

Treatment for MS involves managing current symptoms and slowing progression. Sufferers can often manage symptoms with physical therapy, occupational therapy, exercise, and diet; however, pharmacological intervention is generally required to slow progression.[1,11]

Several drugs successfully alleviate MS symptoms. Corticosteroids reduce inflammation and shorten the duration of relapse. Muscle relaxants are effective for spasticity, or the uncontrollable, often painful contractions of skeletal muscles. Stimulants help combat the generalized fatigue that usually accompanies MS. Additional medications for incontinence, pain, or depression might be necessary as well. Unfortunately, many of these medications cause side effects such as hypertension, osteoporosis, and weakness,[9–11] so additional problems can result.

Beta interferons and glatiramer acetate are the two primary medications used to treat MS. Beta interferon, which resembles the interferon produced naturally in the body by certain white blood cells, prevents the body's T cells from destroying myelin sheath. Additionally, it inhibits inflammation by hindering the movement of additional immune cells to sites of inflammation. As it acts, it can also cause generalized aches, worsen headaches, and enhance feelings of depression.[8] The FDA has approved the use of beta interferon for mobile MS sufferers who experience the relapse-remitting form even though it does not reverse existing damage and cannot prevent permanent disability.[11]

The actions of glatiramer are similar to those of beta interferon. It inhibits T-cell activity and prevents attack of myelin. After injection into the subcutaneous layer, patients often feel flushed and short of breath for up to 15 minutes, but these are the only major side effects.

PRECAUTIONS DURING EXERCISE

Those with MS face many physical challenges on a daily basis, including generalized fatigue, muscle spasticity, poor balance, incoordination, pain, and incontinence. Consequently, they must be cautious when participating in activities since activities might exacerbate these symptoms. This section explores concerns when working with clients who have MS.

FATIGUE

The most common symptom associated with MS is fatigue. Fatigue can range from a general lack of energy to total physical and mental exhaustion. Most MS sufferers claim that their generalized fatigue interferes with normal activities and decreases their quality of life more than any other symptom they experience.[12] For some, fatigue develops suddenly and severely for no apparent reason. For others, it only results from prolonged exertion or overheating. For many others, it is a side effect of antidepressants or other medications used to manage MS. No matter what the cause, personal trainers and other health professionals need to be aware of this symptom and make daily adjustments to the exercise routine based on energy levels. Additionally, moderation in exercise is even more important in this particular population than in any other population since overexertion is a trigger for debilitating fatigue in many MS sufferers.[1,5,8,12,13]

Some experts classify the fatigue seen in MS into two types: fatigability and lassitude. Fatigability occurs within a specific muscle or group of muscles after continual use; it is alleviated with rest. Lassitude, on the other hand, is a persistent feeling of exhaustion that does not subside with rest. Some individuals experience both fatigability and lassitude at the same time, whereas other individuals experience one without the other. Nevertheless, fatigability and lassitude can interfere with exercise ability. Exercise tends to be most effective when fatigue is a secondary symptom of MS that results from inactivity.[14]

> ### QUICK REFERENCE
>
> High-intensity activity and activity in a hot environment can exacerbate MS symptoms and cause debilitating fatigue by dramatically increasing core body temperature. Experts believe that an elevated core body temperature temporarily interferes with the communication between demyelinated axons and their effectors, thereby worsening symptoms.[15]

MUSCLE SPASTICITY

Muscle spasticity is a common complaint among MS sufferers. It often occurs in the lower extremities and can be quite dangerous during exercise. Imagine what might happen if a client is holding a pair of dumbbells overhead when a thigh starts to spasm; severe injury could result. Many sufferers take muscle relaxants to manage spasticity, but these medications can interfere with exercise ability as well. Health professionals should consider these factors when designing exercise programs. Flexibility training seems to reduce the severity and frequency of spasticity and should be a major component of the exercise prescription.[1,8]

MUSCLE WEAKNESS, POOR BALANCE, AND INCOORDINATION

Muscle weakness, poor balance, and incoordination in a person with MS can result from one of two reasons. First, many people with MS become inactive once diagnosed because despite the benefits provided by exercise, several physicians continue to discourage exertion. It is common for doctors to suggest that MS patients avoid stairs and take elevators; that they park close to a store instead of farther away; and that they avoid walking longer than necessary because overexertion can worsen symptoms. These are the exact opposite of what they recommend to the general population! Although the intent is to minimize the risk of triggering symptoms, the result is loss of muscle mass, strength, and flexibility, which ultimately results in overall weakness and imbalance. Health and fitness professionals, therefore, need to stabilize clients with balance problems while they strengthen muscles and joints. A focus on simple movements will likely be necessary for this group.[14]

The second factor that contributes to muscle weakness, poor balance, and incoordination is destruction of the myelin sheath and axons. Unfortunately, exercise cannot improve the loss in functional ability associated with demyelination,[14] but it can preserve and improve muscle function in unaffected areas.

> ### QUICK REFERENCE
> Some researchers believe that exercise prevents degeneration and promotes neurogenesis by increasing the production of neuronal growth factors. Currently, there is very little evidence to support this hypothesis, but research continues.[5,16]

SENSITIVITY TO HEAT

In more than 80% of MS sufferers, an increased core body temperature exacerbates symptoms. The primary reason for this is that high temperature interferes with impulse propagation along demyelinated axons. Therefore, it is imperative to keep exercise intensity low to avoid overheating. It is also important to exercise in a cool environment, perhaps in the water or in an air-conditioned room.[14]

PAIN

Pain levels vary among MS sufferers on a daily basis. Additionally, the medications that MS sufferers use to manage their pain often have numerous side effects. Health professionals need to be aware of these side effects and should modify exercises based on current pain level.

INCONTINENCE

As MS progresses, problems with the urinary system usually develop. This might be exhibited by frequent urges to urinate, it might lead to the inability to completely empty the urinary bladder, it might result in varying degrees of incontinence, or it might cause frequent urinary tract infections. Because of the embarrassment associated with these issues, people with MS often restrict water intake. Limiting water intake is especially dangerous to the MS sufferer because overheating can exacerbate symptoms.[1,8]

Overall, people with MS can safely participate in exercise as long as they are aware of these special precautions. Since both overexertion and overheating can increase symptom severity or promote relapse, the intensity of the activity and the environment in which the activity occurs are important. Avoid exercising outdoors in the heat and drink adequate water to keep that internal body temperature within norm. If symptoms develop, decrease intensity or stop the exercise altogether.

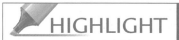

HIGHLIGHT   Gait Problems with MS

According to the National Multiple Sclerosis Society, those suffering from MS often experience difficulty while walking. Many factors compound this problem, but the major contributor is a sedentary lifestyle, which promotes muscle weakness, joint inflexibility, and loss of balance—factors that can cause "foot drag," "foot drop," "vaulting," "hip hike," or "circumduction" of the thigh. These "techniques" help the sufferer compensate for weaknesses on one or both sides of the body. Gait problems are worse for those who experience muscle spasticity because sufferers tend to favor the side of the body not afflicted with involuntary muscle contractions. Additionally, many MS sufferers complain of complete numbness or tingling in the feet—which is the number one cause of foot drop. In some cases, the numbness is so extreme that sufferers cannot feel any contact with the floor—a factor that further impairs balance. Lastly, generalized fatigue interferes with walking because sufferers have the propensity to develop a sloppy gait when fatigue develops.[1,8] The resulting gait can then cause misalignments that eventually result in joint problems.

Overall, weakened muscles and joints can cause balance problems that result in ataxia—a swaying movement that resembles drunkenness. Regular strength training and stretching can certainly help improve walking ability by increasing strength, improving flexibility, enhancing balance and coordination, and maintaining proper communication between the nervous and muscular systems. It cannot, however, repair damaged nerves. Since poor walking mechanics during aerobic training can trigger other musculoskeletal problems that might result in huge setbacks for the client, health professionals should evaluate clients for gait problems. If problems are noted, take time to teach proper walking technique—which consists of a heel first, ball-of-foot second, toes third movement that propels the client forward. Make sure the client does not drift to one side, and encourage a straight posture. In some cases, those with balance and coordination problems might need to use canes or walkers to prevent falls, but in any case, practice proper walking technique to ultimately improve gait.

BARRIERS TO EXERCISE

The fear of worsening symptoms and promoting disease progression are probably the primary barriers to exercise in this population. Sometimes health care professionals instill this fear in their MS patients as they discourage patients from exerting themselves. At other times, those with MS notice an increase in symptom severity following activity, so they avoid activity to prevent symptoms. What some physicians and MS sufferers fail to realize is that exercise done at a moderate intensity and in a cool environment can actually minimize symptoms such as fatigue, incoordination, and muscle spasticity.

The unpredictability of relapse is another common barrier. An MS sufferer who has been exercising and making gains in strength, flexibility, and cardiorespiratory endurance might lose all of these improvements during a relapse. It often takes weeks, sometimes even months, to work through a relapse, and by that time, most exercise-induced improvements are lost. Following a relapse, clients basically have to start from the beginning. In fact, they often require a totally new exercise protocol.[14]

Additional barriers to exercise for those with disabilities include a general lack of energy, decreased self-confidence, limited disease-specific knowledge of fitness center staff, and fear of falling because of muscle weakness and balance problems.[17] The next section describes some of the benefits of exercise for this population and presents current scientific evidence to support it.

BENEFITS OF EXERCISE

As recently as 20 years ago, physicians unequivocally encouraged people suffering from MS to refrain from physical activity because they believed that exertion would worsen fatigue and possibly encourage new symptom development. Over the years, however, researchers have discovered that those with MS not only tolerate exercise well without worsening symptoms, but they also experience several benefits from it. Some benefits experienced by exercisers with MS include reduced risk for several chronic diseases; fewer episodes of debilitating fatigue; improved muscular strength, muscular endurance, flexibility, and balance; and improved mood and confidence level.

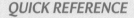

> *QUICK REFERENCE*
> Research has shown that exercise does not reduce the rate of relapse, nor does it slow the progression of MS. Nevertheless, it reduces the overall loss of functional capacity associated with advancing stages of the disease.

REDUCED RISK FOR CERTAIN CHRONIC DISEASES

When they begin exercising, those with MS experience the same reduced risk for heart disease, cancer, stroke, and diabetes as members of the general population. As mentioned

---

Foot drag—a condition where the foot does not move forward in a smooth motion because the brain does not know exactly where the foot is.

Foot drop—occurs during walking when the person's toes contact the floor first, prior to the heel. A healthy walking stride occurs with a heel first, ball-of-foot second, and toes third movement.

Vaulting—occurs during walking when the person raises the heel on the stronger leg to enable the weaker leg to swing through.

Hip hike—a compensatory movement that involves raising the stronger hip to allow movement of the weaker side of the body.

Circumduction—swinging one leg out to the side to permit walking.

in several other chapters, consistent exercise lowers blood pressure, enhances oxygen delivery to body cells, and improves blood lipid levels, all of which benefit the heart and blood vessels.[9,10,12,18] Exercise also helps maintain a healthy weight, which not only improves heart health but also decreases the risk of developing type 2 diabetes (see Chapter 9 for further information). The combination of a healthy weight and a healthy blood lipid profile further protects against colon and breast cancer. Additionally, all weight-bearing exercises promote healthy bone tissue and inhibit bone loss.

EXERCISE AND THE PERCEPTION OF FATIGUE

Numerous studies have investigated the effects of exercise on fatigue level, but the results are conflicting. Some researchers have found that exercise actually decreases the perception of fatigue, but most have discovered that exercise resulted in no change in fatigue levels at all—in the short or long term. Even if physical activity does not reduce fatigue, it is important to note that it does not exacerbate fatigue either. This is encouraging given that many physicians discourage activity fearing that increased exertion intensifies fatigue.[12–15,18,19,20]

IMPROVED MUSCULAR STRENGTH, MUSCULAR ENDURANCE, FLEXIBILITY, AND BALANCE

No one would dispute that exercise improves strength, endurance, flexibility, and balance in the general population, so it should be no surprise that those suffering from MS can experience these same benefits when they become active.[1,14,18] Some would argue that activity is even more important for someone with MS since MS sufferers, who are much more likely to be sedentary than the average person, typically experience a major decline in functional capacity after diagnosis. Consider the cycle of events that are set into motion when someone with MS avoids activity: without stimulation, muscle mass diminishes; as muscle mass diminishes, joint stability decreases; as joints weaken, surrounding ligaments, tendons, and muscles stiffen; and as supportive structures stiffen and muscles weaken, balance and coordination problems result. Furthermore, since the nervous and muscular systems work together to move body parts, they need to regularly communicate with one another to preserve normal functioning. Regular physical activity encourages this interaction and promotes more efficient communication.[21,22]

IMPROVED MOOD AND CONFIDENCE

A diagnosis of MS is a hard blow for most people. It often destroys confidence and impairs mood. It might even lead to depression. In fact, many (but certainly not all) people diagnosed with MS seek out therapy or take medication for depression. In some cases, exercise is a worthy prescription for low self-esteem and a poor mood. It not only promotes the release of powerful chemicals that elevate mood, but it also encourages social interaction and provides a sense of accomplishment for participants, both of which enhance mood. MS clients suffering from depression might still need medical or therapeutic interventions, but physical activity can certainly help. It gives them some sense of control over their bodies, something those with MS often feel that they lack.[12,14,15,18,23]

According to the National Multiple Sclerosis Society, physical activity helps manage MS symptoms. In fact, a study in 1996 at the University of Utah was the first to demonstrate that MS patients who participated in aerobic exercise improved muscular strength, cardiorespiratory functioning, urinary bladder and bowel functioning, and perceived level of fatigue and depression. Furthermore, participants had a more positive attitude about life in general.[1,24] Since then, several studies have confirmed these findings by demonstrating that exercise can be a healthy adjunct to traditional treatment methods for MS.

Health professionals working with this special population need to be even more flexible on a daily basis than they are with their other clients. MS symptoms fluctuate frequently, so be prepared to make adjustments, or possibly even postpone workouts based on client capabilities and limitations *each day*. Pushing through excessive fatigue is not advisable, for this can prompt a relapse.

QUICK REFERENCE
The goal of exercise is to make the participant as personally fit as possible!

RECOMMENDATIONS FOR EXERCISE TESTING AND PRESCRIPTION

The symptoms of MS vary so much among sufferers that it is difficult to make specific exercise recommendations that consider the degrees of limitation of all sufferers. Some people with MS maintain normal functioning and experience infrequent relapse, while others are severely disabled and have frequent relapse. Health professionals need to accommodate their clients' changing capabilities, which often fluctuate on a daily basis. Additionally, physicians, physical therapists, and other rehabilitation specialists should help create exercise prescriptions for clients with MS. Furthermore, health or fitness professionals who plan to work with this special needs group should consider pursuing postrehabilitative specialty training since this condition requires extensive knowledge about disease progression and variability.

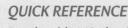

QUICK REFERENCE
People with MS should always consult a physician before beginning an exercise program. In fact, a physician and physical therapist should be involved with exercise testing and prescription.

Currently, there are no standard guidelines for exercise and the MS patient. Nevertheless, organizations such as the National Multiple Sclerosis Society and the National Center on Physical Activity and Disability have made some general recommendations for this special population. Another excellent resource is Brad Hamler's book, *Exercise for Multiple Sclerosis: A Safe and Effective Program to Fight Fatigue, Build Strength, and Improve Balance.*[8] The following exercise suggestions are a compilation of recommendations from these sources.

- Fitness professionals and their MS clients should always check with a physician and/or physical therapist for guidelines on the type, intensity, and duration of workout. This is imperative because the type of exercise most beneficial for the MS client not only depends on current fitness level, but it also depends on the particular symptoms experienced by that client.
- Choose activities that the client enjoys and is capable of executing with proper body alignment. More functional clients can participate in jogging, cycling, or rowing activities, while less functional clients might need to limit activity to walking.
- A 5 to 10 minute low-intensity warm-up with very gradual progression is essential prior to exercise to prepare potentially weakened or spastic muscles and tight joints for activity. Focus on limbering movements. Avoid stretching early in the warm-up since stretching unprepared muscles can lead to muscle spasms or injury in some MS clients.[8] The treadmill or stationary cycle provides good warm-ups.
- Intensity should remain low throughout the workout since overexertion can exacerbate MS symptoms in some MS clients. As Brad Hamler states in his book, "MS patients are recommended not to push too hard...."[8] This is true for both aerobic and resistance training. Overexertion can promote excessive heat production. Excessive heat production raises core temperature. An elevated core temperature can cause extreme fatigue and joint or muscle injuries. Since those with MS have a diminished sweating response to begin with, excessive heat production can be dangerous.[25] Consider using fans to cool the exercise room.
- Encourage clients to drink plenty of cool water before, during, and after exercise. This helps moderate core body temperature and prevents overheating. Clients with MS sometimes avoid drinking recommended amounts of water, especially if they have problems with their urinary systems. They might feel embarrassed about taking frequent bathroom breaks, so fitness professionals need to be sympathetic and emphasize the importance of water intake. Perhaps offer periodic bathroom breaks during the workout.
- Make sure the exercise environment is cool so that the risk for overheating is limited. Avoid physical activities outside during the hottest times of the day or the hottest months of the year.
- Consider water aerobics or swimming for cardiovascular training. The water cools the body and limits the risk of overheating. The water is also excellent for resistance training, especially with the use of special water devices that increase resistance.
- In addition to exercise in the water, tai chi and yoga provide remarkable benefits for the MS client. Both involve slow, deliberate movements that emphasize flexibility, balance, and strength.

> ### QUICK REFERENCE
> According to Brad Hamler, author of *Exercise for Multiple Sclerosis*,[8] those with MS cannot afford to waste energy. Instead, they need to exercise at maximum efficiency and avoid thinking that "more is better."

- Encourage frequent rest periods during the workout. During resistance training, allow a 30 to 90 second rest period in between each set. If clients feel particularly fatigued, offer longer rest periods. Elastic bands, light dumbbells, exercise equipment, and the client's body weight provide safe and effective resistance for this group of clients. A stability ball is also indispensable for improving core strength and balance. Be careful with free weights since many MS patients experience unpredictable muscle spasms that might cause them to drop the weights. Instead, use elastic bands or weight equipment for any overhead resistance exercises.
- Avoid slippery floor surfaces and clear the exercise area of floor hazards since balance is often a problem in this special population. Consider using a body bar or the client's cane to help with balance, and assess balance frequently so that modifications can be made to meet client needs. Clients might need to perform an exercise in the seated position rather than in the standing position. They might have to hold onto a wall or a piece of equipment while performing an exercise to increase stability.
- Ensure adequate lighting since many MS sufferers have eyesight problems. Mark equipment clearly.
- Aerobic training should be done three times per week for approximately 30 minutes at 60% of their VO_{2max}. Most studies suggest that this level of training effectively improves cardiovascular functioning.[14] Water exercise sessions may last up to an hour since the water naturally cools the exerciser and reduces the risk of overheating.
- Full body resistance training may be done two to three times per week and should include one exercise per muscle group. Rest for at least 48 hours in between each workout. Begin with the larger muscle groups first and then work the smaller ones. Use a light resistance, whether it is elastic bands or dumbbells. Choose a resistance that allows for 20 to 30 repetitions.[8]
- Ensure proper body alignment during all exercises. This means maintaining a neutral spine and a full range of motion (if possible) throughout all movements.

> ### QUICK REFERENCE
> If clients with MS notice any new symptoms developing during exertion, they should stop the activity immediately. Only continue if doing so does not elicit the same symptoms again.

SAMPLE RESISTANCE TRAINING PROGRAM FOR THOSE WITH MS

People with MS can benefit from resistance training that uses free weights, weight machines, elastic bands, their own body weight, and several other tools designed for the general population. The key is to vary the mode and to design a program that meets an individual client's capabilities.

WARM-UP

- Before resistance training, do a 5- to 10-minute warm-up on the treadmill or stationary cycle to increase blood flow to muscles before challenging them with resistance.
- Keep in mind that the warm-up should be gradual and of low intensity to avoid overheating.

CORE TRAINING

A strong core improves posture and balance and can improve the functioning of all muscles in the body. Choose one of the following exercises per exercise session and perform 20 to 30 repetitions.

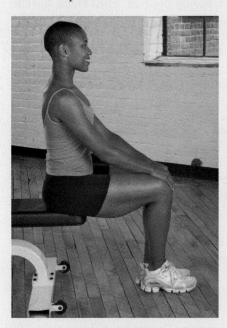 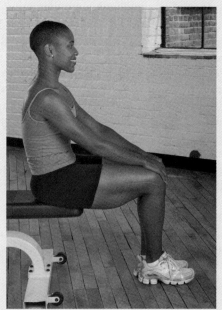

■ **Seated Abdominal Squeezes (Fig. 12.1)**
Sit in a chair with back straight, feet flat on the ground, and arms to the side or on the knees. Squeeze the abdominals and release while breathing. Perform 20 to 30 repetitions. This is an effective exercise for beginners.

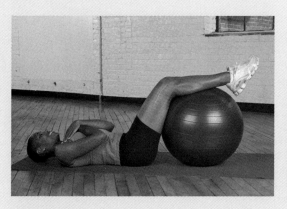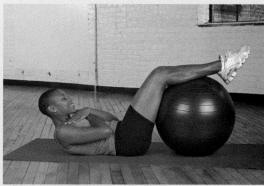

■ **Basic Crunch with a Stability Ball (Fig. 12.2)**

Lie on back with legs propped up on stability ball. Hips and knees should be bent at 90 degrees. Cross arms to front of chest. Slightly raise shoulder blades, head, and neck up from floor by contracting the abdominals. Maintain a neutral spine. Slowly lower the shoulder blades, head, and neck while maintaining tension in the abdominals. Do not touch shoulder blades to floor in between repetitions. Repeat 20 to 30 times.

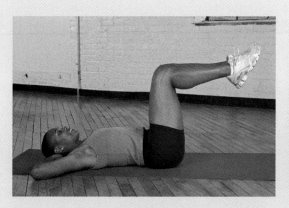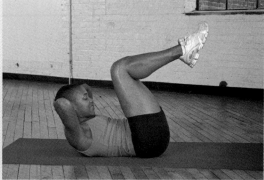

■ **Reverse Crunch (Fig. 12.3)**

Lie on back with hips and knees bent at 90 degrees. Legs should be parallel to the ground and arms should be lying flat on each side. Roll the hips toward the chest while contracting the abdominals. Release and repeat 20 to 30 times.

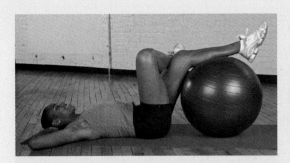 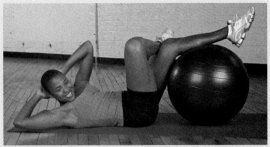

■ Oblique Crunches with a Stability Ball (Fig. 12.4)

Lie on back with legs propped up on stability ball. Hips and knees should be bent at 90 degrees. Cross right leg over left knee. Place left hand behind head and stretch right arm out to the right. Slightly raise left shoulder blade, head, and neck up from floor by contracting the abdominals and rotate to the right. Maintain a neutral spine. Slowly lower the left shoulder blade, head, and neck while maintaining tension in the abdominals. Do not touch shoulder blade to floor in between repetitions. Repeat 20 to 30 times. Perform the same exercise using the right shoulder blade. To make the exercise more difficult, place both hands behind the head as pictured.

LOWER-BODY TRAINING

A strong lower body helps enhance posture, maintain balance, and improve gait. Choose one exercise per muscle group and perform 20 to 30 repetitions of each.

Quadriceps Training

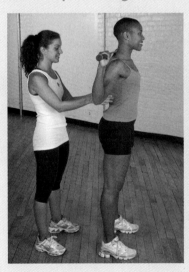 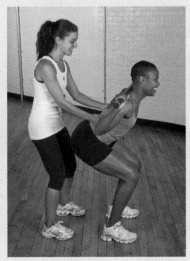

■ Standing Squat (Fig. 12.5)

Stand with feet slightly wider than shoulder width apart. Point toes forward. Clasp hands and flex shoulders at 90 degrees to the front. Keeping the spine neutral, slowly lower the buttocks while keeping the knees over the ankles. Stop when the thighs are parallel to the ground (with knees and hips bent at 90 degree angles). Do not lean forward.

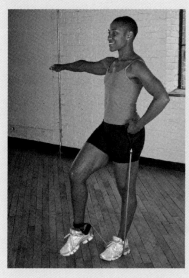
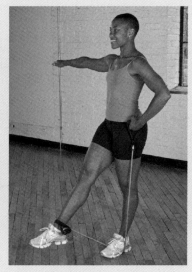

■ **Single-Leg Extension with Elastic Tubing (Fig. 12.6)**
Loop elastic tubing and place securely around right ankle. Hold other handle in left hand; keep left arm extended at side. Step on tubing with left foot. Extend right leg. Pause. Return to start. Perform 20 to 30 times on right. Switch and repeat with left leg.

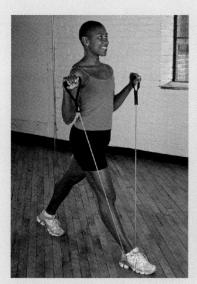
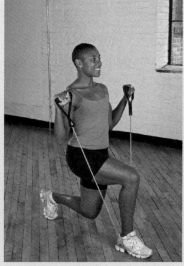

■ **Single-Leg Lunges Using an Elastic Tubing (Fig. 12.7)**
Hold one handle in each hand. Place tubing under right foot. Step back with left foot; elevate left heel. Place hands on waist or on shoulders. Contract abdominals and maintain neutral spine. Keep right knee over right ankle. Drop left knee down toward floor, but do not let knee touch floor. Pause. Return to start. To increase difficulty, lift left leg back after lunging (hyperextend left thigh). Complete 20 to 30 repetitions. Switch sides and repeat.

Hamstrings Training

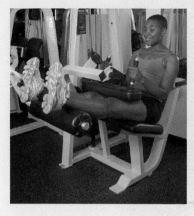 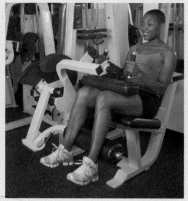

■ Leg Curl Using Weight Machine (Fig. 12.8)

Sit in a leg curl machine with back pressed against pad and hands holding grips. Maintain neutral spinal alignment during entire exercise and contract abdominal muscles to protect lower back. Bend knees to 90 degrees. Pause. Return to starting position. Repeat 20 to 30 times.

Lower-Leg Training

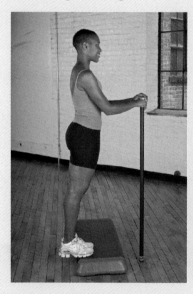 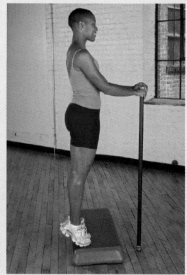

■ Calf Raises on a Platform (Fig. 12.9)

Stand on a step with heels unsupported, and maintain balance with a body bar, cane, or nearby wall if necessary. Slowly lift both heels while contracting calf muscles. Lower and repeat 20 to 30 times. For variation, do one calf at a time. If balance is a problem, sit in a chair with back straight and knees bent at 90 degrees. Lift heels and lower. Place lightweights on thighs for added challenge.

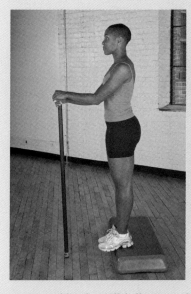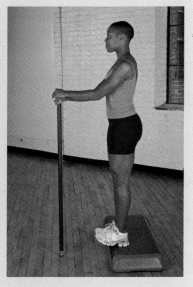

■ Toe Lifts for Tibialis Anterior (Fig. 12.10)

Stand on platform with toes unsupported. Use wall, body bar, or personal trainer for balance if necessary. Begin with toes pointing down. Lift toes toward ceiling and release. Perform 20 to 30 times.

UPPER-BODY TRAINING

Exercises that focus on the upper body improve posture and preserve functional strength. Choose one exercise for each muscle group and perform 20 to 30 repetitions of each.

Chest Training

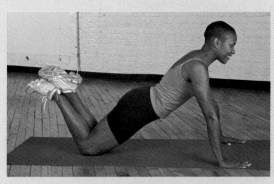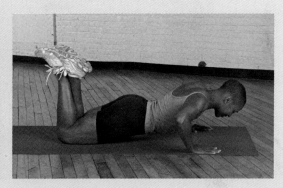

■ Push-Ups on Knees (Fig. 12.11)

Start in push-up position with hands slightly wider than shoulder width apart and knees in contact with the floor. Maintain a neutral spine and contract abdominals throughout movements. Lower the torso until elbows are at a 90 degree angle. Then extend from the elbows to push back into starting position. Repeat 20 to 30 times. Make this exercise more difficult by extending knees and doing a regular push-up.

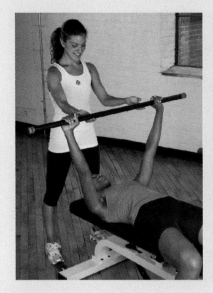
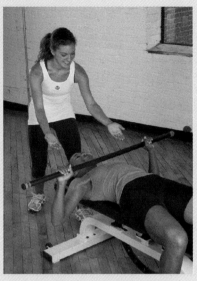

■ **Chest Press Using a Body Bar (Fig. 12.12)**

Lie on a flat bench with feet flat on floor (this position allows for more balance than the feet-up-on-bench position). Grasp a body bar with hands slightly wider than shoulder width apart. Extend elbows while pushing bar up at a slight angle and contracting chest muscles. Lower the bar back toward chest without touching bar to chest. Repeat 20 to 30 times. Modify this exercise by using an incline bench.

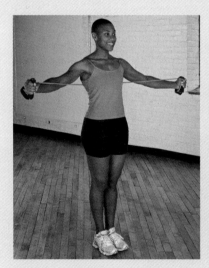
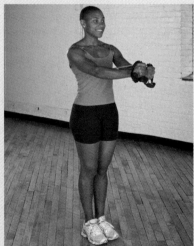

■ **Chest Fly with an Elastic Band (Fig. 12.13)**

Stand with feet slightly wider than shoulder width apart. Contract the abdominals and maintain neutral spinal alignment throughout exercise. Place band around back just below shoulder level. Grasp each end of band with one hand and turn palms to the front. Begin with shoulders abducted and arms parallel to ground. Keeping the elbows slightly bent, bring arms to the front of the body while contracting the chest muscles. Slowly return to starting position. Repeat 20 to 30 times.

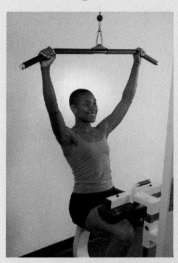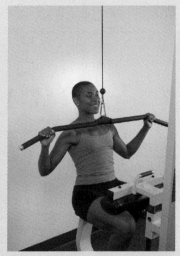

■ **Lateral Pulldown Using Weight Machine (Fig. 12.14)**

Sit on a lat pulldown machine with pad on thighs. Hold the bar with hands placed slightly wider than shoulder width apart. Keep back in neutral alignment while contracting abdominal muscles. Pull the bar down toward the chest while depressing scapulae. Do not pull the bar behind the neck since this can put excessive pressure on the cervical spine and shoulders. Do not try to touch the bar to the chest since this puts excessive pressure on shoulder; simply bring the bar to chin level (or slightly below chin level). Pause. Return to starting position. Repeat 20 to 30 times.

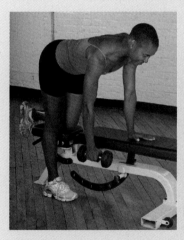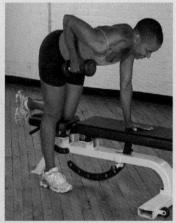

■ **Single-Arm, Bent-Over Row On a Bench (Fig. 12.15)**

Hold a dumbbell in the right hand. Contract abdominals and maintain neutral spine throughout movement. Place left knee and left hand on bench while bending at hip. Extend right hand with weight toward floor. Pull weight up while flexing right elbow. Pause. Slowly lower weight while extending elbow. Repeat 20 to 30 times. Switch sides.

Shoulder Training

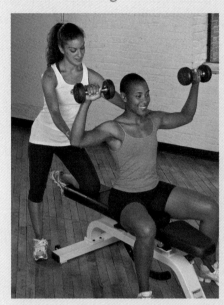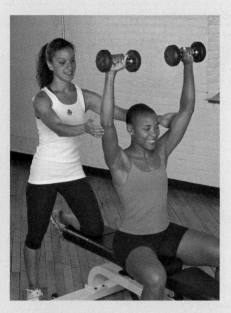

■ **Shoulder Press with Dumbbells (Fig. 12.16)**

Sit on a bench with knees bent, feet on floor, back in neutral alignment. Grasp one dumbbell in each hand and hold them at about ear height with arms parallel to floor. Extend elbows while pushing weights up toward ceiling. Pause. Return to starting position. Repeat 20 to 30 times.

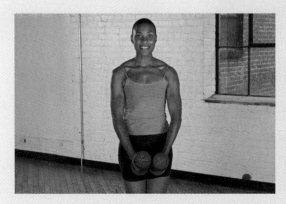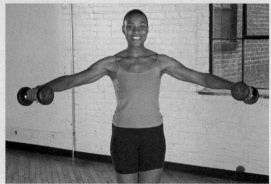

■ **Lateral Shoulder Raises with Dumbbells (Fig. 12.17)**

Stand with feet shoulder width apart, spine in neutral alignment, and abdominals contracted. Hold one dumbbell in each hand, palms facing each other. Slowly abduct arms to about 70 degrees while keeping elbows slightly bent. Pause. Lower to starting position. Repeat 20 to 30 times.

Biceps Training

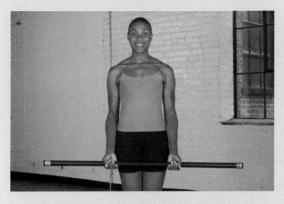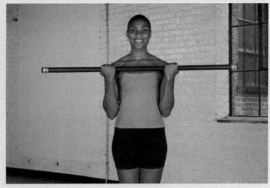

■ **Biceps Curl Using a Body Bar (Fig. 12.18)**

Stand with feet slightly wider than shoulder width apart, spine in neutral alignment, abdominals contracted. Hold body bar in front with both hands, elbows extended. Slowly flex elbows while contracting biceps until bar is at shoulder level. Pause. Return to starting position. Repeat 20 to 30 times. For variation, perform this exercise using elastic bands or dumbbells.

Triceps Training

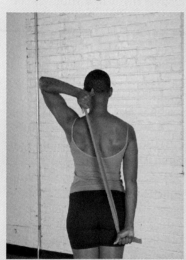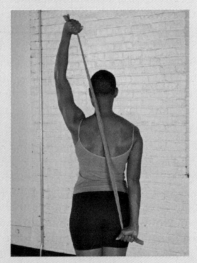

■ **Triceps Extension Using an Elastic Band (Fig. 12.19)**

Stand with feet shoulder width apart, neutral spine, abdominals contracted. The elastic band will be behind the back during this exercise. Hold one end of the elastic band with the right hand and fully extend right arm. Hold the other end of the elastic band with the left hand while left elbow is bent. During this exercise, extend left elbow so that hand moves toward ceiling until left arm is straight (without locking elbow) and perpendicular to floor. Pause. Return to starting position. Repeat 20 to 30 times. Switch hands and repeat on right arm. For variation, use dumbbells to perform this exercise. Alternatively, use a body bar to work both triceps at the same time.

STRETCHING

Stretch all muscles worked during this routine. Either stretch each muscle group following the exercise that focused on that particular muscle group, or stretch all muscles following the entire routine.

NUTRITIONAL CONSIDERATIONS

Some organizations suggest that specific diets can treat MS, but there is currently a relative lack of research into the relationship between nutrition and MS. Based on what *is* known about this disease, however, diet does not appear to cause, prevent, or slow development. Still, some groups suggest that certain nutrients, including dietary fats, antioxidants, vitamin B_{12}, and vitamin D, might improve MS symptoms.[8,26]

Researchers began looking at the relationship between dietary fat intake and MS progression because fat is the major component of the myelin sheath, the part of the neuron attacked by the immune system in MS. Some studies suggest that a higher intake of essential omega-6 fatty acids can actually improve MS symptoms.[27,28] Consequently, the National Institute for Health and Clinical Excellence suggests that those with MS consume in their daily diets 17 to 23 g of omega-6 fatty acids.

Antioxidants are chemicals in the body that fight free radicals (see Chapter 2 for further information). Since some evidence suggests that free radicals are partly responsible for the damage that occurs in MS, various experts recommend increasing antioxidant intake.[8,26,28-30] This, however, is controversial because high levels of antioxidants enhance immunity, and since overactive immune cells destroy myelin sheath, excessive antioxidant intake could worsen MS damage. Overall, further research is necessary before specific recommendations can be made.[26,31]

Vitamin B_{12}, found only in animal-based products, is also needed by the body to make myelin sheath. Interestingly, the neurological symptoms of a vitamin B_{12} deficiency resemble the symptoms associated with MS. If the B_{12} deficiency is caught early, the symptoms are reversible; if caught too late, they become permanent. Because of its role in nervous system functioning, vitamin B_{12} has been the focus of recent research. Some experts believe that vitamin B_{12} supplements should be used to treat MS, but more research is needed before recommendations can be made. The fact that most MS sufferers have adequate B_{12} levels implies that B_{12} supplements will do nothing to improve the symptoms or progression of MS.[26,32]

Because MS is more common in geographical areas with limited exposure to sunlight, some have suggested a link between vitamin D deficiency and MS. (Remember, the body produces vitamin D when exposed to UV radiation.[26,33,34]) They believe that vitamin D supplements might actually slow disease progression in those suffering from deficiencies. Unfortunately, not enough research exists to support this hypothesis, so although adequate vitamin D is necessary to prevent bone loss, intakes in excess of current recommendations are not presently advised for the treatment of MS.[26]

A few organizations suggest that dietry restrictions of gluten, sugar, pectin, and processed foods slows the progression of MS, but current data do not support this.[35,36] In fact, based on what experts *do* know about MS, these particular food components play absolutely no role in MS development.[26]

People with MS benefit from a well-balanced diet just like members of the general population. They usually report that they feel better when they eat healthy foods that comply with basic dietary guidelines (such as those found at www.mypyramid.gov). As long as their diets are varied and provide adequate energy, those with MS do not normally require any special supplements.

SUMMARY

The type and amount of exercise considered safe and effective for MS clients depend solely on how advanced the MS is. Those with mild to moderate MS can usually participate in various exercises and subsequently benefit from increased physical activity. Those with severe MS, however, might be unable to participate in traditional aerobic or resistance exercises because of severe muscle spasticity, muscle weakness, ataxia, or fatigue. This does not mean that they should avoid exercise altogether. Instead, it means that exercise prescriptions need to be carefully structured to work around client capabilities.[14]

The good news is that people with MS do not have to avoid physical activity for fear of worsening their symptoms. Studies show that mild- to moderate-intensity exercise as described in this chapter is well tolerated by MS clients and provides benefits similar to those experienced by the general population. By following safety guidelines and by listening carefully to their bodies, MS sufferers can develop muscular strength, bone density, and cardiorespiratory fitness to avoid the secondary complications associated with a sedentary lifestyle.

CASE STUDY

Greg, a 28-year-old man recently diagnosed with relapsing-remitting MS, is referred to you for training. He was a running back in college but has not been very active since he graduated. Greg's major symptoms are general fatigue and muscle weakness in his right leg that cause him to have a slight limp, but his physician classifies him as highly functional. Despite the fact that he has not been very active over the past 6 years, Greg still looks rather muscular, and he would like to stay that way.

- Design an exercise program for Greg and discuss what he can realistically expect. Be sure to discuss the type, frequency, duration, and intensity of the program.

- Would you offer any nutritional advice? If so, what?

THINKING CRITICALLY

1. Describe some of the symptoms of MS. Do these symptoms suggest any other conditions or diseases?
2. What is an autoimmune disorder? Why is MS classified as one?
3. What is the function of the myelin sheath? Define demyelination and remyelination.
4. List and briefly describe the four different categories of MS. Which is the most common? Which is the least common?
5. List four symptoms of MS that might interfere with exercise ability (these are listed as precautions in this chapter). How does each of these symptoms interfere with the ability to exercise?
6. Why do many MS sufferers develop gait problems? How does this affect their ability to exercise?
7. What are the major barriers to exercise for this particular population? Explain.
8. Describe four benefits of exercise in this population.
9. Why are there no standard exercise guidelines for this special population?
10. Identify three nutrients that are being investigated for their potential in slowing MS development and progression. Explain why some experts believe these nutrients might have therapeutic effects.

REFERENCES

1. National Multiple Sclerosis Society. www.nationalmssociety.org
2. Khan F, Pallant J. Use of the international classification of functioning, disability and health to identify preliminary comprehensive and brief core sets for multiple sclerosis. Disabil Rehabil 2007;29(3):205–213.
3. National Institute of Neurological Disorders and Stroke. www.ninds.nih.gov/disorders/multiple_sclerosis/multiple_sclerosis.htm
4. Compston A, Coles A. Multiple sclerosis. Lancet 2008;372(9684):1502.
5. White L, Castellano V. Exercise and brain health—implications for multiple sclerosis. Part I. Sports Med 2008;38(2):91–100.
6. Antel J. Stem cells: understanding their role in treating MS. MS in Focus 2008;11:4–6.
7. Franklin R. Remyelination, the next treatment for MS? MS in Focus 2008;11:18–20.
8. Hamler B. Exercise for multiple sclerosis. A safe and effective program to fight fatigue, build strength, and improve balance. New York: Hatherleigh Press, 2006.
9. Olenik L. Moving well with multiple sclerosis: PACE model part 1. Palaestra. 2005.
10. Olenik L. Responding to multiple sclerosis: PACE model part 3—movement and the stress response. Palaestra. 2006.
11. Mayo Clinic. www.mayoclinic.org
12. Smith C, Hale L. The effects of non-pharmacological interventions on fatigue in four chronic illness conditions: a critical review. Phys Ther Rev 2007; 12:324–334.
13. McCullagh R, Fitzgerald P, Murphey R, et al. Long-term benefits on quality of life and fatigue in multiple sclerosis patients with mild disability: a pilot study. Clin Rehabil 2008;22:206–214.
14. Karpatkin H. Multiple sclerosis and exercise: a review of the evidence. Int J MS Care 2005;7:36–41.
15. Dodd K, Taylor N, Denisenko S, et al. A qualitative analysis of a progressive resistance exercise programme for people with multiple sclerosis. Disabil Rehabil 2006;28(18):1127–1134.
16. White L, Castellano V. Exercise and brain health—implications for multiple sclerosis. Part II. Sports Med 2008;38(3):179–186.
17. Elsworth C, Dawes H, Sackley C, et al. A study of perceived facilitators to physical activity in neurological conditions. Int J Ther Rehabil 2009;16(1): 17–42.

18. Costello E, Raivel K, Wilson R. The effects of a twelve-week home walking program on cardiovascular parameters and fatigue perception of individuals with multiple sclerosis: a pilot study. Cardiopulm Phys Ther J 2009;20(1):5–12.

19. Smith C, Hale L, Oslon K, et al. How does the experience of fatigue in people with multiple sclerosis change during an eight week exercise programme? J Physiother 2008;36(2):92–93.

20. Fragoso Y, Santana D, Pinto R, et al. The positive effects of a physical activity program for multiple sclerosis patients with fatigue. NeuroRehabilitation 2008;23:153–157.

21. Taylor N, Dodd K, Prasad D, et al. Progressive resistance exercise for people with multiple sclerosis. Disabil Rehabil 2006;28(18):1119–1126.

22. Snook E, Motl R, Gliottoni R, et al. The effects of walking mobility on the measurement of physical activity using accelerometry in multiple sclerosis. Clin Rehabil 2009;23:248–258.

23. Rietberg MB, Brooks D, Uitdehaag BMJ, Kwakkel G. Exercise therapy for multiple sclerosis. Cochrane Database Syst Rev 2004;3: Art. No.: CD003980. Doi: 10.1002/14651858.CD003980.pub2.

24. Petajan J, Gappmaier E, White AT, et al. Impact of aerobic training on fitness and quality of life in multiple sclerosis patients. Ann Neurol 1996; 39:432–441.

25. National Center on Physical Activity and Disability. www.ncpad.org

26. Multiple Sclerosis Society. www.mssociety.org

27. Harbige L, Sharief M. Polyunsaturated fatty acids in the pathogenesis and treatment of multiple sclerosis. Br J Nutr 2007;7:S46–S53.

28. Van Meeteren M, Teunissen C, Dijkstra C, et al. Antioxidants and polyunsaturated fatty acids in multiple sclerosis. Eur J Clin Nutr 2005;59:1347–1361.

29. Anonymous. Multiple sclerosis therapy. Pain and central nervous system weekly. Atlanta. February 9,2009;358.

30. Kaur C, Ling E. Antioxidants and nueroprotection in the adult and developing central nervous system. Curr Med Chem 2008;15(29):3068.

31. Besler H. Serum levels of antioxidant vitamins and lipid peroxidation in multiple sclerosis. Nutr Neurosci 2002;5(3):215–220.

32. Reynolds E. Vitamin B_{12}, folic acid, and the nervous system. Lancet 2006;5:949–960.

33. Cantorna M. Vitamin D and multiple sclerosis: an update. Nutr Rev 2008;66:S135.

34. Kimball S, Ursell M, O'Connor P, et al. Safety of vitamin D_3 in adults with multiple sclerosis. Am J Clin Nutr 2007;86(3):645.

35. Haghighi A, Ansari N, Mokhtari M, et al. Multiple sclerosis and gluten sensitivity. Clin Neurol Neurosurg 2007. Doi:10.1016/j.clineuro.2007.04.011

36. Tengah C, Lock R, Unsworth D, et al. Multiple sclerosis and occult gluten sensitivity. Neurology 2004;62:2326–2327.

SUGGESTED READING

Hamler B. Exercises for Multiple Sclerosis: A Safe and Effective Program to Fight Fatigue, Build Strength, and Improve Balance. New York: Hatherleigh Press, 2006.

Page numbers in "*italics*" denote figures; those followed by "t" denote tables.